New Techniques in
URORADIOLOGY

New Techniques in
URORADIOLOGY

edited by

Sameh K. Morcos
Northern General Hospital
Sheffield, U.K.

Richard H. Cohan
University of Michigan Hospital
Ann Arbor, Michigan, U.S.A.

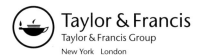

Taylor & Francis
Taylor & Francis Group
New York   London

Taylor & Francis an imprint of the
Taylor & Francis Group, an informa business

Published in 2006 by
Taylor & Francis Group
270 Madison Avenue
New York, NY 10016

© 2006 by Taylor & Francis Group, LLC

No claim to original U.S. Government works
Printed in the United States of America on acid-free paper
10 9 8 7 6 5 4 3 2 1

International Standard Book Number-10: 0-8247-2875-0 (Hardcover)
International Standard Book Number-13: 978-0-8247-2875-5 (Hardcover)
Library of Congress Card Number 2005055937

Library of Congress Cataloging-in-Publication Data

New techniques in uroradiology / edited by Sameh Morcos, Richard H. Cohan.
    p. ; cm.
  Includes bibliographical references and index.
  ISBN-13: 978-0-8247-2875-5 (hardcover : alk. paper)
  ISBN-10: 0-8247-2875-0 (hardcover : alk. paper)
  1. Genitourinary organs--Imaging. 2. Genitourinary organs--Diseases--Diagnosis. 3. Tomography. 4. Magnetic resonance imaging. I. Morcos, Sameh. II. Cohan, Richard H.
  [DNLM: 1. Urogenital Diseases--diagnosis. 2. Diagnostic Imaging--methods. WJ 141 N532 2006]

RC874.N49 2006
616.6'0754--dc22   2005055937

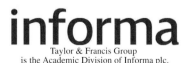
informa
Taylor & Francis Group
is the Academic Division of Informa plc.

Visit the Taylor & Francis Web site at
http://www.taylorandfrancis.com

To the memory of my late parents, Kamel and Monira,
and to my wife and daughters, Sandra, Sarah, Hannah and Rebecca.

SKM

To my wonderful wife, Nina, and to my children, Adam, Alex, Charlie, and Rebeka,
who have kept me young and made me prematurely old both at the same time.

RHC

Preface

This book will cover the modern use of ultrasound, computed tomography, magnetic resonance imaging, and radioisotopes in imaging the urinary tract. It will also offer an insight into new advancements in these modalities, including the fast developing field of functional imaging.

This book offers information about a wide range of uroradiological topics, ranging from the use of magnetic resonance imaging or multislice computed tomography in urography to image-guided ablation of renal tumors. The importance of using helical computed tomography in diagnosing stones of the urinary tract and determining the nature of complicated renal cysts is discussed and the use of the magnetic resonance imaging technique in imaging the prostate and the urinary tract in infants and children. In addition, the use of imaging to guide interventional urological procedures and recent developments in interventional urinary tract radiologic techniques are reviewed. The use of imaging in planning for nephron-sparing surgery and for managing patients with renal artery stenosis is also discussed. Furthermore, as the kidney is the main route of elimination of water-soluble contrast media, which are regularly used in imaging the urinary tract, the safety of these agents is addressed.

This book is primarily intended for practicing radiologists, particularly those with a special interest in the urinary tract. However, it would also prove useful for urologists and renal physicians.

We hope that the information provided in this book will help the readers practice modern uroradiology safely and wisely.

We are most grateful to all the authors of this book for their hard work in preparing the manuscripts and for their expert contributions.

S.K. Morcos
R.H. Cohan

Contents

Contributors

Saroja Adusumilli Division of Abdominal Imaging, Department of Radiology, Section of Magnetic Resonance Imaging, University of Michigan Health System, Ann Arbor, Michigan, U.S.A.

Deniz Altinok Department of Pediatric Imaging, Children's Hospital of Michigan, Detroit, Michigan, U.S.A.

Michele Bertolotto Institute of Radiology, University of Trieste, Trieste, Italy

Elaine M. Caoili Department of Radiology, University of Michigan Health System, Ann Arbor, Michigan, U.S.A.

Richard H. Cohan Department of Radiology, University of Michigan Health System, Ann Arbor, Michigan, U.S.A.

Christian Combe Department of Nephrology, Groupe Hospitalier Pellegrin, and INSERM, University Victor Segalen-Bordeaux 2, Bordeaux, France

Nancy S. Curry Medical University of South Carolina, Charleston, South Carolina, U.S.A.

Yahsou Delmas Department of Nephrology, Groupe Hospitalier Pellegrin, and INSERM, University Victor Segalen-Bordeaux 2, Bordeaux, France

Lorenzo E. Derchi DICMI—Radiology, University of Genova, Genova, Italy

James H. Ellis Department of Radiology, University of Michigan Health System, Ann Arbor, Michigan, U.S.A.

J. Damien Grattan-Smith Department of Pediatric Radiology, Scottish Rite Children's Hospital, Atlanta, Georgia, U.S.A.

Nicolas Grenier Service d'Imagerie Diagnostique et Thérapeutique de l'Adulte, Groupe Hospitalier Pellegrin, and ERT CNRS Imagerie Moléculaire et Fonctionnelle, University Victor Segalen-Bordeaux 2, Bordeaux, France

Robert P. Hartman   Department of Radiology, Mayo Clinic, Rochester, Minnesota, U.S.A.

Olivier Hauger   Service d'Imagerie Diagnostique et Thérapeutique de l'Adulte, Groupe Hospitalier Pellegrin, and ERT CNRS Imagerie Moléculaire et Fonctionnelle, University Victor Segalen-Bordeaux 2, Bordeaux, France

Brian R. Herts   Section of Abdominal Imaging, Division of Diagnostic Radiology and The Glickman Urological Institute, The Cleveland Clinic Foundation, Cleveland, Ohio, U.S.A.

A. J. W. Hilson   Department of Nuclear Medicine, Royal Free Hospital, London, U.K.

J. Louis Hinshaw   Department of Radiology, University of Wisconsin, Madison, Wisconsin, U.S.A.

Akira Kawashima   Department of Radiology, Mayo Clinic, Rochester, Minnesota, U.S.A.

Fred T. Lee Jr.   Department of Radiology, University of Wisconsin, Madison, Wisconsin, U.S.A.

Andrew J. LeRoy   Department of Radiology, Mayo Clinic, Rochester, Minnesota, U.S.A.

Graham J. Munneke   Radiology Department, St. George's Hospital, London, U.K.

Claus Nolte-Ernsting   Department of Diagnostic and Interventional Radiology, University Hospital Hamburg—Eppendorf, Hamburg, Germany

Uday Patel   Radiology Department, St. George's Hospital, London, U.K.

E. Scott Pretorius   Department of Radiology, Section of Magnetic Resonance Imaging, Hospital of the University of Pennsylvania, Philadelphia, Pennsylvania, U.S.A.

Parvati Ramchandani   Department of Radiology, University of Pennsylvania Medical Center, Philadelphia, Pennsylvania, U.S.A.

Erick M. Remer   Section of Abdominal Imaging, Division of Diagnostic Radiology, The Cleveland Clinic Foundation, Cleveland, Ohio, U.S.A.

Joseph C. Veniero   Section of Abdominal Imaging, Division of Diagnostic Radiology, The Cleveland Clinic Foundation, Cleveland, Ohio, U.S.A.

J. Michael Zerin   Department of Pediatric Imaging, Children's Hospital of Michigan, Detroit, Michigan, U.S.A.

1

Radiographic Iodinated Contrast Media: Adverse Reactions, Premedication, and Other Considerations

James H. Ellis
Department of Radiology, University of Michigan Health System, Ann Arbor, Michigan, U.S.A.

ADVERSE REACTIONS TO INTRAVASCULAR RADIOGRAPHIC IODINATED CONTRAST MEDIA

The administration of radiographic iodinated contrast media (RICM) when performing diagnostic and interventional radiologic procedures provides great benefit to patients, and its use is generally straightforward and without complication. This chapter will focus on acute adverse reactions to the intravascular administration of RICM and methods to minimize their occurrence and severity.

Acute adverse reactions to the intravascular administration of RICM are encountered in as many as 3.1% of patients receiving intravenous injections of low-osmolality nonionic contrast media (LOCM) and 12.7% of patients receiving intravenous injections of high-osmolality ionic contrast media (HOCM) (1). Fortunately, the majority of these reactions are mild and clinically insignificant. Severe and very severe reactions (the latter requiring hospitalization) have been noted much less frequently, in only 0.04% and 0.004%, respectively, of patients receiving intravenous injections of LOCM, and 0.22% and 0.04%, respectively, of patients receiving intravenous injections of HOCM (1). The vast majority of patients who have severe, even potentially life-threatening, reactions respond to rapid and aggressive treatment (2). Fatal reactions are exceedingly rare, having been encountered in as few as 1:170,000 patients injected with HOCM or LOCM (1).

Adverse reactions can be broadly classified as idiosyncratic (meaning the mechanism for the initiation of the reaction is not understood) and nonidiosyncratic (2). Idiosyncratic reactions have manifestations indistinguishable from those seen with true allergic reactions. Nonidiosyncratic reactions have manifestations that generally do not resemble allergic reactions but instead are believed to reflect physiologic effects of contrast media or direct toxicity of contrast media on a variety of organ systems.

1

IDIOSYNCRATIC REACTIONS

Idiosyncratic reactions most often begin within 20 minutes of contrast media injection (2). Their occurrence is not related to the dose of contrast material administered. They can be produced by the intravascular injection of even tiny amounts (less than 5 mL) of contrast material. Although the manifestations of idiosyncratic reactions are identical to those seen in patients having true anaphylactic reactions, reactions to contrast material are not true allergic reactions in the vast majority of patients (3,4). The formal definition of an allergic reaction requires prior exposure to the offending agent to sensitize the individual and the development of antibodies against the allergen (2). Neither of these requirements is routinely met in idiosyncratic contrast reactions. Hence idiosyncratic reactions to RICM have been termed anaphylactoid or allergic-like rather than anaphylactic or allergic reactions.

Typical idiosyncratic reactions to contrast media are urticaria (hives), diffuse cutaneous and subcutaneous edema (angioedema), upper airway (laryngeal) edema, bronchospasm, and hypotension with tachycardia. However, there is some overlap with nonidiosyncratic reactions. Subclinical bronchospasm and vasodilatation (which in pronounced cases may produce hypotension) may be detectable in many patients if carefully looked for; these manifestations are probably related to the direct physiologic effects of contrast media rather than an allergic-like response.

Patients at Risk

Certain groups of patients are more likely to have idiosyncratic reactions to RICM. Patients with a history of a prior contrast reaction have about four times the risk of an adverse reaction, and patients with a history of allergies or asthma have about two to three times the risk of an adverse reaction, compared to patients who do not have these histories (1). Shellfish allergy is not a "special" allergy with respect to contrast media injection but should be managed in the same way as other non-contrast allergies (e.g., peanut, bee sting, or penicillin allergies) (5).

In our experience, some patients relate a history of allergy, often to food, that probably is not a true allergy. For example, a stated allergy to milk may, on closer questioning, reflect lactase deficiency and inability to properly digest milk. Some stated food allergies really reflect an earlier episode of food poisoning. There is no evidence that these patients are at increased risk for contrast reactions.

Reducing Risk

Choice of Contrast Medium

Several studies have shown that the frequency of reaction in the general population receiving RICM is reduced when LOCM is administered rather than HOCM (1,6,7). There are approximately one-quarter to one-fifth as many reactions when LOCM is administered intravenously compared to when HOCM is administered intravenously. This reduction applies to idiosyncratic reactions taken as a whole and to the subset of severe reactions (1). Furthermore, in addition to reducing risk in the general population, LOCM reduces risk in patients who are at higher risk for contrast reactions, such as those discussed in the previous section (1,7).

There is insufficient data to determine if iso-osmolality contrast media may reduce the rate of acute idiosyncratic reactions even further than the low rate observed with administration of LOCM. The size of the population that would have to be tested to produce a study with sufficient power to detect a small but important difference is prohibitive. However, if a patient has had a prior severe reaction to a specific contrast agent, switching to another brand of LOCM or to iso-osmolality contrast medium makes common sense even if the utility of such a change in contrast agents has not been scientifically proved.

Premedication

To reduce the risk of an idiosyncratic contrast reaction in high-risk patients, premedication with corticosteroids and H1 antihistamines has been recommended. Other drugs, such as H2 antihistamines and ephedrine, can be added to the regimen but are not widely used (2,8).

Premedication is generally recommended for patients who have a history of: an allergic-like reaction to contrast media; other true allergies, particularly if multiple and/or severe; and true asthma, particularly with frequent or severe attacks. It is also recommended for asthmatic patients who are currently or who have recently been symptomatic. Various premedication protocols have been proposed for high-risk patients. Ours [with the drug schedule adapted from Refs. 9 and 10] is as follows.

For oral administration prior to an elective examination: prednisone 50 mg per oral 13, 7, and 1 hour before the examination and diphenhydramine 50 mg per oral (or i.m.) 1 hour before the examination. Patients should be cautioned not to drive automobiles or perform possibly dangerous tasks after taking diphenhydramine, because it can lead to drowsiness.

For intravenous administration in urgent situations or if the patient cannot take oral medications, the following regimen has been recommended: hydrocortisone 200 mg i.v. stat and q 4 hour until the examination is complete (four total doses for an elective examination) and diphenhydramine 50 mg intravenously one hour before the procedure.

Universal steroid premedication for all patients, regardless of risk status, has been proposed for both HOCM (11) and LOCM (12) administration. When populations as a whole (regardless of risk factors) were premedicated with steroids, rates of reactions fell by approximately one-third to one-half. Although the study (12) involving LOCM administration did not have enough patients to draw statistically significant conclusions about moderate or severe reactions, it did show that the total number of reactions was reduced by steroid administration. Universal steroid premedication for all patients prior to RICM administration has not been widely adopted, however, probably because of logistical problems and the relatively low frequency of acute idiosyncratic reactions to LOCM (13).

NONIDIOSYNCRATIC REACTIONS

Nonidiosyncratic reactions are a diverse group (2,14), ranging from mild symptoms that are typically considered a physiologic effect of contrast media rather than a reaction to severe, even life-threatening, states. Nonidiosyncratic contrast reactions are for the most part dose dependent: they are less likely to occur and, if they do occur, are less likely to be severe when smaller doses of contrast material are employed. In general, nonidiosyncratic reactions occur less often and with less severity when LOCM is administered than when HOCM is administered.

There are a number of commonly encountered nonidiosyncratic effects of RICM. Intravascular injections of RICM normally produce peripheral vessel dilatation, which the patient perceives as a sensation of heat or warmth (15). Nausea and vomiting are probably the result of a transient effect of the contrast material on the central nervous system. Vasovagal reactions are acute nonidiosyncratic hypotensive reactions that typically include nausea, diaphoresis, anxiety, and bradycardia.

Less commonly, RICM produce adverse toxic effects on other systems. RICM, on contact with the central nervous system, lowers the seizure threshold. Seizures can occur from intravascular injection of contrast media, especially if a disease process has resulted in the breakdown of the blood–brain barrier. Contrast media injection results in a temporary decrease in cardiac contractility and may induce arrhythmias. When contrast medium reaches the pulmonary vasculature, it causes increased pulmonary vascular resistance as well as bronchospasm (typically subclinical; thus, when symptomatic bronchospasm occurs, it is not always clear if this represents a nonidiosyncratic or idiosyncratic reaction). Because HOCM and, to a lesser degree, LOCM have osmolality higher than that of human blood, water is drawn into the vascular system, with the consequent expansion of intravascular volume that may not be tolerated well by patients with tenuous cardiac status (15). Rarely, contrast media induce noncardiogenic pulmonary edema, a phenomenon that is poorly understood but is suspected to be due to a toxic effect leading to increased pulmonary capillary permeability.

Contrast-induced nephrotoxicity is another nonidiosyncratic reaction. It will be covered in more detail in a separate section entitled "Contrast-Induced Nephrotoxicity."

Patients at Risk

A variety of diseases can be aggravated by contrast media (2,14,15). In patients with cardiac disease (and rarely in patients without), contrast media administration can induce arrhythmias or precipitate an episode of angina. The osmotic increase in blood volume can result in a worsening of congestive heart failure. HOCM administered to patients who have a pheochromocytoma can result in release of vasoactive substances leading to a hypertensive crisis; however, in comparison, it appears that the risk of this occurrence following the administration of LOCM is very low (16). In patients with myasthenia gravis, acute myasthenic crisis has been reported following injection of HOCM (14) but not LOCM; the acute worsening of the respiratory symptoms of myasthenia usually presents the greatest danger to the patient. Thyroid storm has been reported following contrast media administration to patients with uncontrolled hyperthyroidism. In patients who suffer from sickle cell anemia (but not sickle trait), contrast medium administration may precipitate a sickle cell crisis. As previously mentioned, intravascular RICM administration can lead to seizure activity. However, this is a rare occurrence, with patients with brain lesions that have resulted in the breakdown of the blood–brain barrier at higher risk.

Reducing Risk

Premedication

For some, but not all, of the nonidiosyncratic reactions, it may be possible to reduce risk via premedication. For example, patients who have a pheochromocytoma can be premedicated with phenoxybenzamine to produce alpha blockade (16). This prevents the most clinically significant adverse effects of the release of vasoactive substances if that should occur following contrast media administration but is rarely done when LOCM is administered. Risk can be reduced in patients with hyperthyroidism if their disease can be controlled prior to contrast media administration.

Choice of Contrast Medium

In general, LOCM produces fewer and less severe nonidiosyncratic reactions than HOCM. Regarding iso-osmolality contrast media, there is insufficient evidence to draw conclusions about its use in patients at risk for nonidiosyncratic reactions, though common sense would suggest that it might reduce the risk of worsening active congestive heart failure because it should have a smaller volume expansion effect.

Because nonidiosyncratic reactions in general are dose dependent, the risk can be reduced by lowering the amount of RICM administered to the minimum necessary to answer the clinical question for which the examination is being done. In some cases, this might involve choosing a different study that does not require RICM.

CONTRAST-INDUCED NEPHROTOXICITY

Contrast-induced nephrotoxicity (CIN), a nonidiosyncratic reaction, is often defined on laboratory, rather than clinical, grounds. Although there are a variety of definitions employed in various studies, CIN usually refers to an acute elevation in the level of serum creatinine by >0.5 mg/dL or >50% of baseline. The incidence of this complication is estimated to be 2% to 7% (17), though the incidence varies with the criteria used to define CIN and with the population under study. Direct measurements of creatinine clearance or mathematical estimations of creatinine clearance based on various clinical parameters (18) would likely be more accurate determinants of CIN; however, serum creatinine is the most common value measured in clinical studies. Most clinical studies of CIN suffer from two problems: the clinical significance of the arbitrary choice of the degree of creatinine elevation defining CIN is unknown, and may be too sensitive a marker; and long-term follow-up of patients is not done to quantify the consequence of RICM administration.

In patients who suffer from CIN, serum creatinine elevation is first detectable between one and three days after contrast material injection and peaks by three to seven days (19). The creatinine level usually eventually returns to baseline, most often within 10 to 14 days (17,20); however, in some series, as many as one in four patients who developed CIN suffered a sustained reduction in renal function (17).

Patients at Risk

A number of risk factors for the development of CIN have been described, particularly pre-existing renal insufficiency (21–26). Patients whose renal failure is the result of diabetic nephropathy are at even greater risk, and when renal failure occurs, it is more likely to be irreversible (27). However, the presence of diabetes mellitus alone (in the absence of renal failure) is probably not a risk factor for contrast-induced renal failure (28–30). Other risk factors that have been implicated include American Heart Association class IV congestive heart failure, hyperuricemia, dehydration, concurrent use of such nephrotoxic drugs as aminoglycoside antibiotics and nonsteroidal anti-inflammatory agents, advanced age, and administration of large doses of contrast media for one or multiple contrast–enhanced studies performed within a short period of time (14,19,31,32). Multiple myeloma has long been considered a risk factor but may not be important if the patient is hydrated (14,33). The incidence of contrast-induced renal failure is greatest when multiple risk factors are present (17).

Reducing Risk

Because the only treatment for CIN is at best supportive, prevention is the key. Avoiding large or closely repeated doses of contrast media and discontinuing other nephrotoxic drugs (when possible) reduces the risk.

Premedication

Hydration of the patient (commonly beginning 12 hours before and continuing two hours after contrast media administration) has long been used to reduce the risk of CIN. For intravenous hydration, normal saline has been shown to be more efficacious as a hydrating agent than half-normal saline (34). A preliminary study (35) of 119 patients suggests that hydration with sodium bicarbonate solutions may be even more effective than hydration with normal saline in reducing CIN risk.

Over the years, many drug therapies have been proposed to reduce the incidence of CIN. Attempts to improve upon saline administration alone by adding other drugs such as mannitol, furosemide, theophylline, calcium antagonists, dopamine, endothelin receptor blockers, prostaglandin E1, and atrial natriuretic peptide have not proven uniformly successful (36–38). Many of these drugs have side effects the significance of which are not yet fully understood. The search for pharmaco-therapeutic agents that might mitigate the nephrotoxic effects of contrast media continues, however.

Tepel et al. (37), relying on evidence (39) that reactive oxygen species may play a causative role in CIN, administered the antioxidant acetylcysteine in a prospective, placebo-controlled, randomized trial in high-risk patients and demonstrated a protective effect of the drug. In patients with chronic renal insufficiency, oral acetyl-cysteine combined with intravenous hydration was better than placebo and hydration in reducing the incidence of CIN. (Acetylcysteine is better known by its various trade names, including Mucomyst, Mucosil, Fluimucil, Genac, and many others).

Some questions about this study can be raised. The amount of contrast agent administered to the patients for computed tomography (CT) scans was relatively small (75 mL of a 300 mgI/mL nonionic agent). For reasons not fully explained, patients with serum creatinine as low as 1.2 mg/dL (which would be within the range of normal at many institutions) were included as "chronic renal failure" patients. The number of patients in the study was small (83 in total), especially given the low incidence of clinically significant renal failure caused by RICM. None of the patients in this series required dialysis, and no long-term outcome information about any of the patients was reported. Thus, the cost-effectiveness and clinical significance of this intervention remained undetermined. Because patients with acute renal failure were excluded, the study provided no evidence as to whether acetylcys-teine may protect patients in acute renal failure from CIN.

Since the publication of the Tepel study, a number of other studies have been performed in an attempt to replicate the results and perhaps overcome some of the deficiencies of the initial work. Results from these studies have been mixed. Some (40–44) have supported the use of acetylcysteine to reduce CIN risk and others

(45–50) have not. In an attempt to resolve these differences, meta-analyses of the data from multiple studies have been performed. Two such meta-analyses (51,52) have indicated that acetylcysteine is effective in reducing CIN risk in patients with chronic insufficiency. Both meta-analyses were performed on the same seven studies (37,40–42,45–47), of which four showed that acetylcysteine reduced risk in patients with chronic renal insufficiency and three did not show a reduction in risk. When the results of those studies were combined as a meta-analysis of 805 patients, the combination of hydration and acetylcysteine reduced relative risk by 56% ($P = 0.02$) compared to hydration alone (51). One meta-analysis (51) noted that the results might have been limited by publication bias, whereas the other (52) found no evidence of publication bias. Both meta-analyses noted that the studies they reviewed did not give much insight into the clinical significance of the reduction of CIN (as CIN was defined in the studies, an issue discussed previously in this chapter). The incidence of dialysis was the same (0.75%) in the drug and placebo groups (52), and the studies did not investigate such clinical endpoints as in-hospital morbidity and mortality (51). The optimum dose of acetylcysteine is not known; for example, preliminary evidence (53) suggests that doubling the dose used in many earlier studies might be more effective.

Another drug that was proposed to have protective action against contrast nephropathy is fenoldopam (trade name: Corlopam®). Fenoldopam is a selective dopamine-1-receptor agonist for intravenous use as an antihypertensive. It is a vasodilator that increases renal perfusion but does not have the unwanted systemic effects of dopamine (54). In dogs, fenoldopam blunted the decrease in renal blood flow and glomerular filtration rate caused by contrast media, but the study did not prove whether it would reduce clinical nephrotoxicity (55). In a small study of 46 angiography patients with minimum serum creatinine values of 1.5 mg/dL who were treated with fenoldopam, contrast nephropathy occurred in 13%; the authors employed published data to suggest that 38% should have been expected to demonstrate nephrotoxicity (56). This study, weakened by the lack of a true control group, demonstrates why confirmatory controlled studies are important before the wholesale adoption of new approaches. In a subsequent randomized, controlled, sufficiently powered study of 315 patients, Stone et al. (57) showed no positive effect of fenoldopam in the prevention of CIN. Thus, at present, the use of fenoldopam cannot be recommended.

Choice of Contrast Medium

While it is now well accepted that LOCM are less nephrotoxic than HOCM in patients with pre-existing renal impairment (30,58), two studies have suggested that the use of iso-osmolality agents may further reduce the risk of CIN from RICM administration. In a randomized comparison (59) of iodixanol (iso-osmolality contrast medium) and iohexol (LOCM) in 102 patients with serum creatinine of more than 1.7 mg/dL, only 15% of the patients in the iodixanol group showed a rise of greater than 10% in serum creatinine, compared to 31% of patients in the iohexol group ($P < 0.05$). Similarly, in a study (60) of 129 patients with serum creatinine in the range of 1.5 to 3.5 mg/dL, an increase in serum creatinine of at least 0.5 mg/dL occurred in only 3% of the iodixanol group, compared to 26% in the iohexol group ($P = 0.002$). The peak increase in serum creatinine within three days of RICM administration averaged 0.13 mg/dL in the iodixanol group compared to 0.55 mg/dL in the iohexol group ($P = 0.001$). Comparable studies comparing iodixanol with other LOCM are not yet available.

THE PATIENT AT HIGHER RISK FOR A DELAYED REACTION

Delayed reactions, observed after administration of both ionic and nonionic contrast media, are usually defined as reactions that occur more than one hour after contrast material injection. The maximum amount of time delay between contrast injection and an accepted delayed reaction varies with the study, but following patients beyond one week is rare.

Many such delayed reactions produce very nonspecific symptoms, including fever, chills or rigors, rash, pruritus, flushing, dizziness, arthralgia, diarrhea, nausea, vomiting, headache, and, rarely, hypotension (61–64). The incidence of delayed reactions has been reported to be 0.5% to 23% (64). However, in a study that surveyed both patients undergoing nonenhanced CT and patients undergoing enhanced CT, delayed adverse reactions were reported in 10.3% of the patients who did not receive contrast material (and in 12.4% of those who did) (65). Other studies showed similar results; thus many so-called delayed reactions are not the consequence of the contrast media (63,64) but are likely related to daily life and/or the illness for which the patient is being imaged. It appears that most true delayed reactions are skin reactions (65). A contrast media–specific T-cell response has been postulated as a possible mechanism (63).

Patients at Risk

There may be an increased incidence of skin reactions when nonionic dimers (iso-osmolality contrast media) are administered, though not all studies have found a difference (64). Delayed reactions to contrast material have also been encountered with increased frequency (12–29%) and increased severity in patients who are currently receiving or who have recently (within two years) received intra-arterial or intravenous interleukin-2 (IL-2) immunotherapy for treatment of metastatic cancer (61,66). To reduce the risk of a second delayed reaction, switching to another brand of contrast medium and premedication with oral corticosteroids has been recommended (64). However, steroids should be avoided in patients treated with IL-2 immunotherapy unless the immunotherapist agrees (because steroids could blunt the therapeutic effects of the immunotherapy).

OTHER CONSIDERATIONS

The Patient Taking Metformin

Metformin (generic, alone or in combination in trade name drugs Glucophage®, Glucovance®, Avandamet®, Metaglip®, and many others) is an oral antihyperglycemic medication that is being prescribed with increased frequency. Although metformin itself is not nephrotoxic, patients who are taking this drug and who happen to develop renal failure (as a result of a contrast material injection or other renal insult) may rarely develop lactic acidosis, which can be fatal (67–69). The U.S. Food and Drug Administration (FDA) approved drug package insert for metformin states that metformin should be discontinued at the time that a contrast-enhanced study is performed and should not be restarted until the patient's renal function is documented to be normal a minimum of 48 hours after that study (70). Some referring physicians may want their patients to have alternate glucose control during this period. Some European authors have suggested that if the patient has normal renal function at the time of the examination, metformin need not be stopped (71–73).

The Pregnant Patient

RICM crosses the placenta (74). In general, intravenous contrast material should be avoided, when possible, in pregnant women so as to eliminate any theoretical adverse effects on the fetus. However, if contrast media administration is required, it can probably be safely injected (at least in the third trimester) (75). The risk of radiation exposure from the examination is generally the greater issue than is RICM administration. If the radiation exposure can be justified, withholding contrast material is reasonable only if the absence of RICM would not compromise examination quality and lead to a nondiagnostic examination.

The Patient Who Is Breast Feeding

A number of studies have shown that the amount of contrast material excreted in breast milk is minimal. In one study, it was determined that the amount of nonionic iohexol-350 ingested by a breast-fed baby within 24 hours of maternal contrast media injection (at a volume of 1 mL/kg) would equal only 0.2% of the allowed pediatric dose for that infant (76). Excretion of the magnetic resonance imaging contrast agent gadopentatate dimeglumine is even lower (77). These studies indicate that there is no definite reason for a lactating mother to stop breast-feeding after a contrast media injection. Nonetheless, as an extra precaution, some researchers (and the FDA package inserts) recommend that infants be fed formula and that the mother use a breast pump for 24 hours following maternal contrast administration (77). The American College of Radiology suggests that the mother be informed about the safety of continuing to breast-feed but be allowed to make her own choice (15).

CONCLUSION

Problematic patients present with a variety of conditions, but most can be managed effectively. The risk of an acute idiosyncratic reaction to contrast material can be reduced in high-risk patients through the use of nonionic RICM and the use of premedication with steroids and antihistamines. In patients at risk for acute nonidiosyncratic reactions, caution should be employed in the administration of RICM, and other diagnostic tests should be considered. Hydration is widely accepted as an intervention to reduce the risk of CIN. As premedication to lower the risk of CIN, acetylcysteine has a favorable cost and adverse event profile although definitive proof of effectiveness awaits additional investigations. Other CIN premedication regimens remain to be proved effective, and some are complicated by a relatively high number of adverse events. Delayed reactions are nonspecific and it is often unclear if they truly are caused by RICM administration; fortunately serious delayed reactions are rare. Patients taking metformin, pregnant patients, and patients who are breast-feeding can be managed by relatively simple interventions.

REFERENCES

1. Katayama H, Yamaguchi K, Kozuka T, et al. Adverse reactions to ionic and nonionic contrast media. A report from the Japanese Committee on the Safety of Contrast Media. Radiology 1990; 175:621–628.

2. Cohan RH, Leder RA, Ellis JH. Treatment of adverse reactions to radiographic contrast media in adults. Radiol Clin North Am 1996; 34:1055–1076.
3. Carr DH, Walker AC. Contrast media reactions: experimental evidence against the allergy theory. Br J Radiol 1984; 57:469–473.
4. Shehadi WH. Contrast media adverse reactions: occurrence, recurrence, and distribution patterns. Radiology 1982; 143:11–17.
5. Coakley FV, Panicek DM. Iodine allergy: an oyster without a pearl? AJR 169; 1997:951–952.
6. Wolf GL, Arenson RL, Cross AP. A prospective trial of ionic vs nonionic contrast agents in routine clinical practice: comparison of adverse effects. AJR 1989; 152:939–944.
7. Palmer FJ. The RACR survey of intravenous contrast media reactions final report. Australas Radiol 1988; 32:426–428.
8. Marshall GD Jr, Lieberman PL. Comparison of three pretreatment protocols to prevent anaphylactoid reactions to radiocontrast media. Ann Allergy 1991; 67:70–74.
9. Greenberger PA, Halwig JM, Patterson R, Wallemark CB. Emergency administration of radiocontrast media in high-risk patients. J Allergy Clin Immunol 1986; 77:630–634.
10. Greenberger PA, Patterson R. The prevention of immediate generalized reactions to radiocontrast media in high-risk patients. J Allergy Clin Immunol 1991; 87:867–872.
11. Lasser EC, Berry CC, Talner LB, et al. Pretreatment with corticosteroids to alleviate reactions to intravenous contrast material. N Engl J Med 1987; 317:845–849.
12. Lasser EC, Berry CC, Mishkin MM, et al. Pretreatment with corticosteroids to prevent adverse reactions to nonionic contrast media. AJR 1994; 162:523–526.
13. Ellis JH, Cohan RH, Sonnad SS, Cohan NS. Selective use of radiographic low-osmolality contrast media in the 1990s. Radiology 1996; 200:297–311.
14. Cohan RH, Dunnick NR. Intravascular contrast media: adverse reactions. AJR 1987; 149:665–670.
15. Committee on Drugs and Contrast Media. Manual on Contrast Media. Version 5.0. Reston, VA: American College of Radiology, 2004.
16. Mukherjee JJ, Peppercorn PD, Reznek RH, et al. Pheochromocytoma: effect of nonionic contrast medium in CT on circulating catecholamine levels. Radiology 1997; 202:227–231.
17. Porter GA. Radiocontrast-induced nephropathy. Nephrol Dial Transplant 1994; 9(suppl 4):146–156.
18. Ashley JB, Millward SF. Contrast agent-induced nephropathy: a simple way to identify patients with preexisting renal insufficiency. AJR 2003; 181:451–454.
19. Idee JM, Beaufils H, Bonnemain B. Iodinated contrast media-induced nephropathy: pathophysiology, clinical aspects and prevention. Fundam Clin Pharmacol 1994; 8:193–206.
20. Teruel JL, Marcen R, Onaindia JM, et al. Renal functional impairment caused by intravenous urography: a prospective study. Arch Intern Med 1981; 141:1271–1274.
21. Lautin EM, Freeman NJ, Schoenfeld AH, et al. Radiocontrast-associated renal dysfunction: incidence and risk factors. AJR 1991; 157:49–58.
22. Lautin EM, Freeman NJ, Schoenfeld AH, et al. Radiocontrast-associated renal dysfunction: a comparison of lower osmolality and conventional high-osmolality contrast media. AJR 1991; 157:59–65.
23. Porter GA. Contrast-associated nephropathy. Am J Cardiol 1989; 64:22E–26E.
24. Porter GA. Experimental contrast-associated nephropathy and its clinical implications. Am J Cardiol 1990; 66:18F–22F.
25. Porter GA. Contrast-associated nephropathy: presentation, pathophysiology and management. Miner Electrolyte Meta 1994; 20:232–243.
26. Schwab SJ, Hlatky MA, Pieper KS, et al. Contrast nephropathy: a randomized controlled trial of a nonionic and an ionic radiographic contrast agent. N Engl J Med 1989; 320:149–153.
27. Manske CL, Sprafka JM, Strony JT, Wang Y. Contrast nephropathy in azotemic diabetic patients undergoing coronary arteriography. Am J Med 1990; 89:615–629.
28. Barrett BJ. Contrast nephrotoxicity. J Am Soc Nephrol 1994; 5:125–137.
29. Tommaso CL. Contrast-induced nephrotoxicity in patients undergoing cardiac catheterization. Cathet Cardiovasc Diagn 1994; 31:316–321.

30. Rudnick MR, Goldfarb S, Wexler L, et al. Nephrotoxicity of ionic and nonionic contrast media in 1196 patients: a randomized trial. Kidney Int 1995; 47:254–261.
31. Taliercio CP, Vlietstra RE, Fisher LD, Burnett JC. Risk for renal dysfunction with cardiac angiography. Ann Int Med 1986; 104:501–504.
32. Morcos SK. Prevention of contrast media nephrotoxicity—the story so far. Clin Radiol 2004; 59:381–389.
33. McCarthy CS, Becker JA. Multiple myeloma and contrast media. Radiology 1992; 183:519–521.
34. Mueller C, Buerkle G, Buettner HJ, et al. Prevention of contrast media-associated nephropathy: randomized comparison of 2 hydration regimens in 1620 patients undergoing coronary angioplasty. Arch Intern Med 2002; 162:329–336.
35. Merten GJ, Burgess WP, Gray LV, et al. Prevention of contrast-induced nephropathy with sodium bicarbonate: a randomized controlled trial. JAMA 2004; 291:2328–2334.
36. Solomon R. Contrast-medium-induced acute renal failure. Kidney Int 1998; 53:230–242.
37. Tepel M, van der Giet M, Schwarzfeld C, et al. Prevention of radiographic-contrast-agent-induced reductions in renal function by acetylcysteine. N Engl J Med 2000; 343:180–184.
38. Gleeson TG, Bulugahapitiya S. Contrast-induced nephropathy. AJR 2004; 183:1673–1689.
39. Safirstein R, Andrade L, Vieira JM. Acetylcysteine and nephrotoxic effects of radiographic contrast agents—a new use for an old drug. N Engl J Med 2000; 343:210–212.
40. Diaz-Sandoval LJ, Kosowsky BD, Losordo DW. Acetylcysteine to prevent angiography-related renal tissue injury (the APART trial). Am J Cardiol 2002; 89:356–358.
41. Shyu KG, Cheng JJ, Kuan P. Acetylcysteine protects against acute renal damage in patients with abnormal renal function undergoing a coronary procedure. J Am Coll Cardiol 2002; 40:1383–1388.
42. Kay J, Chow WH, Chan TM, et al. Acetylcysteine for prevention of acute deterioration of renal function following elective coronary angiography and intervention: a randomized controlled trial. JAMA 2003; 289:553–558.
43. Baker CS, Wragg A, Kumar S, et al. A rapid protocol for the prevention of contrast-induced renal dysfunction: the RAPPID study. J Am Coll Cardiol 2003; 41:2114–2118.
44. MacNeill BD, Harding SA, Bazari H, et al. Prophylaxis of contrast-induced nephropathy in patients undergoing coronary angiography. Catheter Cardiovasc Interv 2003; 60:458–461.
45. Briguori C, Manganelli F, Scarpato P, et al. Acetylcysteine and contrast agent-associated nephrotoxicity. J Am Coll Cardiol 2002; 40:298–303.
46. Allaqaband S, Tumuluri R, Malik AM, et al. Prospective randomized study of N-acetyl-cysteine, fenoldopam, and saline for prevention of radiocontrast-induced nephropathy. Catheter Cardiovasc Interv 2002; 57:279–283.
47. Durham JD, Caputo C, Dokko J, et al. A randomized controlled trial of N-acetylcysteine to prevent contrast nephropathy in cardiac angiography. Kidney Int 2002; 62:2202–2207.
48. Boccalandro F, Amhad M, Smalling RW, Sdringola S. Oral acetylcysteine does not protect renal function from moderate to high doses of intravenous radiographic contrast. Catheter Cardiovasc Interv 2003; 58:336–341.
49. Oldemeyer JB, Biddle WP, Wurdeman RL, et al. Acetylcysteine in the prevention of contrast-induced nephropathy after coronary angiography. Am Heart J 2003; 146:E23.
50. Fung JW, Szeto CC, Chan WW, et al. Effect of N-acetylcysteine for prevention of contrast nephropathy in patients with moderate to severe renal insufficiency: a randomized trial. Am J Kidney Dis 2004; 43:801–808.
51. Birck R, Krzossok S, Markowetz F, et al. Acetylcysteine for prevention of contrast nephropathy: meta-analysis. Lancet 2003; 362:598–603.
52. Isenbarger DW, Kent SM, O'Malley PG. Meta-analysis of randomized clinical trials on the usefulness of acetylcysteine for prevention of contrast nephropathy. Am J Cardiol 2003; 92:1454–1458.
53. Briguori C, Colombo A, Violante A, et al. Standard vs double dose of N-acetylcysteine to prevent contrast agent associated nephrotoxicity. Eur Heart J 2004; 25:206–211.

54. Murphy MB, Murray C, Shorten GD. Fenoldopam: a selective peripheral dopamine-receptor agonist for the treatment of severe hypertension. N Engl J Med 2001; 345:1548–1557.

55. Bakris GL, Lass NA, Glock D. Renal hemodynamics in radiocontrast medium-induced renal dysfunction: a role for dopamine-1 receptors. Kidney Int 1999; 56:206–210.

56. Madyoon H, Croushore L, Weaver D, Mathur V. Use of fenoldopam to prevent radio-contrast nephropathy in high-risk patients. Catheter Cardiovasc Interv 2001; 53:341–345.

57. Stone GW, McCullough PA, Tumlin JA, et al. Fenoldopam mesylate for the prevention of contrast-induced nephropathy: a randomized controlled trial. JAMA 2003; 290:2284–2291.

58. Barrett BJ, Carlisle EJ. Metaanalysis of the relative nephrotoxicity of high- and low-osmolality iodinated contrast media. Radiology 1993; 188:171–178.

59. Chalmers N, Jackson RW. Comparison of iodixanol and iohexol in renal impairment. Br J Radiol 1999; 72:701–703.

60. Aspelin P, Aubry P, Fransson SG, et al. Nephrotoxic effects in high-risk patients undergoing angiography. N Engl J Med 2003; 348:491–499.

61. Choyke PL, Miller DL, Lotze MT, et al. Delayed reactions to contrast media after interleukin-2 immunotherapy. Radiology 1992; 183:111–114.

62. Donnelly PK, Williams B, Watkin EM. Polyarthropathy—a delayed reaction to low osmolality angiographic contrast medium in patients with end stage renal disease. Eur J Radiol 1993; 17:130–132.

63. Christiansen C, Pichler WJ, Skotland T. Delayed allergy-like reactions to x-ray contrast media: mechanistic considerations. Eur Radiol 2000; 10:1965–1975.

64. Webb JA, Stacul F, Thomsen HS, et al. Late adverse reactions to intravascular iodinated contrast media. Eur Radiol 2003; 13:181–184.

65. Yasuda R, Munechika H. Delayed adverse reactions to nonionic monomeric contrast-enhanced media. Invest Radiol 1998; 33:1–5.

66. Shulman KL, Thompson JA, Benyunes MC, Winter TC, Fefer A. Adverse reactions to intravenous contrast media in patients treated with interleukin-2. J Immunotherapy 1993; 13:208–212.

67. Assan R, Heuclin C, Ganeval D, et al. Metformin-induced lactic acidosis in the presence of acute renal failure. Diabetologia 1977; 13:211–217.

68. Bailey CJ, Turner RC. Metformin. N Engl J Med 1996; 334:574–579.

69. Dachman AH. New contraindication to intravascular iodinated contrast material. Radiology 1995; 197:545.

70. Rasuli P, French GJ, Hammond DI. Metformin hydrochloride all right before, but not after, contrast medium administration. Radiology 1998; 209:586–587.

71. Nawaz S, Cleveland T, Gaines PA, Chan P. Clinical risk associated with contrast angiography in metformin treated patients: a clinical review. Clin Radiol 1998; 53:342–344.

72. McCartney MM, Gilbert FJ, Murchison LE, et al. Metformin and contrast media—a dangerous combination? Clin Radiol 1999; 54:29–33.

73. Landewe-Cleuren S, van Zwam WH, de Bruin TW, de Haan M. Prevention of lactic acidosis due to metformin intoxication in contrast media nephropathy [in Dutch]. Ned Tijdschr Geneeskd 2000; 144:1903–1905.

74. Moon AJ, Katzberg RW, Sherman MP. Transplacental passage of iohexol. J Pediatrics 2000; 136:548–549.

75. Bona G, Zaffaroni M, Defilippi C, Gallina MR, Mostert M. Effects of iopamidol on neonatal thyroid function. Eur J Radiol 1992; 14:22–25.

76. Nielson ST, Matheson JN, Skinnemoen K, Andrew E, Hafsahl G. Excretion of iohexol in human breast milk. Acta Radiologica 1987; 28:523–526.

77. Schmiedl U, Maravilla KR, Gerlach R, Dowling CA. Excretion of gadopentatate dimeglumine in human breast milk. AJR 1990; 154:1305–1306.

2

Helical CT in the Diagnosis of Urolithiasis

Robert P. Hartman, Akira Kawashima, and Andrew J. LeRoy
Department of Radiology, Mayo Clinic, Rochester, Minnesota, U.S.A.

INTRODUCTION

Urinary stone (calculus) disease is one of the most common urinary tract abnormalities. Although small renal stones are often asymptomatic, clinical presentations in affected patients include hematuria, pain, urinary obstruction, infection, and renal functional impairment, the last occasionally being irreversible. Because of the frequent recurrence of renal stones and their complications, imaging studies play an important role in the diagnosis and management of both patients with acute and patients with chronic urinary stone disease (1–4). The introduction of helical computed tomography (CT) technology in 1990 changed the urologic evaluation of patients with urinary calculi. Since Smith et al. first reported the use of unenhanced CT for the evaluation of patients with acute flank abdominal pain (5), CT has become the imaging modality of choice at the vast majority of emergency centers in the United States. Many studies have documented the unmatched accuracy of CT in the detection of urinary stones when compared to plain abdominal radiography [kidney, ureters, and bladder (KUB) radiographs], excretory urography (EU), ultrasonography (US), and magnetic resonance imaging (MRI).

BACKGROUND

The first radiograph of a urinary calculus was obtained by John McIntyre in 1896 within months of Roentgen's original report (6). In the following century, many reports in the radiologic and urologic literature overestimated the ability of plain abdominal radiographs or KUBs to detect ureteral calculi (3). In 1962, Herring examined the composition of 10,000 urinary calculi and found that approximately 90% of these contained calcium (7). This report has been cited as evidence that 90% of ureteral calculi therefore are visible on KUB radiographs (8). However, in studies by Roth et al. (9) and Mutgi et al. (10), in which radiographs in patients with known urinary tract calculi were retrospectively reviewed, sensitivities of 62% and 58% for plain film detection of urinary tract calculi were reported. Given this relatively low sensitivity, reliance on the KUB film alone has not been recommended (unless it is obviously positive). Therefore, currently, the KUB examination alone has a limited role in initial clinical stone diagnosis.

The primary factors that affect the detection of ureteral stones on KUBs include stone size, composition, and location. Stone size has the greatest effect on clinical detection on plain radiographs. Smaller stones are more difficult to identify than larger ones. The radiopacity of ureteral calculi also affects the detectability of any stone on plain radiographs. Stones composed of calcium phosphate have the greatest density of common stones, followed by slightly less opaque stones of calcium oxalate

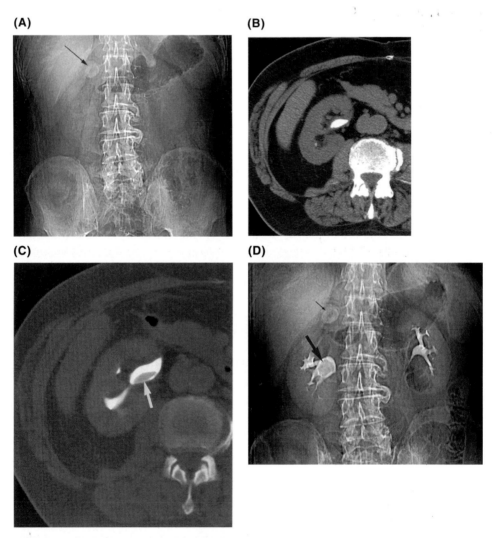

Figure 1 Uric acid stones (**A**) CT SPR image obtained at 80 kVp and 300 mA reveals no opaque renal stones. A large calcified gallstone (*arrow*) projects over the right-upper quadrant of the abdomen. (**B**) Unenhanced CT scans demonstrate a 2 cm stone in the right renal pelvis and a tiny caliceal tip renal stone. (**C**) Renal pelvic stone appears as a filling defect (*arrow*) on the bone window setting of the pyelographic phase image of a subsequently performed enhanced CT. (**D**) CT SPR image obtained eight minutes after intravenous contrast administration shows the large uric acid stone as a filling defect (*large arrow*) in the right renal pelvis (calcified gallstone, *small arrow*). *Abbreviations*: CT, computed tomography; SPR, scanned projection radiography.

and magnesium ammonium phosphate. Uric acid stones are radiolucent (Fig. 1), and small cystine stones are frequently radiolucent. Cystine stones that grow larger than 1.5 cm in size become faintly radiopaque. The accumulation of calcium and other mineral salts within larger cystine and uric acid stones also increases the likelihood of their detection on plain radiographs. Rarely encountered matrix stones are usually radiolucent. This relative opacity scale for various stones has been derived from film radiograph interpretations, including the term *radiolucent*. (A similar stone composition analysis based on CT appearances is not yet available.) The position of the stone also can lead to difficulty in detection either by obscuring overlying bowel contents or bone, or from misinterpretation of calcific densities in the abdomen or pelvis such as arterial calcifications, calcified lymph nodes, calcified masses, or phleboliths. The detection of stones located in the soft tissues of the pelvis is a particularly common clinical problem because of the presence of pelvic phleboliths. The dilemma of confusing a pelvic phlebolith with a distal ureteral stone was noted as a limitation of plain radiography as early as 1908 in a study by Orton (11).

In 1929, Swick first introduced EU as a practical procedure (12). Urographic opacification of the ureter permitted the determination of the ureteral position in relation to the calcification seen on the plain radiograph of the abdomen and pelvis to determine whether the opacity was a ureteral stone or an extraureteral calcification. In addition to delineating the course of the ureter to the level of stones, signs of stone-induced ureteral obstruction could be detected, including delayed nephrogram, delayed excretion of contrast material, dilatation of the intrarenal collecting system, forniceal rupture with perinephric contrast extravasation, and dilatation of the ureter down to the presumed stone seen on the plain radiograph. Of course, there are occasional limitations. Excretion into the obstructed renal collecting system can be delayed. An EU may take hours to complete in patients with moderate or high-grade obstructions. Also, EU cannot be performed in patients with contraindications for intravascular injection of iodinated contrast material.

CT EVALUATION

Application of Unenhanced Helical CT to the Evaluation of Flank Pain

Since Smith et al. first reported the use of unenhanced CT in the evaluation of patients with flank pain in 1995, CT has become the study of choice for the evaluation of suspected ureterolithiasis (5). The sensitivity of noncontrast helical CT detection of urinary calculi has been reported to range from 97% to 100%, with specificities between 92% and 100% (13–16). Stone size and location can be accurately defined.

In addition to the superior accuracy of noncontrast helical CT compared to other imaging modalities for stone detection and localization, both the rapid speed of the CT examination and the detection of nonstone disease have positioned CT as the primary diagnostic examination in acutely symptomatic patients. A modern multidetector row helical CT (MDCT) scan can be obtained in less than 20 seconds or a single breath-hold compared with at least 40 to 60 minutes for an EU examination (3). Unenhanced CT examination is currently well accepted by patients because iodinated contrast injection or bowel preparation is not needed.

Because CT exams are not limited to visualizing only the urinary tracts (in contrast to EU), the detection of nonurinary tract disease is an important advantage of CT in the evaluation of acute abdominal pain. Alternative diagnoses were made in

14% of cases in a series by Smith et al. (13). Fielding et al. reported noncalculus urinary pathology in 14% and nonurinary diagnoses in 11% of cases (14). Commonly encountered extraurinary causes for abdominal or pelvic pain—including diverticulitis, appendicitis, inflammatory bowel disease, ruptured abdominal aneurysm, and ovarian masses thought to have undergone torsion—can all be detected with CT, as well as nonstone related urinary tract disorders such as pyelonephritis and renal masses (17).

An additional advantage of using CT for stone detection is in the evaluation of patients with complex body physiques that prevent detection on using traditional radiographic techniques. Those patients with severe scoliosis or obesity are readily studied with CT, while EU and US are often indeterminate because of physical limitations. In patients with renal transplants, CT not only defines the status of stone disease in the transplanted kidney but also permits evaluation of the native, minimally functioning kidneys for stones or collecting system obstruction.

The utilization of CT for stone disease evaluation has several disadvantages. An inexpensive and accurate way of following small stones identified on an emergency room (ER) CT scan is yet to be defined. As already stated, often, follow-up KUB radiographs are indeterminate. Nonvisualization of a calculus previously identified on a CT on a subsequent KUB film could indicate that the stone has been passed in the urine or that it is still in place but merely is not detectable on conventional radiographs to begin with. Repeated CT scans in this setting may not be cost efficient. Additionally, the detection of innumerable tiny calculi within the kidneys in asymptomatic patients has created a new class of patients who have radiographically definable stone disease, but no clinical sequelae. Patients with medullary sponge kidney and associated stone disease (Fig. 2) and those with chronic stone disease who undergo regular metabolic reevaluations may be difficult to evaluate with serial CT scanning compared to a KUB because their multiple tiny stones may change in position from study to study. In patients with chronic stone disease, major clinical decisions about stone therapy options are based on stone growth, movement, and composition. In many patients, the traditional KUB may address these specific issues equally well as the more expensive CT examination.

Comparison with Urinalysis, KUB, EU, US, and MR Urography

Recent comparison of CT with other clinical and imaging diagnostic methods, including urinalysis and other radiographic studies, has confirmed unenhanced CT's unrivaled position as the most accurate method for urinary stone detection. For example, one study has shown that reliance on the presence or absence of hematuria in deciding whether urolithiasis may be present is frequently not helpful. Luchs et al. reported an 84% sensitivity of hematuria on microscopic urinalysis in 587 patients with ureteral stones revealed by unenhanced CT (18). However, the specificity and negative predictive value were much lower, at 48% and 65%, respectively (18).

The more traditional imaging techniques of conventional radiography and EU have also proven much less sensitive. In a retrospective study by Levine et al. in 1997 comparing the sensitivity of KUB with unenhanced CT, a sensitivity of 59% was found for detecting ureteral calculi on the KUB (8). In a study by Jackman et al., only 22 of 46 (48%) ureteral stones shown on CT were visible on KUB (19). Out of 20 patients with renal colic, Smith et al. reported that both unenhanced CT and EU demonstrated ureteral obstruction in 12 patients (5). Of these 12 patients, a ureteral stone was demonstrated in five on both CT and EU, a stone was depicted

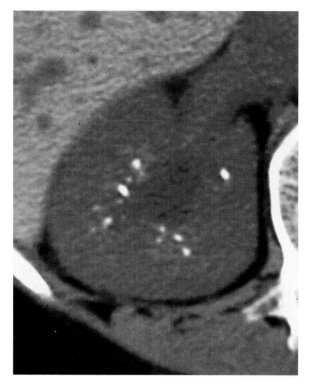

Figure 2 Unenhanced CT of the right kidney demonstrates medullary nephrocalcinosis and ne-phrolithiasis in a patient with medullary sponge kidney. *Abbreviation*: CT, computed tomography.

in six on CT only, and a stone could not be delineated definitively in one patient on CT or EU. In a report by Sourtzis et al., CT was also shown to be more accurate in identifying ureteral stones than EU (20).

Pfister et al. have shown unenhanced CT to be more effective in evaluating patients with acute renal colic than EU (21). In a study of 115 patients with asymptomatic microscopic hematuria, urinary calculi were revealed by CT in 24 patients (22). Stones were identified on EU in only 13 of these 24 patients. Calculi missed on EU tended to be relatively small. They ranged in size from 1 to 5 mm. In this series, one false positive CT for ureteral stone could have been avoided if the protocol had included unenhanced imaging of the entire ureters (22).

In a recent study of combined imaging utilizing both KUB and US compared with unenhanced CT for diagnosing ureteral stones by Catalano et al. in 2002, combining KUB and US had a stone detection sensitivity of 77% as against 92% with unenhanced CT (23). Acute ureteral obstruction detection with US is compromised because it may take many hours following onset of symptoms before identifiable distension of the upper urinary tract develops. The use of intrarenal Doppler US can improve the detection of early obstruction based on measurement of an elevated resistive index (RI). In a 2001 study by Shokeir and Abdulmaaboud, detection of a change in RI facilitated diagnosis of ureteral obstruction in 47 (90%) of 52 patients with obstructing ureteral stones shown on EU. Unenhanced CT demonstrated ureteral stones in 50 (96%) of these patients (24). US has the advantage of avoiding patient radiation exposure, but the US examination is much more time consuming and its quality is very dependent both on the operator's skills and on the patient's body habitus.

There are only a few studies that have compared the ability of MRI to diagnose urolithiasis with that of unenhanced CT. In a study of 49 patients with acute flank pain who were imaged with unenhanced CT, magnetic resonance (MR) urography with and without gadolinium, and EU, ureteral stones were found in 32 patients. The sensitivities of MR urography in detecting ureteral stones and obstruction were 94% to 100% and 100%, respectively, whereas those of CT were 87% to 91% and 94%, respectively (25). In the same study, stone size was more accurately assessed on CT than MR urography, and all small caliceal renal stones shown on CT were not defined on MR urography. MR urography does not involve radiation exposure but is more expensive, less readily available in the ER setting, and is a much longer examination than unenhanced CT.

CT Techniques

No patient preparation is required for unenhanced renal stone CT. The usual method of scanning uses 120 to 140 peak kilovolt (kVp) with 5 mm collimation and pitch of 1.0 to 1.5. At many institutions, renal stone CT is performed using reduced mA (<100 mA rather than the more standard exposure of >200 mA). Issues related to the choice of mA will be discussed further in section 3.5. After the patient's basic abdominal anatomy is defined on the initial CT scanned projection radiograph, referred to as CT scout (GE Healthcare, Milwaukee, Wisconsin, U.S.A.) or topogram (Siemens Medical Systems, Iselin, New Jersey, U.S.A.), axial scanning proceeds from just cephalad to the kidneys (usually at the level of T12) to just below the bladder base (at the level of pubic symphysis) in one or two breath-holds in most patients. With the increased speed and tube heat capacity of the more recently introduced MDCT scanners, the entire scan can be obtained comfortably during one suspension of respiratory motion. Some authors have advocated scanning the patient in the prone position, but this often is not possible in the ER setting because patients with severe abdominal pain are too uncomfortable to lie prone. Occasionally, selective additional lateral or prone images may be helpful in determining if a stone is impacted in the ureter at the ureterovesical junction or if it has passed into the bladder (Fig. 3). An indeterminate opacity in the region of the ureter can be further assessed with retrospective scan reconstructions in 2 to 3 mm slice increments and thinner slice thicknesses through the limited region containing the opacity.

Soft copy interpretation at a workstation is more efficient and accurate than hardcopy interpretation. Curved 2-D reformation paralleling the course of the ureter has been suggested as a helpful diagnostic tool (26), but creation of these images can be time-intensive for the physician. Any reformatted images of the ureters can be generated from the axially acquired dataset on a dedicated CT workstation.

It is frequently advantageous to have a radiologist review the images while the patient is still on the CT table. Sometimes, intravenous administration of iodinated contrast material can determine if the opacity of interest lies within the ureter when unenhanced CT findings are indeterminate. Such intravenous contrast enhancement may be necessary in 12% of cases (3). Opacification of the ureters usually can be displayed on CT images obtained five minutes after starting intravenous contrast administration. The concept of "indication creep" has been defined where some physicians request CT for stone detection as a general screening test for all patients with abdominal pain (27). Close interactions between CT radiologists and ER physicians

(A)

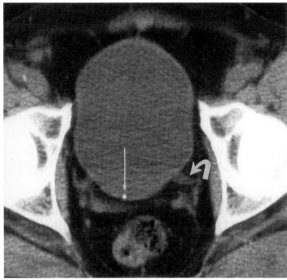

(B)

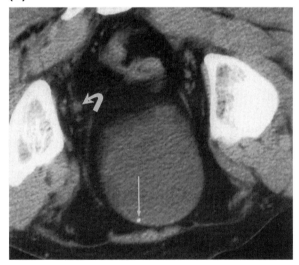

Figure 3 Tiny bladder calculus recently passed from the left ureter. (**A**) Unenhanced CT scan reveals a stone in the posterior aspect of the urinary bladder (*small arrow*). Occasionally, it is difficult to determine whether stones in this location are in a distal ureter near the ureterovesical junction or have passed into the bladder ureterclasis present (*curved arrow*). (**B**) Repeat CT scan obtained in the prone position confirms that this stone is mobile within the bladder (*small arrow*). Left ureterectasis is seen on both the supine and the prone CT images (*curved arrow*). *Abbreviation*: CT, computed tomography.

can help determine when intravenous contrast administration may be helpful after a nondiagnostic unenhanced scan to further evaluate for noncalculus renal pathology [e.g., acute pyelonephritis, infected hydronephrosis (pyonephrosis), renal infarct, renal vein thrombosis, tumor] and nonurinary pathology in patients with somewhat nonspecific symptoms (Fig. 4) (3,28,29).

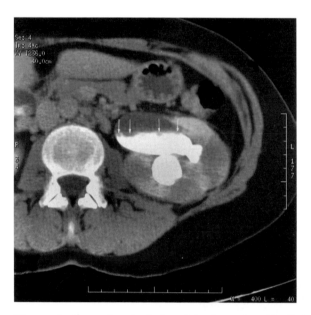

Figure 4 Pyonephrosis (infected hydronephrosis). Enhanced CT scan demonstrates left pyelocaliectasis with irregular urine-contrast level (*arrows*) due to collecting system debris. Coarse hypoattenuating areas in the left renal parenchyma are characteristic of acute pyelonephritis. CT scans at a lower level displayed an obstructing stone in the left ureter (not shown). *Abbreviation*: CT, computed tomography.

Although the KUB has a limited value for the initial diagnosis of urinary stones, it may still be useful for following patients with stones documented by non-contrast CT. CT scanned projection radiography (SPR) images primarily are obtained as the initial anatomic reference to prescribe the subsequent axial CT scan parameters, but the performance and role of CT SPR images have been studied in evaluating CT-detected urinary stones. Chu et al. (30) and Assi et al. (31) reported 49% and 47% sensitivities, respectively, of CT SPR images obtained at 120 to 140 kVp and 80 mAs for the detection of ureteral stones. In a study from our institution, 7 (30%) to 11 (48%) of 23 ureteral stones were prospectively identified on CT SPR images obtained at 80 kVp and 300 mA, without the prior knowledge of unenhanced CT findings (32). When correlated with the unenhanced CT findings, 16 (70%) of 23 ureteral stones were visible on CT SPR images, a sensitivity comparable to that of KUB, where 17 (74%) of the ureteral stones were identified. Therefore, a review of the CT SPR image in patients with diagnosed ureteral stones may be useful in determining if the affected patient can be followed with KUB rather than by serial CT exams. In some instances, axial CT image characteristics of a detected calculus can be used to predict the likelihood of stone visibility on a KUB radiograph. Zagoria et al. found that 95% of stones measuring greater than 300 Hounsfield Units (HU) on axial CT images obtained using 5 mm thickness could be seen on KUB films, whereas only 7% of calculi measuring less than 200 HU could be detected (33). Nearly 80% of calculi measuring 5 mm or larger on the axial CT images could be detected on KUB films, as opposed to only 37% measuring less than 5 mm (33).

CT urography recently has evolved as the primary radiologic examination for the evaluation of patients with common and uncommon urologic conditions (34,35). Excretory phase-enhanced CT is an essential part of CT urography protocols.

When pyelonephritis is suspected in a febrile patient with a ureteral stone revealed by noncontrast CT, contrast-enhanced CT can help estimate the degree of urinary obstruction and demonstrate changes of acute renal inflammation. Excretory phase-enhanced CT scans are useful in determining whether an indeterminate calcification lies in the intrarenal collecting system or ureter and in differentiating parapelvic cysts from hydronephrosis (36). Excretory phase-enhanced CT can also establish a diagnosis of a caliceal diverticulum complicated with stones or better delineate other complex stone diseases with associated distortion of the intrarenal collecting system.

Interpretation

The primary sign of ureterolithiasis on unenhanced CT is the identification of a focus of increased attenuation located within the ureteral lumen. The ureter can be followed on axial CT slices from the renal pelvis as it courses caudally, anterior to the psoas muscle, and initially lateral to the gonadal vein. Lower in the abdomen, the gonadal vein crosses the ureter, and the ureter courses medially. In the pelvis, the ureter over-rides the iliac vessels, courses through the mid-pelvis laterally, and then turns medially to the ureterovesical junction through the space anterior to the seminal vesicle and posterior to the posterolateral aspect of the bladder. Calculi commonly become lodged at several typical sites along the course of the ureter: at the ureteropelvic junction, as the ureter crosses the iliac vessels, and at the ureterovesical junction.

Secondary signs have been described for aiding the diagnosis of ureteral stones in difficult cases (5,13,37,38). These signs include pyelocaliectasis and ureterectasis proximal to a stone, perinephric edema, and nephromegaly on the symptomatic side. The contralateral kidney and ureter can be used as an intrinsic reference. Perinephric edema consists of stranding in the perinephric fat, perinephric fluid collections, and/ or thickening of the renal fascia (Fig. 5) (39). In a study by Katz et al. (38), dilatation

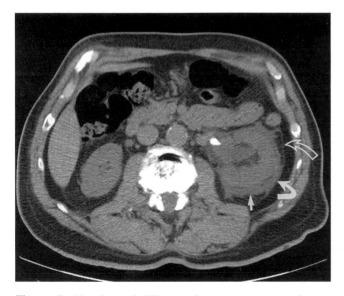

Figure 5 Unenhanced CT scan demonstrates a renal stone at the ureteropelvic junction associated with a perinephric fluid collection (*straight arrow*). The fluid collection extends to Gerota's fascia (*curved arrow*). Gerota's fascia is also thickened (*open arrow*). *Abbreviation*: CT, computed tomography.

of the ipsilateral renal collecting system was present in 69% of patients with ureteral stones, ureteral dilatation in 67%, perinephric edema in 65%, and periureteric edema in 65%. When several secondary signs are seen together, however, the positive predictive value increases dramatically. For example, the combination of perinephric edema and ureteral dilatation for the diagnosis of ureteral obstruction has been reported to occur in 99% of cases (37). Because the presence of secondary signs on the symptomatic side is highly indicative of a stone in the ureter, careful scrutiny to identify a stone is necessary. An indeterminate opacity in the region of the ureter should strongly suggest a ureteral stone if the secondary signs are present.

Perinephric edema seen on CT manifests the physiologic changes in the kidney secondary to acute obstruction. Increased pressure in the intrarenal collecting system in the acute phase of obstruction causes increased lymphatic flow in the perinephric space. In addition, there can be pyelotubular, pyelolymphatic, pyelosinus, and pyelovenous backflow, and elevated intrarenal venous pressure. The perinephric edema seen on CT probably represents resorbed urine and lymphatic fluid infiltrating the perinephric space along the renal capsule, the bridging septa of Kunin, and the pararenal fascia. A perinephric fluid collection probably represents a later phase of the same process, with confluent fluid collections most frequent on CT along the renal capsular surface. Occasionally, excretory phase-enhanced CT scans can document urinary extravasation from caliceal rupture secondary to an obstructing ureteral stone (Fig. 6). The amount of perinephric edema has been reported to correlate with the degree of ureteral obstruction as shown on EU (39). However, other studies have not found this to be the case. When limited perinephric edema is found, low-grade obstruction is likely to be found with EU. Extensive perinephric edema on CT is highly predictive of the calculus causing high-grade obstruction on EU (39). In a report with contrary results by Bird et al., the secondary CT findings alone were not helpful in differentiating high-grade obstruction from low-grade obstruction as evidenced by furosemide diuretic scintirenography (40). In a study by Varanelli et al., the presence of secondary signs on CT increased in frequency related to the prolongation of the duration of patient symptoms (41). It also remains controversial whether the presence and severity of the secondary CT signs of obstruction can predict the likelihood of spontaneous stone passage. Takahashi et al. reported that, in addition to stone size, the degree of perinephric fat stranding and perinephric fluid collection was helpful in predicting the stone passage (42), whereas Boulay et al. (43) and Fielding et al. (44) reported that secondary CT signs of obstruction were not useful in predicting the clinical outcome.

Stone size is the single most reliable indicator of spontaneous ureteral stone passage. In a 2002 study by Coll et al., the spontaneous passage rate for stones measured on axial CT at 1 mm in diameter was 87%; for stones 2 to 4 mm, 76%; for stones 5 to 7 mm, 60%; for stones 7 to 9 mm, 48%; and for stones larger than 9 mm, 25% (45). The spontaneous passage rate as a function of stone location was 48% for proximal ureter stones, 60% for mid-ureteral stones, 75% for distal stones, and 79% for ureterovesical junction stones. In general, stones 6 mm or greater in size have usually required intervention. In an experimental phantom study by Olcott et al., three-dimensional (3-D) maximal intensity projection images have been shown to be more accurate in determining stone size than conventional radiography and nephrotomography (46). Coronally reformatted images have also been shown to more accurately predict stone size than axial CT images alone in a clinical study (47). Both 3-D and coronal reformatted images likely allow for more accurate determination of stone size along the z-axis, which is often the longest stone diameter.

(A)

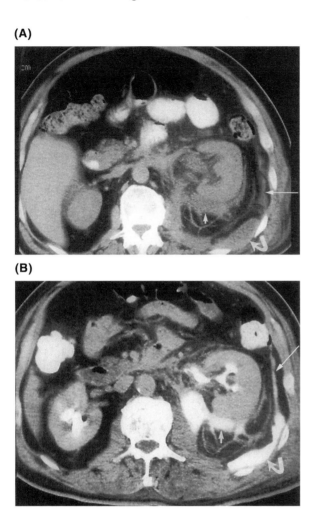

(B)

Figure 6 Urinary extravasation due to an obstructing ureteral stone. (**A**) Unenhanced CT scans demonstrate stranding of the perinephric fat on the left and a large amount of perinephric (*short straight arrow*) and pararenal (*curved arrow*) fluid. Gerota's fascia is thickened (*long straight arrow*). (**B**) Excretory phase-enhanced CT scan reveals urinary extravasation into the left perinephric (*short straight arrow*) and posterior pararenal (*curved arrow*) spaces. Thickening of Gerota's fascia (*long straight arrow*). *Abbreviation*: CT, computed tomography.

Georgiades et al. have reported that differences in renal parenchymal attenuation on unenhanced CT between an acutely obstructed kidney and the nonobstructed contralateral normal kidney is a reliable secondary sign of acute renal obstruction (48). The attenuation of the "pale" kidney secondary to renal parenchymal edema from obstruction is less than that of the normal side and the difference in attenuation is usually more than 5 HU. This sign is not completely specific for an acute obstruction. The "pale" kidney sign may also be caused by interstitial edema from acute pyelonephritis and by venous congestion from renal vein thrombosis.

A major pitfall in the interpretation of unenhanced CT in the evaluation of patients with suspected ureterolithiasis is the frequent inability to identify accurately the ureter amongst periureteral vessels and to differentiate with certainty ureteral stones from extraurinary calcifications (e.g., renal artery calcification, iliac artery calcification, phleboliths, and calcified vas deferens). In some cases, intrinsic morphologic features of a pelvic calcification can be used to help determine whether it is within or merely adjacent to the urinary tract.

While it has long been known that on KUB films phleboliths are typically round and may contain a central area of lucency, this lucency is only rarely seen on CT (Fig. 7). Whereas most phleboliths are round or oval, most ureteral calculi are slightly angular in shape (49).

The "soft tissue rim" sign, a 1 mm to 2 mm halo of soft tissue attenuation around a focus of increased attenuation on unenhanced CT, has been described as a useful sign in diagnosing ureteral stones and in differentiating a ureteral stone from a pelvic phlebolith (Fig. 8). The rim is considered to represent the edematous ureteral wall surrounding an impacted stone. The sensitivity and specificity of this sign have been reported in one study to be 76% and 92%, respectively (50). In another study, the rim sign was positive in 50% of ureteral stones, indeterminate in 34% (because of the lack of a periureteral fat plane), and negative in 16% (51). Therefore, the absence of the soft tissue rim sign does not preclude the diagnosis of ureteral stone. The soft tissue rim is present around only 0% to 20% of phleboliths (50–52). Larger (greater than 5 mm) stones less commonly exhibit a "rim" sign, likely due to stretching of the ureteral wall. In a study by Guest et al., the presence of a positive "rim" sign only without associated secondary signs was found in only 1 of 37 patients with ureteral stones (53). The rim sign is rarely the sole indicator of the presence or absence of ipsilateral ureterolithiasis.

The "comet-tail" sign, an eccentric tapering of soft tissue extending from one surface of a calcification (analogous to the appearance of a comet), has been reported as a useful sign in diagnosing phleboliths (52,54) (Fig. 9). The presence

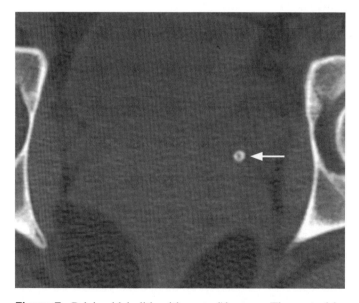

Figure 7 Pelvic phlebolith with central lucency. The central lucency of a phlebolith in the left side of the pelvis (*arrow*) on a 2.5 mm slice thickness CT scan that was retrospectively generated from the original 5 mm slice thickness CT scan. *Abbreviation*: CT, computed tomography.

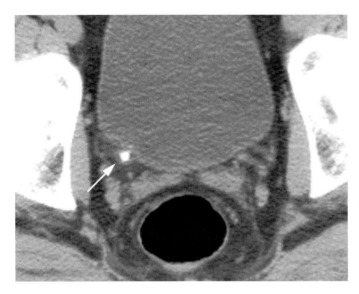

Figure 8 Unenhanced CT scan reveals a small stone in the distal right ureter (*arrow*) associated with the "soft tissue rim" sign, a halo of soft tissue attenuation surrounding the stone. *Abbreviation*: CT, computed tomography.

of the tail sign has been reported in 21% of pheboliths and 0% of ureteral stones (52). Identification of a positive "comet-tail" sign does not preclude the coexistence of ureterolithiasis because the sign is occasionally present adjacent to calculi or in patients with ipsilateral calculi located elsewhere in the pelvis (53).

The complications of urinary stone disease are better defined with CT than competing imaging modalities. Renal and perinephric abnormalities secondary to

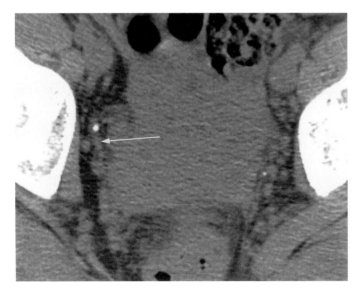

Figure 9 Unenhanced CT scan shows the "comet-tail" sign (*arrow*), an eccentric tapering soft tissue extension from one surface of calcification as from a comet, characteristic of a phlebolith. *Abbreviation*: CT, computed tomography.

acute stone disease are described above. Renal abscess formation secondary to inf-ected stone material is well defined on CT (28). CT is also the radiologic examination of choice for delineating chronic urinary tract abnormalities related to underlying stone disease, such as renal parenchymal atrophy, renal sinus replacement lipomato-sis (Fig. 10), and xanthogranulomatous pyelonephritis (Fig. 11) (28).

Radiation Exposure

Physician and patient concerns remain about the radiation exposure that results from widespread and often repeated use of CT. The target population with sympto-matic stone disease is generally young and has a nonfatal illness (3). Although unen-hanced CT provides diagnostic advantages and does not require intravenous iodinated contrast material, the radiation exposure accompanied by CT has been reported to be two to three times higher than that of EU (21). In one study, Denton et al. reported exposure of CT as 4.7 mSv versus 1.5 mSv for a three-film EU (55). Homer et al. reported an average effective dose of 4.95 mSv for unenhanced CT per-formed with 5 mm thick images, a 2.0 pitch, 120 kV, and 280 mA versus 1.48 mSv for EU (56). In a study by Pfister et al., the mean radiation dose was 6.5 mSv for unen-hanced CT with 5 mm collimation, 1.5 pitch, 120 kV, and 260 mAs versus 3.3 mSv for EU (21).

For patients undergoing a CT examination, the absorbed radiation dose depends on the CT technique. Scanning techniques utilizing reduced mAs (decreased from typically used values exceeding 200 mA to well under 100 mA) still allow for detection of most stones, while exposing patients to less radiation. Studies on mod-ifying CT techniques to maintain accurate detection of stones with reduced radiation dosage are in progress (57–60). Newer CT scanners include better collimators, detec-tors, and processors so that the dose from a single noncontrast helical CT is

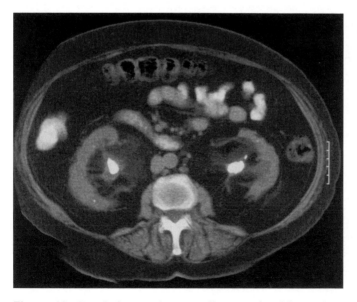

Figure 10 Renal sinus replacement lipomatosis with renal stones. Unenhanced CT scan reveals calculi in the renal pelvis with associated renal parenchymal loss, increased amount of renal sinus fat, and renal sinus fat stranding. *Abbreviation*: CT, computed tomography.

(A)

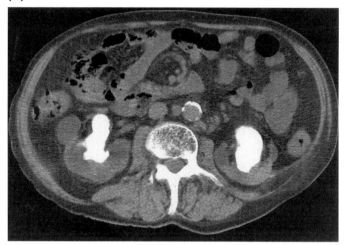

(B)

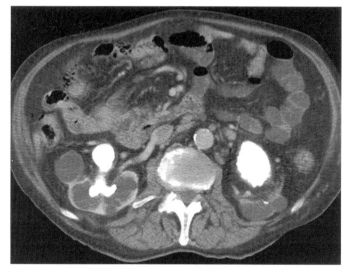

Figure 11 Bilateral xanthogranulomatous pyelonephritis. (**A**) Unenhanced CT scan demonstrates large branching calculi in the renal pelvis bilaterally. (**B**) Enhanced CT scan demonstrates hydronephrotic-appearing areas of decreased attenuation in the renal parenchyma. *Abbreviation*: CT, computed tomography.

approaching that of a standard six-film EU examination. However, performing multiple CT acquisition series, such as precontrast and postcontrast, or rescanning with thinner collimation considerably increases the patient dose. More recently, automatic tube current modulation techniques on MDCT scanners have been shown to maintain acceptable image quality regardless of patient attenuation characteristics while substantially reducing patient radiation exposure (61).

The imaging of suspected stone disease in pregnant patients causes considerable anxiety in both the patient and her imaging physician about potential adverse affects on the fetus. Symptomatic stones affect about 0.25% of all pregnancies, usually in the

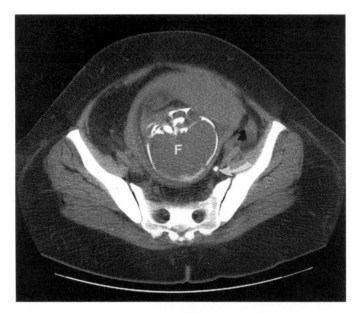

Figure 12 Unenhanced CT scan obtained through the pelvis reveals a stone (*arrow*) in the distal left ureter. Note a fetus (F) in the gravid uterus. *Abbreviation*: CT, computed tomography.

third trimester, usually pass without intervention and are the most common nonobstetric cause for a pregnant patient's hospitalization. Although most patients can be managed clinically without imaging, in those patients with prolonged pain or the development of infectious complications, imaging may become necessary (62). Serial examinations with US, including transvaginal imaging, often are not diagnostic for stone disease. Rather than perform a "limited urogram," we have switched to CT (Fig. 12) in this setting based on the lower radiation dose to the fetus calculated by our physicists compared to the serial films required for a urogram (63). The ability of CT to detect nonurinary tract diseases in this setting is an important clinical consideration. The utilization of MR imaging is also evolving in this setting of pregnancy.

CT Characterization of Stone Composition

The vast majority of renal and ureteral calculi can be detected on unenhanced CT. To some degree the visibility relates to stone size and composition (64). Stones that are not visible on KUB but visible on CT include small stones and plain film–radiolucent stones, such as uric acid stone, xanthine, triamterene (65), ephedrine, and guifenesin (66). Rarely encountered small matrix stones (67) and stones composed of excreted protease-inhibitor drugs (namely indinavir, nelfinavir, and sulfadiazine) for the treatment of HIV-infected patients (68) are not opaque on unenhanced CT and appear as filling defects in the renal collecting system on excretory phase-enhanced CT scans. In a series by Bani Hani et al., CT showed an egg-shaped mass with a thin outer rim of calcification surrounding a soft-tissue density center in three of five patients with matrix stones (69).

Stone composition is one factor in determining the mechanical properties of how stones fragment when exposed to lithotripter shock waves (70). Attempts have been made by many investigators to determine stone composition using CT attenuation value measurements of stones in vitro (71–73) and in vivo (74–77). Most of the in vivo studies were able to differentiate uric acid stone from at least one other stone type. In a recent in vitro study by Zarse et al., high-resolution MDCT yielded no overlapping range in attenuation value of various stones including uric acid stones (566–632 HU), struvite (862–944 HU), calcium oxalate (1416–1938 HU), and hydroxyapatitie (2150–2461 HU) (73).

Future Developments

CT is now well established as the primary radiological examination in the detection of urinary tract stone disease. Several potential applications of CT technology hold promise for further increasing the clinical value of CT in stone evaluation. An accurate CT-based method of defining overall stone volume would be helpful both in determining the choice of stone therapy and in assessing the results of that therapy. This would be particularly advantageous in those patients with medically treatable stones such as those composed of cystine or uric acid. A simple CT software program to provide accurate stone composition analysis from CT scans would offer similar clinical benefits. The development of sophisticated techniques utilizing measurement of coherent scatter data from X-ray diffraction studies may facilitate this composition analysis (78). Continued reduction in radiation exposure from diagnostic CT is a progressive application needed in all aspects of imaging.

CONCLUSIONS

CT is highly accurate in detecting urinary stones. As MDCT technology evolves, CT applications in the evaluation of urinary calculi continue to increase in clinical practice.

REFERENCES

1. Preminger GM, Vieweg J, Leder RA, Nelson RC. Urolithiasis: detection and management with unenhanced spiral CT—a urologic perspective. Radiology 1998; 207:308–309.
2. Smith RC, Levine J, Rosenfeld AT. Helical CT of urinary tract stones. Epidemiology, origin, pathophysiology, diagnosis, and management. Radiol Clin North Am 1999; 37:911–952.
3. Kenney PJ. CT evaluation of urinary lithiasis. Radiol Clin North Am 2003; 41:979–999.
4. Sandhu C, Anson KM, Patel U. Urinary tract stones—Part I: role of radiological imaging in diagnosis and treatment planning. Clin Radiol 2003; 58:415–421.
5. Smith RC, Rosenfield AT, Choe KA, et al. Acute flank pain: comparison of non-contrast-enhanced CT and intravenous urography. Radiology 1995; 194:789–794.
6. Macintyre J. Roentgen rays: photography of renal calculus. Description of an adjustable modification in the focus tube. Lancet 1896; 2:118.
7. Herring LC. Observations on the analysis of ten thousand urinary calculi. J Urol 1962; 88:545–562.
8. Levine JA, Neitlich J, Verga M, Dalrymple N, Smith RC. Ureteral calculi in patients with flank pain: correlation of plain radiography with unenhanced helical CT. Radiology 1997; 204:27–31.
9. Roth CS, Bowyer BA, Berquist TH. Utility of the plain abdominal radiograph for diagnosing ureteral calculi. Ann Emerg Med 1985; 14:311–315.
10. Mutgi A, Williams JW, Nettleman M. Renal colic. Utility of the plain abdominal roentgenogram. Arch Intern Med 1991; 151:1589–1592.

11. Orton GH. Some fallacies in the X-ray diagnosis of renal and ureteral calculi. BMJ 1908; 2:716–719.

12. Swick M. Darstellung der Niere und Harnwege im Röntgenbild durch intravenöse Einbringung eines neuren Kontrastoffes, des Uroselectans. Klin Wschr 1929; 8: 2087–2089.

13. Smith RC, Verga M, McCarthy S, Rosenfield AT. Diagnosis of acute flank pain: value of unenhanced helical CT. AJR 1996; 166:97–101.

14. Fielding JR, Steele G, Fox LA, Heller H, Loughlin KR. Spiral computerized tomography in the evaluation of acute flank pain: a replacement for excretory urography. J Urol 1997; 157:2071–2073.

15. Chen MYM, Zagoria RJ. Can noncontrast helical computed tomography replace intravenous urography for evaluation of patients with acute urinary tract colic? J Emerg Med 1999; 17:299–303.

16. Niall O, Russell J, MacGregor R, Duncan H, Mullins J. A comparison of noncontrast computerized tomography with excretory urography in the assessment of acute flank pain. J Urol 1999; 161:534–537.

17. Talner L, Vaughan M. Nonobstructive renal causes of flank pain: findings on non-contrast helical CT (CT KUB). Abdom Imaging 2003; 28:210–216.

18. Luchs JS, Katz DS, Lane MJ, et al. Utility of hematuria testing in patients with suspected renal colic: correlation with unenhanced helical CT results. Urology 2002; 59:839–842.

19. Jackman SV, Potter SR, Regan F, Jarrett TW. Plain abdominal X-ray versus computerized tomography screening: sensitivity for stone localization after nonenhanced spiral computerized tomography. J Urol 2000; 164:308–310.

20. Sourtzis S, Thibeau JF, Damry N, et al. Radiologic investigation of renal colic: unenhanced helical CT compared with excretory urography. AJR 1999; 172:1491–1494.

21. Pfister SA, Deckart A, Laschke S, et al. Unenhanced helical computed tomography vs intravenous urography in patients with acute flank pain: accuracy and economic impact in a randomized prospective trial. Eur Radiol 2003; 13:2513–2520.

22. Gray Sears CL, Ward JF, Sears ST, et al. Prospective comparison of computerized tomography and excretory urography in the initial evaluation of asymptomatic microhematuria. J Urol 2002; 168:2457–2460.

23. Catalano O, Nunziata A, Altei F, Siani A. Suspected ureteral colic: primary helical CT versus selective helical CT after unenhanced radiography and sonography. AJR 2002; 178:379–387.

24. Shokeir AA, Abdulmaaboud M. Prospective comparison of nonenhanced helical computerized tomography and Doppler ultrasonography for the diagnosis of renal colic. J Urol 2001; 165:1082–1084.

25. Sudah M, Vanninen RL, Partanen K, et al. Patients with acute flank pain: comparison of MR urography with unenhanced helical CT. Radiology 2002; 223:98–105.

26. Sommer FG, Jeffrey RB Jr, Rubin GD, et al. Detection of ureteral calculi in patients with suspected renal colic: value of reformatted noncontrast helical CT. AJR 1995; 165: 509–513.

27. Chen MY, Zagoria RJ, Saunders HS, Dyer RB. Trends in the use of unenhanced helical CT for acute urinary colic. AJR 1999; 173:1447–1450.

28. Kawashima A, Sandler CM, Goldman SM, Raval BK, Fishman EK. CT of renal inflammatory disease. Radiographics 1997; 17:851–866.

29. Kawashima A, Sandler CM, Ernst RD, et al. CT evaluation of renovascular disease. Radiographics 2000; 20:1321–1340.

30. Chu G, Rosenfield AT, Anderson K, Scout L, Smith RC. Sensitivity and value of digital CT scout radiography for detecting ureteral stones in patients with ureterolithiasis diagnosed on unenhanced CT. AJR 1999; 173:417–423.

31. Assi Z, Platt JF, Francis IR, Cohan RH, Korobkin M. Sensitivity of CT scout radiography and abdominal radiography for revealing ureteral calculi on helical CT: implications for radiologic follow-up. AJR 2000; 175:333–337.

32. Hartman RP, Kawashima A, King BF, LeRoy AJ, Vrtiska TJ. Sensitivity of original CT scanned projection radiographs (OCT-SPRs), new-enhanced CT scanned projection radiographs (ECT-SPRs), and film-screen radiographs (FSRs) for the detection of ureteral calculi. In: The Annual Meeting of the Society of Uroradiology, Cancun, Mexico, 2003.

33. Zagoria RJ, Khatod EG, Chen MY. Abdominal radiography after CT reveals urinary calculi: a method to predict usefulness of abdominal radiography on the basis of size and CT attenuation of calculi. AJR 2001; 176:1117–1122.

34. Caoili EM, Cohan RH, Korobkin M, et al. Urinary tract abnormalities: initial experience with multi-detector row CT urography. Radiology 2002; 222:353–360.

35. Kawashima A, Vrtiska TJ, LeRoy AJ, et al. CT urography. Radiographics 2004; 24(suppl. 1):S35–S54.

36. Fielding JR, Silverman SG, Rubin GD. Helical CT of the urinary tract. AJR 1999; 172:1199–1206.

37. Smith RC, Verga M, Dalrymple N, McCarthy S, Rosenfield AT. Acute ureteral obstruction: value of secondary signs of helical unenhanced CT. AJR 1996; 167:1109–1113.

38. Katz DS, Lane MJ, Sommer FG. Unenhanced helical CT of ureteral stones: incidence of associated urinary tract findings. AJR 1996; 166:1319–1322.

39. Boridy IC, Kawashima A, Goldman SM, Sandler CM. Acute ureterolithiasis: non-enhanced helical CT findings of perinephric edema for prediction of degree of ureteral obstruction. Radiology 1999; 213:663–667.

40. Bird VG, Gomez-Marin O, Leveillee RJ, et al. A comparison of unenhanced helical computerized tomography findings and renal obstruction determined by furosemide 99m technetium mercaptoacetyltriglycine diuretic scintirenography for patients with acute renal colic. J Urol 2002; 167:1597–1603.

41. Varanelli MJ, Coll DM, Levine JA, Rosenfield AT, Smith RC. Relationship between duration of pain and secondary signs of obstruction of the urinary tract on unenhanced helical CT. AJR 2001; 177:325–330.

42. Takahashi N, Kawashima A, Ernst RD, et al. Ureterolithiasis: can clinical outcome be predicted with unenhanced helical CT? Radiology 1998; 208:97–102.

43. Boulay I, Holtz P, Foley WD, White B, Begun FP. Ureteral calculi: diagnostic efficacy of helical CT and implications for treatment of patients. AJR 1999; 172:1485–1490.

44. Fielding JR, Silverman SG, Samuel S, Zou KH, Loughlin KR. Unenhanced helical CT of ureteral stones: a replacement for excretory urography in planning treatment. AJR 1998; 171:1051–1053.

45. Coll DM, Varanelli MJ, Smith RC. Relationship of spontaneous passage of ureteral calculi to stone size and location as revealed by unenhanced helical CT. AJR 2002; 178:101–103.

46. Olcott EW, Sommer FG, Napel S. Accuracy of detection and measurement of renal calculi: in vitro comparison of three-dimensional spiral CT, radiography, and nephro-tomography. Radiology 1997; 204:19–25.

47. Nadler RB, Stern JA, Kimm S, Hoff F, Rademaker AW. Coronal imaging to assess urinary tract stone size. J Urol 2004; 172:962–964.

48. Georgiades CS, Moore CJ, Smith DP. Differences of renal parenchymal attenuation for acutely obstructed and unobstructed kidneys on unenhanced helical CT: a useful secondary sign? AJR 2001; 176:965–968.

49. Traubici J, Neitlich JD, Smith RC. Distinguishing pelvic phleboliths from distal ureteral stones on routine unenhanced helical CT: is there a radiolucent center? AJR 17; 172:13–17.

50. Heneghan JP, Verga M, Dalrymple NC, Rosenfield AT, Smith RC. "Rim sign" in the diagnosis of ureteric calculi at unenhanced. CT. Radiology 1997; 202:709–711.

51. Kawashima A, Sandler CM, Boridy IC, et al. Unenhanced helical CT of ureterolithiasis: value of the tissue rim sign. AJR 1997; 168:997–1000.

52. Bell TV, Fenlon HM, Davison BD, Ahari HK, Hussain S. Unenhanced helical CT criteria to differentiate distal ureteral calculi from pelvic phleboliths. Radiology 1998; 207:363–367.

53. Guest AR, Cohan RH, Korobkin M, et al. Assessment of the clinical utility of the rim and comet-tail signs in differentiating ureteral stones from phleboliths. AJR 2001; 177:1285–1291.

54. Boridy IC, Nikolaidis P, Kawashima A, Goldman SM, Sandler CM. Ureterolithiasis: value of the tail sign in differentiating phleboliths from ureteral calculi at nonenhanced helical CT. Radiology 1999; 211:619–621.

55. Denton ER, Mackenzie A, Greenwell T, Popert R, Rankin SC. Unenhanced helical CT for renal colic—is the radiation dose justifiable? Clin Radiol 1999; 54:444–447.

56. Homer JA, Davies-Payne DL, Peddinti BS. Randomized prospective comparison of non-contrast enhanced helical computed tomography and intravenous urography in the diagnosis of acute ureteric colic. Australas Radiol 2001; 45:285–290.

57. Liu W, Esler SJ, Kenny BJ, et al. Low-dose nonenhanced helical CT of renal colic: assessment of ureteric stone detection and measurement of effective dose equivalent. Radiology 2000; 215:51–54.

58. Spielmann AL, Heneghan JP, Lee LJ, Yoshizumi T, Nelson RC. Decreasing the radiation dose for renal stone CT: a feasibility study of single- and multi-detector CT. AJR 2002; 178:1058–1062.

59. Meagher T, Sukumar VP, Collingwood J, et al. Low dose computed tomography in suspected acute renal colic. Clin Radiol 2001; 56:873–876.

60. Hamm M, Knopfle E, Wartenberg S, et al. Low dose unenhanced helical computerized tomography for the evaluation of acute flank pain. J Urol 2002; 167:1687–1691.

61. Kalra MK, Maher MM, Toth TL, et al. Techniques and applications of automatic tube current modulation for CT. Radiology 2004; 233:649–657.

62. Boridy IC, Maklad N, Sandler CM. Suspected urolithiasis in pregnant women: imaging algorithm and literature review. AJR 1996; 167:869–875.

63. McCollough CH, Atwell TD, King BF, LeRoy AJ. Evaluation of renal colic during pregnancy: a comparison of radiation dose from radiographic and CT exams. In: The Annual Meeting of the Society of Uroradiology, Kauai, HI, 2000.

64. Tublin ME, Murphy ME, Delong DM, Tessler FN, Kliewer MA. Conspicuity of renal calculi at unenhanced CT: effects of calculus composition and size and CT technique. Radiology 2002; 225:91–96.

65. Guevara A, Springmann KE, Drach GW, Hillman BJ. Triamterene stones and computerized axial tomography. Urology 1986; 27:104–106.

66. Assimos DG, Langenstroer P, Leinbach RF, et al. Guaifenesin- and ephedrine-induced stones. J Endourol 1999; 13:665–667.

67. Liu CC, Li CC, Shih MC, Chou YH, Huang CH. Matrix stone. J Comput Assist Tomogr 2003; 27:810–813.

68. Blake SP, McNicholas MM, Raptopoulos V. Nonopaque crystal deposition causing ureteric obstruction in patients with HIV undergoing indinavir therapy [see comment]. AJR 1998; 171:717–720.

69. Bani Hani AH, Segura JW, LeRoy AJ. Urinary matrix calculi: our experience at a single institution. J Urol 2005; 173:120–123.

70. Williams JC Jr, Saw KC, Paterson RF, et al. Variability of renal stone fragility in shock wave lithotripsy. Urology 2003; 61:1092–1096; discussion 1097.

71. Mostafavi MR, Ernst RD, Saltzman B. Accurate determination of chemical composition of urinary calculi by spiral computerized tomography. J Urol 1998; 159:673–675.

72. Williams JC Jr, Paterson RF, Kopecky KK, Lingeman JE, McAteer JA. High resolution detection of internal structure of renal calculi by helical computerized tomography. J Urol 2002; 167:322–326.

73. Zarse CA, McAteer JA, Tann M, et al. Helical computed tomography accurately reports urinary stone composition using attenuation values: in vitro verification using high-resolution micro-computed tomography calibrated to Fourier transform infrared microspectroscopy. Urology 2004; 63:828–833.

74. Nakada SY, Hoff DG, Attai S, et al. Determination of stone composition by noncontrast spiral computed tomography in the clinical setting. Urology 2000; 55:816–819.
75. Dretler SP, Spencer BA. CT and stone fragility. J Endourol 2001; 15:31–36.
76. Motley G, Dalrymple N, Keesling C, Fischer J, Harmon W. Hounsfield unit density in the determination of urinary stone composition. Urology 2001; 58:170–173.
77. Pareek G, Armenakas NA, Fracchia JA. Hounsfield units on computerized tomography predict stone-free rates after extracorporeal shock wave lithotripsy. J Urol 2003; 169:1679–1681.
78. Batchelar DL, Chun SS, Wollin TA, et al. Predicting urinary stone composition using X-ray coherent scatter: a novel technique with potential clinical applications. J Urol 2002; 168:260–265.

3

New Developments in Ultrasound Imaging of the Urinary Tract

Michele Bertolotto
Institute of Radiology, University of Trieste, Trieste, Italy

Lorenzo E. Derchi
DICMI—Radiology, University of Genova, Genova, Italy

INTRODUCTION

Ultrasonography (US) is probably the most commonly used technique for imaging the urinary tract. It is widely used to identify, confirm, and/or characterize specific lesions and to guide biopsy and interventional procedures. Furthermore, lack of ionizing radiation makes it the first imaging technique in the study of the female pelvis and the pediatric age group.

The technology of US is advancing rapidly and is aimed at both increasing image quality and opening new fields of applications. This chapter will review the main advances in US technology and address the clinical impact they have had or are likely to have in the future in the field of uroradiology. Advances in the quality and presentation of US images will be discussed as well as new development in portable US machines.

ADVANCES IN IMAGE QUALITY AND IMAGE PRESENTATION

Research in the field of US has been always aimed at obtaining high spatial resolution, good penetration of the US beam, and reduction of signal-to-noise ratio. This has been possible from basic research in the behavior of US in tissues, the physical principles underlying piezoelectric materials, and from progress in the construction and miniaturization of electronic components. The new developments include modern piezoelectric materials with lower characteristic acoustic impedance and greater electromechanical coupling coefficients, production of multiple layer transducers of ceramic materials of variable thickness and shape, better understanding of the behavior of small transducers, and the development of a variety of pulse-characteristic modulation processes that allow accurate control of transmission frequency, amplitude, phase, and pulse length (1–4). These advances have increased the ability of US in demonstrating anatomic and pathological details (Fig. 1). In the following section,

35

(A)   (B)

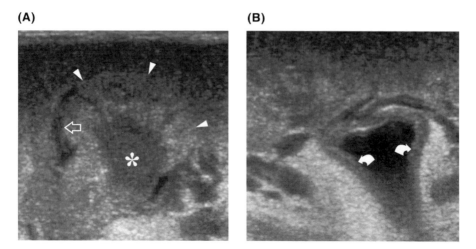

Figure 1 Gray scale US of renal allografts using a broadband, high-frequency linear transducer. (**A**) Normal appearance of a renal pyramid. The excellent spatial and contrast resolution allows differentiation between the outer (*arrowheads*) and inner (*∗*) medulla. Open arrow
indicates an arcuate vessel. (**B**) Renal allograft infection. High-resolution US shows thickening
of the wall of a renal calix (*curved arrows*). *Abbreviation*: US, ultrasonography.

new techniques that caused marked improvement in the quality of US imaging
will be discussed. These include tissue harmonic imaging, compound imaging, the
extended field-of-view technique, three-dimensional (3-D) imaging, and the use of
US contrast media.

Tissue Harmonic Imaging

Increased knowledge in acoustic harmonics has led to a marked improvement in
general ultrasonic imaging. The use of tissue harmonic imaging has led to a marked
improvement in image quality, particularly in large, difficult-to-scan patients (1,3,4).
        At the level of the kidneys and in patients with pelvic masses, harmonic ima-
ging facilitates the differentiation between solid and cystic lesions (Fig. 2), allows
better delineation of intracystic septa and vegetations (Fig. 3), and improves visualization of stones within dilated ureters by providing better delineation of the acoustic shadow (Fig. 4). At present, tissue harmonic imaging is suggested as the standard
setting to be used in abdominal and pelvic US examination, especially when a fluid-
filled lesion is under evaluation and its characteristics have to be analyzed (5–8).

Compound Imaging

Compound imaging is a relatively new technique that allows combining echoes
obtained from US beams oriented along different directions. Electronic steering of
US beams from an array transducer is used to image the same tissue multiple times
from different directions; then the echoes from these multiple acquisitions are averaged
together into a single composite image (1,4). This is possible at a real-time rate,
although the frame-rate is slightly lower than that of conventional imaging. Compound
imaging improves image quality by reducing speckle, without any loss in spatial resolution, and can provide better delineation of lesion contours (Fig. 5). Another approach
to compounding, called "frequency compound," uses simultaneous emission of two US

(A) **(B)**

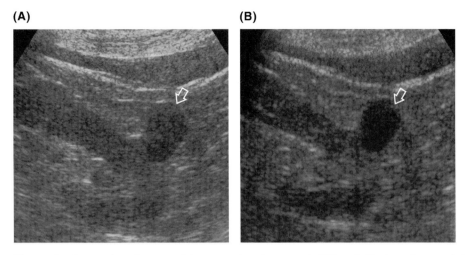

Figure 2 Comparison between (**A**) conventional gray scale US and (**B**) tissue harmonic imaging. A small renal cyst (*arrow*) is better characterized using tissue harmonic imaging due to reduced image artifacts. *Abbreviation*: US, ultrasonography.

beams of different frequencies, again resulting in better image quality, with less noise, reduced speckle, and good contrast resolution (7,8).

In clinical practice, the simultaneous use of tissue harmonic imaging and image compounding is often regarded as the standard setting for abdominal and pelvic US examinations. It must be noted, however, that the acoustic shadow posterior to small calcifications or stones can be less evident when using the image compounding technique, and this can be a drawback in some cases. Hence, switching between standard setting and compound imaging to allow delineation of acoustic shadows is suggested in difficult cases.

(A) **(B)**

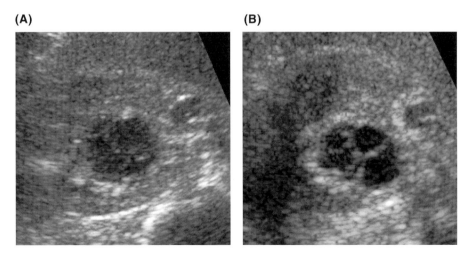

Figure 3 Comparison between (**A**) conventional gray scale US and (**B**) tissue harmonic imaging. The internal septa of this small complex renal cyst are better visible using tissue harmonic imaging because of reduced image artifacts leading to increased contrast resolution between the liquid and solid components of the lesion. *Abbreviation*: US, ultrasonography.

(A)   **(B)**

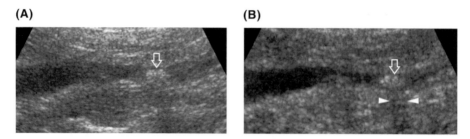

Figure 4 Comparison between (**A**) conventional gray scale US and (**B**) tissue harmonic imaging. Reduced artifacts allow better identification of an uretheral stone (*arrow*) and of its
acoustic shadow (*arrowheads*) in the harmonic image. *Abbreviation*: US, ultrasonography.

Extended Field-of-View

US images have a field-of-view that is limited by the probe width. During the study,
the examiner moves the probe over the area of interest to acquire information on
large volumes of tissues and reconstructs in his/her mind the spatial relationships
between parts of anatomy by memorizing many small image frames (9). This is a
distinct disadvantage of US compared to other imaging methods and is a major
drawback in conveying the information of the study to clinicians. The extended
field-of-view technique has been developed to overcome these limitations and allows
the reconstruction of wide images by progressive addition of data during a hand
sweep with the conventional real-time small probe (Fig. 6). The information about
position is obtained directly from the ultrasound images themselves, using an image
registration–based position-sensing technique, estimating probe position by combining multiple local motion vectors (1,9).

A number of papers have shown the clinical usefulness of this technique in the
evaluation of large pelvic and abdominal lesions as well as in providing anatomic

(A)   **(B)**

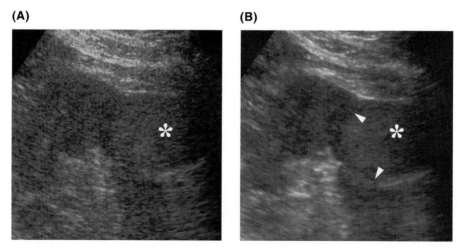

Figure 5 Comparison between (**A**) conventional gray scale US and (**B**) compound imaging.
Improved image quality of compound imaging allows better visualization of a small renal
tumor (*). A thin peripheral hypoechoic rim (*arrowheads*), which is visible only in the compound image, suggests presence of tumor pseudocapsule. *Abbreviation*: US, ultrasonography.

(A)   **(B)**

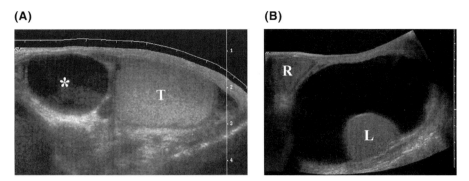

Figure 6   Extended field-of-view images of the scrotal content in two patients. (**A**) Simultaneous visualization of the testis (T) and of a large cyst of the head of the epididymis (*). (**B**) Simultaneous visualization of right (R) and left (L) testes and of hydrocele surrounding the left testis.

context that was not possible with the small field-of-view of the real-time probe (10,11). This is a distinct advantage when explaining the ultrasound images to referring clinicians. It must be noted that the accuracy of measurements obtained with the extended field-of-view system has been proven accurate and repeatable (9,12), thus providing the capability to follow-up volume changes of large lesions during therapy.

3-D Imaging

The development of high-speed computing and the increase in storage capacity of hardware have opened the possibility of applying 3-D technologies to diagnostic ultrasound. Presenting the entire volume of data in a single image can overcome the problems in understanding difficult anatomy, clarify exact spatial relationships, and help sharing information with referring clinicians and patients (1,13).

To acquire volume data sets, it is necessary to obtain a series of contiguous 2-D image planes of the volume under evaluation. The position of each slice within the volume has to be precisely assessed, and this can be obtained through different techniques (13).

Special transducers have been developed integrating the position sensing system within the transducer housing. These "volume transducers" are larger than standard probes and can be more difficult to use; however, they can provide exact knowledge of each scan plane, eliminating distortions in the resultant images. After each slice the transducer plane is automatically moved to the next location, which is then exactly known by the machine. These transducers are usually integrated with the ultrasound equipment, and 3-D images can be immediately displayed after acquisition.

Position sensor devices can be attached to 2-D conventional transducers to obtain data about scan position. At present, small electromagnetic sensors mounted on the transducer are the most used technique for this purpose and, although susceptible to distortion from adjacent metallic objects, have proven able in producing accurate measurements.

The display of 3-D information gathered by US techniques is not simple, and it may be difficult to separate adjacent structures. 3-D ultrasound images, in fact, cannot be classified and processed like computed tomography (CT) and magnetic resonance imaging (MRI) data because they do not represent well-defined parameters, such as density, but are rather a measure of how the acoustic impedance changes as sound waves travel through tissues.

Slice projection from the volume data of images of arbitrary orientation is the most common method to review 3-D ultrasound data. This technique allows retrospective evaluation of anatomy along planes different from the one along which the data themselves have been obtained and has been proven to be useful in a variety of clinical settings.

There are many clinical applications of 3-D ultrasound imaging, particularly in assessing intrauterine fetal anatomy and gynecological imaging (13). In the urinary tract, volume estimation of the urinary bladder with 3-D ultrasound has been shown to be accurate, reliable, and clinically useful (14–16). Volume measurements have also proven accurate in assessing prostatic cancer and benign hyperplasia, with better identification of extraglandular spread (17,18). However, better identification did not result in increased accuracy in cancer staging (17). Ultrasound 3-D imaging can also be used for accurate measurements of renal volume and for monitoring progress in patients with renal diseases. In addition, it can offer useful anatomical information about the renal pelvis and its relation to the branches of the renal artery (19–21).

Ultrasound Contrast Media

The possibility of enhancing visualization of the vascular system with US reflectors after the injection of a variety of fluids was originally described in 1968 (22). Shortly afterwards, it was understood that the source of the observed intravascular echoes was microbubbles developing during the injection process. Since then, the pharmaceutical industry has worked to develop safe and nontoxic, intravenously injectable products made of microbubbles stable enough to cross the pulmonary capillary bed after injection in a peripheral vein and to provide vascular enhancement for the whole duration of the clinical examination (23). The technology adopted has been that of encapsulated bubbles of gas, smaller than the red blood cells (24), with the capability to flow freely in the vascular system. A variety of gases have been used, from air to less diffusible compounds, such as perfluorocarbons or sulfur hexafluoride. A variety of shells with different thicknesses and stiffnesses have been used to encapsulate the microbubbles.

US contrast agents behave as an active source of sound, modifying the characteristic signature of the echo from blood. When properly insonated with a high-power ultrasound beam, microbubbles collapse, producing a high intensity, broadband transient signal. When the power of the ultrasound beam is lower, microbubbles undergo complex oscillation in the ultrasound field and work by resonating, rapidly contracting and expanding in response to the pressure changes of the sound wave, producing multiple harmonic signals.

Microbubble contrast agents are neither filtered by the kidney nor able to enter the interstitial spaces and act as "blood pool agents" until metabolized. However, some have recently been shown to exhibit specific hepatosplenic uptake after their disappearance from the blood pool (24–26).

US contrast agents were originally developed to increase vascular signals during Doppler studies in "difficult" patients and rescue otherwise failed examinations. As a consequence, early clinical experience in uroradiology was mainly focused on visualization of renal arteries and identifying small or deep vessels within parenchymal lesions. These early clinical studies have demonstrated that the success rate of Doppler visualization of the main renal arteries and of accessory renal arteries improves significantly after the administration of microbubbles (27–30).

A variety of softwares have been developed by the manufacturers of US equipment to detect signals from microbubbles. There are basically two imaging approaches that can be used: "destructive contrast-specific modes," which collect the signal from bubble destruction produced using a high-power US beam, and "nondestructive contrast-specific modes," which collect the harmonic signals from bubble insonation with US beams of lower power.

Contrast-specific destructive modes allow excellent depiction of renal vascularity and perfusion defects from different causes, such as renal infection, focal ischemia, or trauma, and differential diagnosis between renal neoplasm and pseudotumors (31–33). Heterogeneous contrast enhancement usually suggests malignancy. In addition, cystic renal tumors can be differentiated from complex benign cystic masses in most cases when contrast enhancement is appreciable within the lesion wall (Fig. 7) or within intracystic septa (33). However, inflammatory cysts can occasionally simulate malignancy (34).

Contrast-specific destructive modes have been also used successfully to evaluate cancer of the prostate gland. Detection of isoechoic tumors and cancers of both the peripheral and central regions of prostate improves using contrast-specific modes, with better guidance to biopsy (35–38).

A technique that allows evaluation of vesico-ureteral reflux has also been developed. After catheterization, the bladder is filled in with saline until the patient has the urge to micturate, and then the US contrast medium is added. Reflux is diagnosed when microbubbles are detected in the ureter or the renal pelvis. The results show good correlation with conventional micturating cystourethrogram and with radionuclide studies (39–42).

The major disadvantage of contrast-specific destructive modes is that intermittent scanning with a limited number of insonations is needed to minimize bubble destruction. Hence, prolonged evaluation of contrast enhancement cannot be performed. This limitation can be overcome by performing nondestructive low–acoustic

(A)   **(B)**

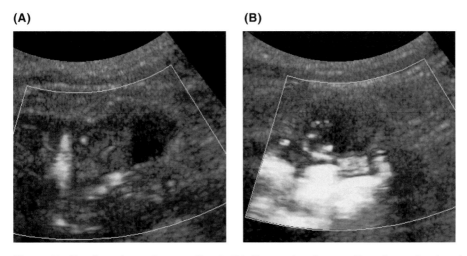

Figure 7 Small cystic renal tumor (2 cm). (**A**) Conventional power Doppler evaluation shows no vascular signals in the tumor wall. (**B**) Power Doppler image obtained with the same imaging parameters during Levovist infusion shows vascularity of tumor wall.

power US scanning after intravenous administration of US contrast agents. This technique allows imaging both kidneys in real time with excellent evaluation of vascularity and reduces artifacts even at unfavorable Doppler angles. Clinical evidence is accumulating that nondestructive scanning is more effective than destructive methods to evaluate all renal pathologies (43,44). Real-time imaging improves the visualization of small focal renal lesions and of perfusion defects (Fig. 8). Improved temporal resolution may allow visualization of segmental areas with delayed enhancement, permitting the diagnosis of segmental renal artery stenosis (Fig. 9) or atheroembolic renal disease. Detection of isoechoic renal tumors remains very difficult because these lesions often appear hyperechoic only in the early arterial phase (Fig. 10), while in the other vascular phases they are isoechoic to the normal renal parenchyma (43,44). However, identification of such tumors is better with nondestructive modes when compared with the destructive imaging mode. Moreover, real-time contrast-specific imaging is effective in improving the sonographic visualization of tumoral pseudocapsule, which appears after microbubble injection as a rim of perilesional enhancement, increasing in the latter phase of the examination (45).

Microbubble contrast agents can also be used as vascular tracers to assess renal perfusion. Preliminary studies performed with Doppler techniques on renal allografts showed that measuring the arteriovenous transit time after bolus injection of microbubbles allows differentiation between normally functioning grafts and kidneys with biopsy-proven rejection (46). Other preliminary investigations showed that analysis of time–intensity curves drawn from the renal cortex after a bolus injection of microbubbles can improve identification of hemodynamically significant renal artery stenosis (47,48).

Renal perfusion can also be assessed using a different approach. If microbubbles are administered with infusion technique, a steady state is reached in which contrast blood concentration can be considered to be constant. When this state has

(A)   **(B)**

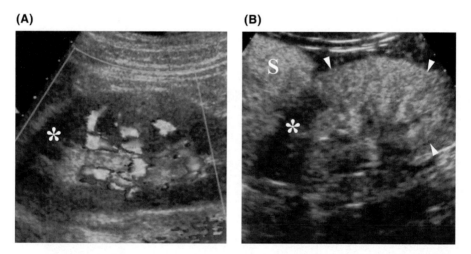

Figure 8 Seventy-two-year-old diabetic patient who presented with left flank pain. (**A**) Color Doppler US (shown here in gray scale): a hypoperfused area at the upper pole of the left kidney is suspected (∗), but with low diagnostic confidence due to unfavorable Doppler angle. Microbubble administration allows to confirm with high diagnostic confidence that the upper portion of the left kidney is ischemic (∗). (**B**) Note excellent contrast enhancement with high spatial resolution of the remaining portions of the left kidney (*arrowheads*) and of the spleen (S). *Abbreviation*: US, ultrasonography.

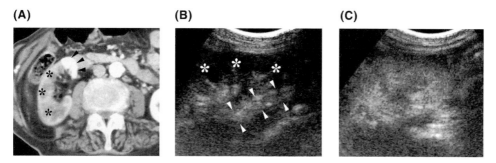

Figure 9 Segmental renal artery stenosis of the right kidney. (**A**) Contrast enhanced CT shows delayed contrast enhancement in the affected portion of the kidney (*) compared with the normally perfused portion (*arrowheads*). (**B** and **C**) Contrast enhanced US. (**B**) Ten seconds after microbubble injection a similar delayed enhancement can be appreciated in the territory perfused by stenotic artery (*), compared with the normally perfused portion (*arrowheads*). (**C**) Forty seconds after microbubble administration renal vascularity appears normal. *Abbreviations*: CT, computed tomography; US, ultrasonography.

been reached, the bubbles within an imaged slice can be destroyed by applying a high-intensity frame to create an inflow void or "negative bolus" (49,50). When the next destructive beam is transmitted, the intensity of the echoes depends on the number of bubbles that have flown into the slice and so increases with longer intervals. If the process is repeated at a series of intervals, a time–intensity curve can be created. The slope of this curve is related to the speed of blood moving into the slice, the maximum signal intensity level relates to the vascular volume, and their product reflects the volume flow rate and approximates perfusion (49,50). This method to evaluate perfusion can be applied to any tissue. Attempts have been made to use it to detect changes in renal blood flow in animals with flow-limiting renal artery stenosis and

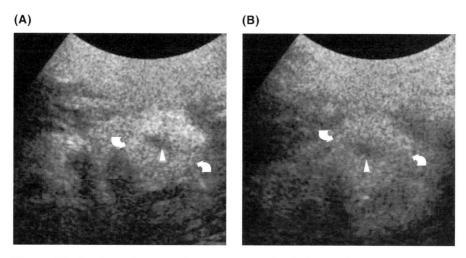

Figure 10 Small renal tumor. Contrast enhanced US. (**A**) During the early arterial phase (18 seconds after microbubble injection) the lesion (*curved arrows*) appears hyperechoic. (**B**) Forty seconds after microbubble injection the lesion (*curved arrows*) appears nearly isoechoic to kidney. A central nonenhancing area (*arrowhead*), probably necrotic, is appreciable in both vascular phases. *Abbreviation*: US, ultrasonography.

(A)   **(B)**

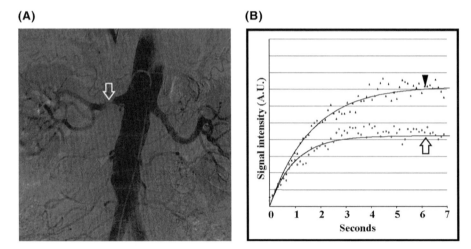

Figure 11 Right renal artery stenosis. (**A**) Angiographic demonstration of the stenosis (*arrow*). (**B**) Time–intensity curve of the right kidney (*arrow*) in comparison with the contralateral kidney (*arrowhead*) obtained with real time, nondestructive imaging during microbubble infusion. A region of interest was placed in the cortex of both kidneys. The curve of the stenotic kidney shows slower rising and reduced plateau signal intensity reflecting reduced speed of blood, percent blood volume, and blood flow. Dots represent experimental data that are fitted to exponential functions (*lines*). Note that the use of real-time imaging allows acquisition of the curves in seven seconds.

during infusion of vasoactive drugs (51). In humans, an excellent correlation was found between perfusion measurements obtained using microbubbles, para-amino-hippurate clearance, and radionuclide studies (52). The major disadvantage of this method is that it is time consuming and is sensitive to relative movement between the probe and the tissue (48,50). Such movement exposes a new slice of tissue that contains bubbles that have not been removed by the previous frame, thus introducing errors. This limitation has been overcome using nondestructive contrast-specific modes. After producing a steady blood concentration of microbubbles as previously described, microbubbles are destroyed in the scan volume using high-power US shots; then reperfusion is observed in real time without destroying microbubbles (49,50). Real-time evaluation markedly reduces movement artifacts, because reperfusion curves from the renal cortex can be obtained in less than 10 seconds (Fig. 11).

Finally, microbubble contrast agents allow evaluation of renal medullary vessels. Medullary enhancement can be detected immediately after cortical enhancement starting from the outer portion, and progressing to the inner portion. Although at present, the evaluation of medullary blood flow has no clinical applications, it offers a useful research tool to evaluate relative changes between the cortical and the medullary blood flow, which could be useful in assessing renal perfusion in diabetic patients and in response to vasoactive drugs.

SMALL, PORTABLE US EQUIPMENT

Electronic miniaturization and the availability of powerful and fast laptop computers have resulted in the development of high-performance, truly portable, high-quality ultrasound scanners. Such machines have been introduced into the market with basic imaging capabilities; however, they have been rapidly expanded to color and spectral Doppler techniques and have proven useful as a fast and accurate means to provide portable ultrasound examinations in the intensive care units and at the bedside. Furthermore, they can be easily integrated into radiology suites to provide alternative guidance to interventional procedures (1,4,53). This trend toward lower cost and a truly portable US system has a great potential to change radically the overall role of US imaging in medicine (4) and may lead to the use of US in the future by clinicians as part of the physical examination of the patient.

REFERENCES

1. Claudon M, Tranquart F, Evans DH, Lefevre F, Correas J-M. Advances in ultrasound. Eur Radiol 2002; 12:7–18.
2. Wittingham TA. Broadband transducers. Eur Radiol 1999; 9(suppl 3):S298–S303.
3. Wittingham TA. Modern developments in diagnostic ultrasound—I. Transducer and signal processing developments. Radiography 1995; 1:61–73.
4. Hangiandreou NJ. AAPM/RSNA physics tutorial for residents: topics in US. B-mode US: basic concepts and new technology. Radiographics 2003; 23:1019–1033.
5. Tranquart F, Grenier N, Eder V, Pourcelot L. Clinical use of ultrasound tissue harmonic imaging. Ultrasound Med Biol 1999; 25:889–894.
6. Choudry S, Gorman B, Charboneau JW, et al. Comparison of tissue harmonic imaging with conventional US in abdominal disease. Radiographics 2000; 20:1127–1135.
7. Schmidt T, Hohl C, Haage P, et al. Diagnostic accuracy of phase-inversion tissue harmonic imaging versus fundamental B-mode sonography in the evaluation of focal lesions of the kidney. AJR 2003; 180:1639–1647.
8. Oktar SO, Yucel C, Ozdemir H, Uluturk A, Isk S. Comparison of conventional sonography, real time compound sonography, tissue harmonic sonography and tissue harmonic compound sonography of abdominal and pelvic lesions. AJR 2003; 181:1341–1247.
9. Weng L, Tirumalai AP, Lowery CM, et al. US extended-field-of view imaging technology. Radiology 1997; 203:877–880.
10. Sauerbrei EE. Extended field-of-view sonography: utility in clinical practice. J Ultrasound Med 1999; 18:335–341.
11. Henrich W, Fuchs I, Schnider A, Buhling KJ, Dudenhausen JW. Transvaginal and transabdominal extended field-of-view (EFOV) and power Doppler EFOV sonography in gynecology. J Ultrasound Med 2002; 21:1137–1144.
12. Fornage BD, Atkinson EN, Nock LF, Jones PH. US with extended field of view: phantom-tested accuracy of distance measurements. Radiology 2000; 214:579–584.
13. Nelson TR, Pretorius DH. Three-dimensional ultrasound imaging. Ultrasound Med Biol 1998; 24:1243–1270.
14. Riccabona M, Nelson TR, Pretorius DH, Davidson TE. In vivo three-dimensional sonographic measurement of organ volume: validation in the urinary bladder. J Ultrasound Med 1996; 15:627–632.
15. Marks LS, Dorey FJ, Macairan ML, et al. Three-dimensional ultrasound device for rapid determination of bladder volume. Urology 1997; 50:341–348.
16. Byun SS, Kim HH, Lee E, et al. Accuracy of bladder volume determinations by ultrasonography: are they accurate over the entire bladder volume range? Urology 2003; 62:656–660.
17. Sedelaar JPM, van Roermund JCH, van Leenders GLJH, et al. Three-dimensional gray scale ultrasound: evaluation of prostate cancer compared with benign prostatic hyperplasia. Urology 2001; 57:914–920.
18. Hamper UM, Trapanotto V, DeJong R, Sheth S, Caskey CI. Three-dimensional US of the prostate: early experience. Radiology 1999; 212:719–723.

19. Gilja OH, Smievoll AI, Thune N, et al. In vivo comparison of 3D ultrasonography and magnetic resonance imaging in volume estimation of human kidneys. Ultrasound Med Biol 1995; 21:25–32.

20. Riccabona M, Fritz G, Ring R. Potential applications of three-dimensional ultrasound in the pediatric urinary tract: pictorial demonstration based on preliminary experience. Eur Radiol 2003; 13:2680–2687.

21. Mohaupt MG, Perrig M, Vogt B. 3D ultrasound imaging—a useful non-invasive tool to detect AV fistulas in transplanted kidneys. Nephrol Dial Transplant 1999; 14:940–943.

22. Gramiak R, Shah PM. Echocardiography of the aortic root. Invest Radiol 1968; 3:356–366.

23. Correas JM, Bridal L, Lesavre A, et al. Ultrasound contrast agents: properties, principles of action, tolerance and artefacts. In: Derchi LE, Grenier N, eds. Ultrasound. Categorical Course ECR 2002. Berlin: Springer-Verlag, 2002:62–74.

24. Burns PN. Microbubble contrast for ultrasound imaging: where, how and why? In: Rumack CM, Wilson SR, Charboneau JW, eds. Diagnostic Ultrasound. 3rd ed. St. Louis: Elsevier Mosby, 2005:55–73.

25. Blomley MJK, Albrecht T, Cosgrove DO, et al. Improved imaging of liver metastases with stimulated acoustic emission in the late phase of enhancement with the US contrast agent SH U 508A: early experience. Radiology 1999; 210:409–416.

26. Lim AKP, Patel N, Eckersley RJ, et al. Evidence for spleen-specific uptake of a microbubble contrast agent: a quantitative study in healthy volunteers. Radiology 2004; 231:785–788.

27. Claudon M, Plouin PF, Baxter GM, Rohban T, Maniez Devos D. Renal arteries in patients at risk of renal arterial stenosis: multicenter evaluation of the echo-enhancer SHU584A at color and spectral Doppler US. Radiology 2000; 214:739–746.

28. Hortling N, Strunk H, Wilhelm K, Hofer U, Schild HH. Visualization of renal arteries and value of color-coded duplex sonography in renal artery stenoses using an ultrasound signal enhancing agent. Rofo 1998; 169:397–401.

29. Melany ML, Grant EG, Dueerinkx AJ, Watts TM, Levine BS. Ability of a phase shift US contrast agent to improve imaging of the main renal arteries. Radiology 1997; 205:147–152.

30. House MK, Dowling RJ, King P, et al. Doppler ultrasound (pre- and post-contrast enhancement) for detection of recurrent stenosis in stented renal arteries: preliminary results. Australas Radiol 2000; 44:36–40.

31. Ascenti G, Zimbaro G, Mazziotti S, et al. Contrast-enhanced power Doppler US in the diagnosis of renal pseudotumors. Eur Radiol 2001; 11:2496–2499.

32. Yücel C, Ozdemir H, Akpek S, et al. Renal infarct: contrast-enhanced power Doppler sonographic findings. J Clin Ultrasound 2001; 29:237–242.

33. Kim B, Lim HK, Choi MH, et al. Detection of parenchymal abnormalities in acute pyelonephritis by pulse inversion harmonic imaging with or without microbubble ultrasonographic contrast agent: correlation with computed tomography. J Ultrasound Med 2001; 20:5–14.

34. Quaia E, Siracusano S, Bertolotto M, Monduzzi M, Pozzi Mucelli R. Characterization of renal tumours with pulse inversion harmonic imaging by intermittent high mechanical index technique: initial results. Eur Radiol 2003; 13:1402–1412.

35. Frauscher F, Klauser A, Halpern EJ, Horninger W, Bartsch G. Detection of prostate cancer with a microbubble ultrasound contrast agent. Lancet 2001; 357:1849–1850.

36. Halpern EJ, Rosenberg M, Gomella LG. Prostate cancer: contrast-enhanced US for detection. Radiology 2001; 219:219–225.

37. Halpern EJ, McCue PA, Aksnes AK, et al. Contrast-enhanced US of the prostate with Sonazoid: comparison with whole-mount prostatectomy specimens in 12 patients. Radiology 2002; 222:361–366.

38. Halpern EJ, Frauscher F, Rosenberg M, Gomella LG. Directed biopsy during contrast-enhanced sonography of the prostate. AJR 2002; 178:915–919.

39. Bosio M. Cystosonography with echocontrast: a new imaging modality to detect vesicoureteric reflux in children. Pediatr Radiol 1998; 28:250–255.

40. Darge K, Troeger J, Duetting T, et al. Reflux in young patients: comparison of voiding US of the bladder and retrovesical space with echo enhancement versus voiding cystourethrography for diagnosis. Radiology 1999; 210:201–207.

41. Darge K, Zieger B, Rohrschneider W, et al. Contrast-enhanced harmonic imaging for the diagnosis of vesicoureteral reflux in pediatric patients. AJR 2001; 177:1411–1415.

42. Kmetec A, Bren AF, Kandus A, Fettich J, Buturovic-Ponikvar J. Contrast-enhanced ultrasound voiding cystography as a screening examination for vesicoureteral reflux in the follow-up of renal transplant recipients: a new approach. Nephrol Dial Transplant 2001; 16:120–123.

43. Robbin ML, Lockhart ME, Barr RG. Renal imaging with ultrasound contrast: current status. Radiol Clin North Am 2003; 41:963–978.

44. Nilsson A. Contrast enhanced ultrasound of the kidney. Eur Radiol 2004; 14(suppl 8): P104–P109.

45. Ascenti G, Gaeta M, Magno C, et al. Contrast-enhanced second-harmonic sonography in the detection of pseudocapsule in renal cell carcinoma. AJR 2004; 182:1525–1530.

46. Blomley M, Albrect T, Eckersley R, et al. Renal arterio-venous transit time measured noninvasively using bolus injection of microbubble contrast [abstr]. Radiology 1998; 209(P):461.

47. Derchi LE, Martinoli C, Pretolesi G, Crespi G, Buccicardi D. Quantitative analysis of contrast enhancement. Eur Radiol 1999; 9(suppl 3):S372–S376.

48. Lencioni R, Pinto S, Napoli V, Bartolozzi C. Noninvasive assessment of renal artery stenosis: current imaging protocols and future directions in ultrasonography. J Comput Assist Tomogr 1999; 23(suppl 1):S95–S100.

49. Harvey CJ, Pilcher JM, Eckersley RJ, Blomley MJK, Cosgrove DO. Advances in ultrasound. Clin Radiol 2002; 57:157–177.

50. Cosgrove DO, Eckersley R, Blomley M, Harvey C. Quantification of blood flow. In: Derchi LE, Grenier N, eds. Ultrasound. Categorical Course ECR 2002. Berlin: Springer-Verlag, 2002:84–90.

51. Wei K, Le E, Bin JP, et al. Quantification of renal blood flow with contrast enhanced-ultrasound. J Am Coll Cardiol 2001; 37:1135–1140.

52. Hosotani Y, Takahashi N, Kiyomoto H, et al. A new method for evaluation of split renal cortical blood flow with contrast echocardiography. Hypertens Res 2002; 25:77–83.

53. Lewin PA. Quo vadis medical ultrasound? Ultrasonics 2004; 42:1–7.

4

CT of Complex Renal Cysts

Nancy S. Curry
Medical University of South Carolina, Charleston, South Carolina, U.S.A.

INTRODUCTION

Complex renal cysts of benign or malignant etiology may be discovered on a computed tomography (CT) scan of patients with urinary tract symptomatology or incidentally discovered in the evaluation of nonrenal disorders of the upper abdomen. Sometimes, sonographic or magnetic resonance (MR) examinations for unrelated clinical problems (e.g., biliary disorders or lumbar disk disease) reveal atypical cystic renal lesions, which are then usually further investigated with dedicated renal CT. Clinical decision-making is heavily dependent on the radiologist having an under-standing of cystic lesions of the kidney and their imaging features. With advanced CT technology, proper protocol selection and guidance from an accumulating body of literature on the subject, the radiologist plays a key role in directing the appropri-ate management of patients with complex renal cysts.

Renal cysts are encountered daily on imaging examinations. They are rare in children and young adults and begin to appear around the age of 30; by the age of 50, half the population has one or more renal cysts, as necropsy series have shown (1). They mostly originate from the cortex and are thought to be related to tubular obstruction and ischemia. Uncomplicated cysts contain a plasma-like fluid and are lined by low cuboidal epithelium with thin, smooth, fibrous walls only 1 to 2 mm thick. Whereas most are unilocular, some contain fibrous septations dividing them fully or partially. About 10% to 15% of cysts contain hemorrhagic fluid and 1% to 2% show plaques of calcium in the wall (2).

Renal cysts are usually asymptomatic even when very large but may come to clinical attention when they become infected or traumatized. The cysts themselves are not of significance. What is important is making the distinction between complex but benign cysts and cystic or solid neoplasms requiring intervention.

Cystic renal neoplasms include cystic nephroma and multilocular cystic renal cell carcinoma (3). These masses usually have a benign clinical course and do not metas-tasize if strict pathologic criteria are applied to make the diagnosis. Cystic nephroma is a benign neoplasm composed of stroma and epithelium that is usually seen in children under the age of four, with male children predominating by a ratio of approximately 2:1. When it presents in adults over the age of 30, it has an 8:1 ratio of female to male predominance. Although almost always benign in behavior, there have been a small number of reported cases of sarcoma developing from cystic nephromas.

These multilocular tumors usually present as encapsulated masses with numerous cysts and septa but no associated expansile solid nodularity. If there are any solid elements, the lesion in question may in fact be a clear cell renal cell carcinoma with a cystic growth pattern, or a cystic Wilms tumor. Because the gross appearances of benign and malignant multilocular masses are similar, they are not distinguishable by imaging features.

CT TECHNIQUE

CT is currently the imaging "gold standard" for characterizing renal masses because of long experience with its use and its wide availability. The newest generation of multidetector, multirow CT machines allows for very rapid multiphasic, very thin section image acquisition. Shortened gantry rotation times and increased number of rows of simultaneously irradiated detectors allow for faster coverage and thinner collimation. Lengthy respiratory suspension is no longer necessary, and image misregistration due to breathing and other motion artifacts is considerably reduced. Multiphasic scans through the kidneys can be acquired very rapidly, each taking only a few seconds to accomplish. The resulting improvement in image quality helps minimize some of the technique-related pitfalls in the evaluation of complex renal masses.

A dedicated renal investigation conducted on a multislice CT produces numerous helical data sets. Although manufacturers use different types of detector arrays, a typical scan from a 16-slice machine might utilize a 16×1.25 mm detector configuration, 27.5 mm/rotation table speed, 0.5 second gantry rotation speed, and a pitch of 1.37. Because multiphasic, multislice scanning can generate many hundreds of images, the thin section acquisitions are reconstructed into thicker sections (5 mm) for electronic display and archival. If necessary, the original thin sections can be exported to a workstation for multiplanar reformatting, volume rendering, and region of interest analysis.

Serial fast scans capture the progressive flow of intravenous contrast material from the renal arteries through the cortex and medulla and ultimately into the collecting structures after concentration and excretion has occurred. The first scan, obtained before any contrast is administered, is essential because it serves as a baseline for recording attenuation changes in a mass during post–contrast enhancement phases. Even without intravenous enhancement, however, the contrast resolution capability of CT allows the distinction of a water density cyst from the adjacent soft tissue of the renal parenchyma. The unenhanced image also discloses any associated calcifications.

After a bolus intravenous injection of iodinated contrast material (300–350 mgI/mL, 3–4 cc/sec), scans can be obtained in any of four visibly distinct temporal phases: the vascular/early corticomedullary (CM) phase, the late CM phase, the tubular–nephrographic or nephrographic phase, and the excretory phase (4). Multiple repeat scans increase radiation dose significantly, so it is important to select only those phases that are likely to be of highest diagnostic yield. Unless a renal cell carcinoma is highly likely, such as in a patient who has had an ultrasound examination suggestive of solid neoplasm, the vascular phase or early CM phase may be omitted. Images obtained in this phase show a brightly enhancing cortex and poorly enhancing medulla. The homogeneously dense nephrographic phase is achieved later, when the cortex and medulla are evenly enhanced. Transiently, in the nephrographic phase, the medulla may eventually even be of higher attenuation than the cortex. Shortly thereafter, the excretory phase begins when the collecting structures begin to fill as the nephrogram decreases in intensity.

CT EVALUATION OF RENAL CYSTS

After administration of intravenous contrast, simple cysts will have no perceptible wall, have a sharply defined interface with the normal renal parenchyma, be of homogeneously low attenuation, and show no enhancement with intravenous contrast material. Lesions that fulfill these criteria may confidently be considered simple benign cysts and follow-up imaging is unnecessary. These characteristics are easily assessed, especially when the cyst is larger than 3 cm in diameter.

Cystic masses may initially be encountered in a standard contrast-enhanced study performed for reasons unrelated to the kidneys. With slice thickness of 5 mm on multislice helical scanners, even some subcentimeter cysts can be determined to be benign and inconsequential. If not characterized on a standard single-phase survey CT, however, a lesion greater than 2 cm should be further evaluated by a dedicated renal CT, ultrasound, or MR imaging. Lesions of 1 to 2 cm are pursued on a limited basis dependent on critical patient information. Advanced age or serious comorbidities may preclude lengthy follow-up or invasive procedures. There is much better reason in younger patients with hereditary syndromes, such as von Hippel–Lindau disease or familial renal tumors, to justify the expense and effort to characterize these smaller lesions.

One of the key features utilized for distinguishing benign cysts from neoplasms is the documentation of enhancement with contrast. To determine whether or not a lesion enhances, region of interest attenuation measurements must be obtained on unenhanced and enhanced CT images. To optimize the validity of statistical sampling of the region of interest, the cursor should be as large as possible and placed at the epicenter of the cyst both in the axial plane and along the z-axis. Any visible heterogeneous areas should be sampled separately, however. Obviously, a similar-sized cursor should be placed in corresponding locations on the pre- and postcontrast scans with all scanning technical parameters and patient positioning held constant between the two series. Reconstructed, overlapping images can be selectively obtained, as needed, to better evaluate the attenuation characteristics of small lesions.

Although an exact value of the minimum attenuation change required to identify true enhancement has not been established, most investigators would agree that a rise in Hounsfield attenuation value of 10 units or more over baseline is suspicious for microvascularity and incompatible with simple cysts (5).

Caution should be taken when assessing small intrarenal lesions, because pseudoenhancement can be an issue. The densely enhancing surrounding renal parenchyma may artificially raise the attenuation of a cyst. Coulam et al. have shown that this is usually not a problem with masses more than 2 cm in diameter, but the attenuation change over baseline may exceed 10 HU in as many as a fourth of masses smaller than 2 cm, thereby mimicking true enhancement (6).

Thin section scanning in the uniform nephrographic stage, when the cortex and medulla are of equal density, detects a larger number of lesions than the earlier CM phase imaging. The exact timing varies from patient to patient depending on circulation time and contrast flow rates. It generally requires scanning approximately 20 to 30 seconds later than standard portal venous phase imaging, which is utilized in most nonfocused abdominal CT. Generally speaking, a scan performed at 90 to 100 seconds is ideal. It is important not to image too early for two reasons: The nonenhanced medulla can easily mask a hypodense mass, and hypovascular masses may be slow to demonstrate enhancement. Cysts also tend to stand out on excretory phase images, but the excretion of dense contrast media into the collecting structures may cause problems with beam-hardening artifacts.

The selection of appropriate scanning protocols and careful region of interest measurements on pre- and postcontrast images are critical factors in the proper assessment of complex cystic renal lesions as will be discussed below.

CT FEATURES OF COMPLEX CYSTS

Benign cysts may have slightly thickened walls or contain septa or calcifications that can blur their distinction from cystic neoplasms. Some cystic lesions will fulfill the criteria for simple cysts with the exception that their contents will have higher attenuation than expected. Due to the relative frequency of these complicating characteristics, the radiologist should provide an opinion on the clinical significance of these findings and try to sort out those that can be safely ignored or followed up from those that require surgical intervention. The referring physician is unlikely to be satisfied with a "malignancy cannot be excluded" disclaimer and, not unexpectedly, will seek guidance from the radiologist regarding the likelihood of malignancy to establish a management plan.

As an aid to distinguishing imaging characteristics of those cystic masses most likely to be benign from those that require surgery, Morton A. Bosniak developed a descriptive categorization system in 1986 (7). He ascribed increasingly complex features to four categories of cysts from I to IV, ranging from simple cysts to cystic neoplasm. Cysts in Categories I and II were considered benign, while the more complex lesions in Categories III and IV mandated surgery.

It was a reasonable expectation that assigning simple cysts into Category I and grossly obvious cystic tumors into Category IV would not be difficult. Not surprisingly, the greatest challenge in using the system was separating the mildly complex Category II lesions, which could be ignored, from the Category III lesions, many of which were malignancies. In 1993, Bosniak modified the classification system to include a group of lesions that were not of sufficient complexity to warrant surgery but which deserved imaging follow-up to assure stability (8,9). These he deemed Category IIF lesions, the "F" standing for the follow-up imaging that he recommended in these instances.

Although based primarily on CT features, the Bosniak cyst classification system is aided by and can be extended to MR with some caution. Experience derived from more recent series of Bosniak's followed group of patients has further refined the system, and recommendations that stem from its use are described below (10–13).

BOSNIAK CLASSIFICATION OF CYSTIC RENAL MASSES

Category I

The simple benign cyst has uniform water density attenuation. There is no calcification, septation, solid elements, or enhancement [increase in attenuation of 10 Hounsfield units (HU) or more] with intravenous contrast. Its wall, if perceptible at all, is hairline thin and the interface with the adjacent parenchyma is sharply defined (Fig. 1).

Category II

Thin, filamentous septation may be present in these benign renal cysts. Also, fine calcification or even short segments of slightly thickened calcification can be found in the wall or septa (Fig. 2). Included in this category are sharply defined, small (less than 3 cm) homogeneously high-attenuation lesions ("hyperdense" cysts) that do not enhance with intravenous contrast (Fig. 3).

Category IIF

These cysts have a greater number of hairline thin septa, minimal wall or septal thickening, or minimal wall or septal enhancement (Fig. 4). Calcification can be thick and nodular (Fig. 5). Totally intrarenal, well-marginated, nonenhancing hyperdense cysts 3 cm in size or larger are included in this category.

Category III

This group is composed of the truly indeterminate cystic masses that have enhancing, thickened, irregular walls or septa. Multilocular masses fall within this group (Figs. 6–8).

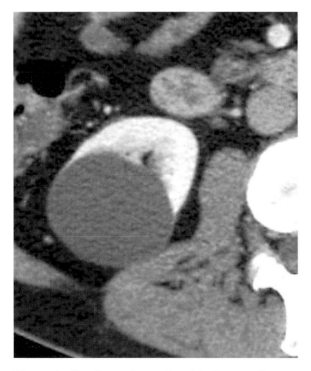

Figure 1 Simple renal cyst, Bosniak Category I.

(A)   **(B)**

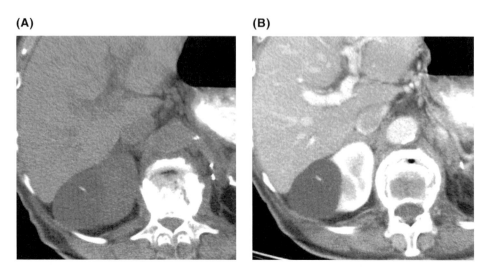

Figure 2 Bosniak Category II cyst. (**A**) Curvilinear calcification within a thin septum, unenhanced scan. (**B**) Lesion remains otherwise cystic after intravenous contrast.

Category IV

These lesions have the characteristics of Category III group with the addition of definable, enhancing soft tissue elements separate from the walls or septa (Figs. 9 and 10).

CALCIFICATIONS

Calcifications can be present in Category II or Category III cystic masses and are a source of uncertainty in assigning a classification to a cystic renal mass. In an analysis of calcifications associated with 81 cystic renal masses, Israel and Bosniak

(A)   **(B)**

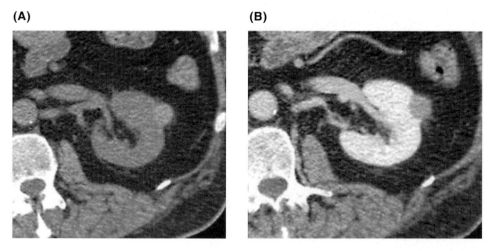

Figure 3 Bosniak Category II hyperdense cyst. (**A**) Homogeneously hyperdense mass measuring 60 HU without intravenous contrast. (**B**) After intravenous contrast the mass did not enhance (61 HU). *Abbreviation*: HU, Hounsfield unit.

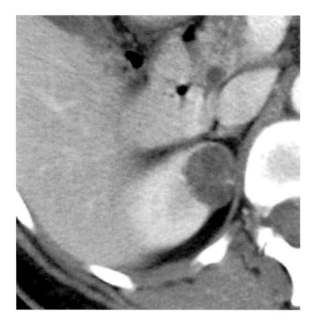

Figure 4 Bosniak Category IIF cyst. Cyst with several internal septations and a minimally thickened wall.

subjectively graded the extent of calcification on a four-point scoring system of minimal, mild, moderate, and severe (12). A score of 1 equaled hairline-thin calcification, 2 indicated some thickness and minimal nodularity, 3 meant further thickness and/or a grossly nodular appearance, and 4 was reserved for grossly thickened, nodular, and extensive calcification. The 21 Category II lesions had the lowest average calcium

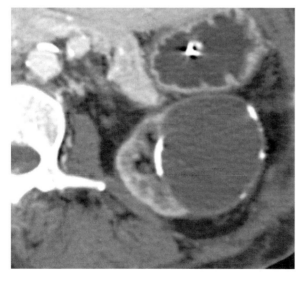

Figure 5 Bosniak Category IIF cyst. Cyst with uniform, mild wall thickening and short, interrupted calcifications. Internally, the lesion was homogeneous, was of low attenuation, and did not enhance with intravenous contrast.

(A)   **(B)**

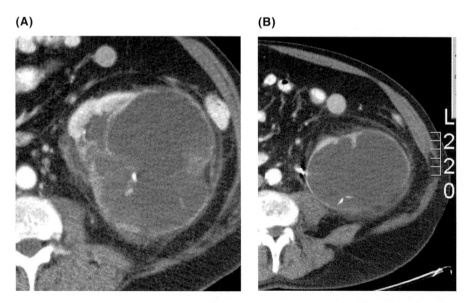

Figure 6 Bosniak Category III. (**A**) A 63-year-old male with microhematuria, left flank pain, and a history of prostate carcinoma. CT shows a cystic mass with irregular wall thickening and associated heterogeneous nonenhancing elements. (**B**) Scan caudal to (**A**) shows thickened internal septa with associated calcifications, a calculus in the proximal ureter, and perinephric stranding. Xanthogranulomatous pyelonephritis at surgery. *Abbreviation*: CT, computed tomography.

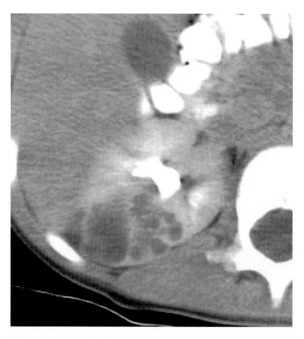

Figure 7 Bosniak Category III complex cyst. Four-year-old male with gross hematuria and a multilocular, encapsulated mass. Multilocular cystic nephroma at surgery.

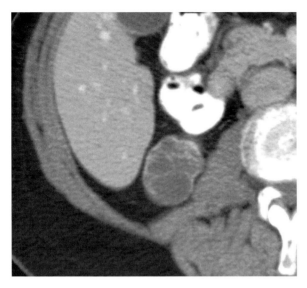

Figure 8 Bosniak Category III complex cyst. A 66-year-old female with incidental mass. Thick-walled, encapsulated, multilocular cystic mass with enhancing septa. Clear cell carcinoma at surgery.

score of 1.4. Nineteen Category IIF lesions scored the highest at 3.1. Twenty-five Category III lesions were intermediate at 2.1. Five of the 22 Category II and IIF followed-up group showed slow increases in the extent of calcification over an average of five years. The pathologic correlation available for 21 calcified Category III lesions yielded 11 benign hemorrhagic or infected cysts, nine renal cell carcinomas, and one multilocular cystic nephroma.

The conclusion of the study was that calcification in a cystic renal mass, even if thick and nodular, is not as important as the presence of solid enhancing elements associated with it. If no soft tissue components are present, even relatively heavily calcified cystic masses can be followed safely (Fig. 11). Neither slow growth nor increase in amounts of calcification should cause concern (Fig. 12).

INCIDENTAL HYPERDENSE MASSES ON NONFOCUSED CT

Occasionally a patient is scanned for a nonurologic reason and an incidental renal lesion is detected that has all the characteristic features of a simple cyst, except that its attenuation is above water density. On contrast-enhanced CT examinations, both hypovascular solid renal masses and hyperdense cysts will appear less dense than the adjacent highly enhancing renal parenchyma. Comparison to other water-density structures, such as the gallbladder or urinary bladder, is a simple method to make sure the high attenuation number is not a machine calibration problem. Routine, frequent water phantom checks of the scanners should prevent drifting of the attenuation numbers. If the high attenuation is not due to artifact and if only postcontrast images are available, the critical issue of whether renal mass enhancement has occurred cannot be assessed.

If not spurious, these "hyperdense" cysts may have achieved their high internal HU values by virtue of increased protein content related to prior hemorrhage or

(A)   (B)

(C)   (D)

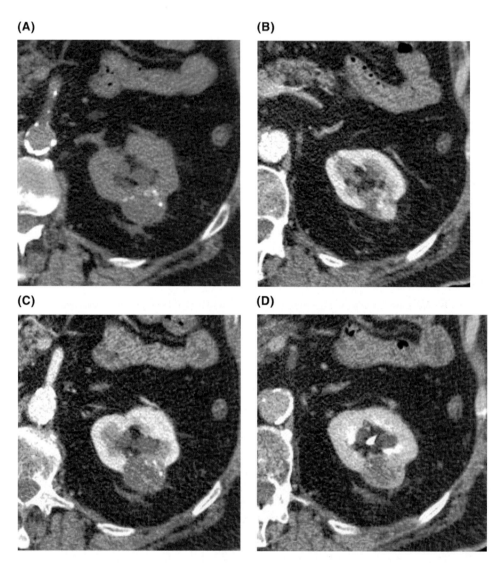

Figure 9 Bosniak Category IV cystic neoplasm. (**A**) A 67-year-old male with gross hematuria and history of prostate carcinoma. Precontrast scan shows interrupted calcifications at the
cyst/parenchymal interface. (**B**) After intravenous contrast, a nodule within the cyst enhances
from 27 to 154 HU. (**C**) The center of the mass remains at low attenuation (11–17 HU). (**D**)
Delayed image shows heterogeneity of the periphery of the mass. An encapsulated renal
cell carcinoma was found at surgery. *Abbreviation*: HU, Hounsfield unit.

another undetermined process (14–20). New and Aronow found that blood with a
hematocrit of 45% measures 58 HU on CT, rising to 60 to 80 HU after blood clot
retraction with the protein component being responsible for the high attenuation (21).
This appears to be consistent with the frequent finding of hemorrhagic cysts in the
range of 70 to 90 HU (19,20).

The importance of hemorrhagic cysts lies in distinguishing them from high
attenuation solid renal tumors (Fig. 13) (22). Ultrasound may not be helpful because
the contents (blood or debris) that make the cyst high in attenuation may also generate internal echoes indistinguishable from a solid tumor. Generally speaking, cysts

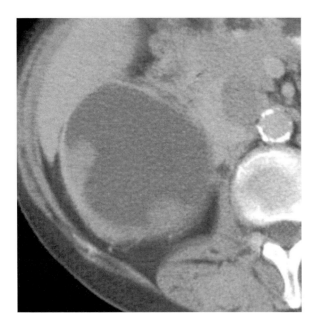

Figure 10 Bosniak Category IV cystic neoplasm. A 65-year-old female with a left neck mass and a 3 cm mass in the right lung. CT shows a thick-walled cystic renal mass with enhancing mural nodules. Core biopsies consistent with renal cell carcinoma. Patient expired five months after diagnosis. *Abbreviation*: CT, computed tomography.

detected on enhanced CT examinations that are only mildly hyperdense, with CT attenuation numbers in the range of 20 to 40 HU, often are anechoic on ultrasound, and, with the help of subsequent ultrasonography, can safely be assigned to Category II or IIF, depending on location, size, and the presence or absence of other

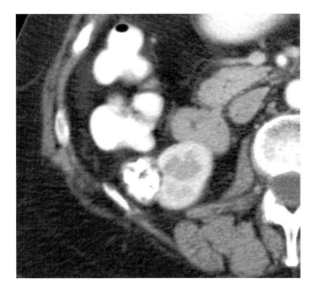

Figure 11 Bosniak Category IIF cyst. Nearly completely calcified mass with no obvious enhancing elements. A benign chronic inflammatory mass was resected. *Source*: Case courtesy of Dr. Frank Muto, Charleston, WV.

(A)   **(B)**

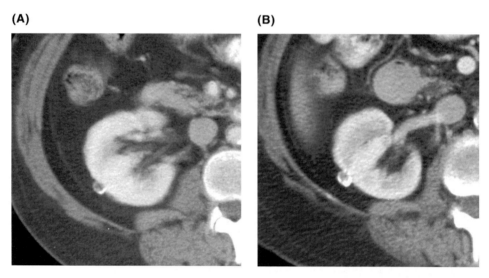

Figure 12 (**A**) A 51-year-old female with breast carcinoma and a subcentimeter rim calcified renal cyst, Bosniak Category II. (**B**) Five years later the lesion has not grown but shows some increase in extent of calcification.

minor complexities (Fig. 14). In comparison, the more highly attenuating masses are more likely to have internal echogenic material that may convincingly mimic carcinoma.

Another way of handling this situation is to obtain delayed CT images at the time of discovery (Fig. 15). The added scan demonstrates whether the high attenuation is a fixed feature of the mass due to its non-neoplastic content or is a temporary

(A)   **(B)**

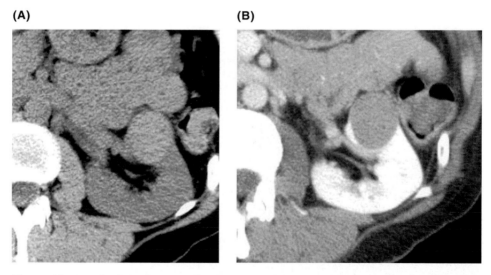

Figure 13 Renal cell carcinoma. (**A**) A 42-year-old female with back pain, hematuria, and a renal mass discovered by lumbar spine MR. CT without intravenous contrast shows mildly hyperdense (55 HU) 3 cm mass. (**B**) After intravenous contrast, the masses enhance to 88 HU, consistent with solid, not cystic character. *Abbreviations*: CT, computed tomography; HU, Hounsfield unit; MR, magnetic resonance.

(A)

(B)

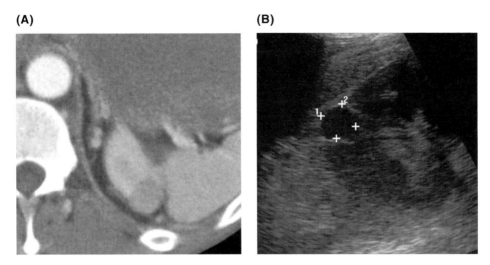

Figure 14 Bosniak Category II hyperdense cyst. (**A**) A 47-year-old male with a pancreatic pseudocyst and incidental high attenuation (72 HU), homogeneous 1.8 cm mass in the posterior upper pole. Bosniak Category II hyperdense cyst versus solid, enhancing renal neoplasm. (**B**) Ultrasound examination shows no internal echoes. *Abbreviation*: HU, Hounsfield unit.

manifestation of its internal vascularity, implying a tumor. This concept of "de-enhancement" was suggested by Macari and Bosniak in 1999 (23). They investigated patients with both known and incidentally discovered high attenuation masses with 15-minute-delayed CT scans. Seventeen hyperdense lesions showed a mean de-enhancement of 32 HU (range 15–67), from an initial mean attenuation of about 82 HU on nephrographic phase images down to 50 HU on the delayed scans.

(A)

(B)

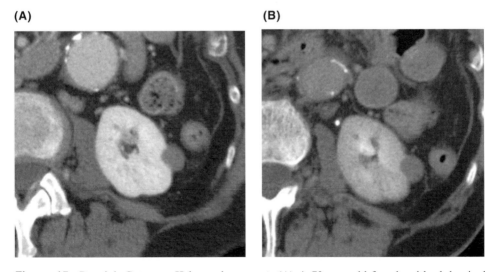

Figure 15 Bosniak Category II hyperdense cyst. (**A**) A 73-year-old female with abdominal aortic aneurysm. CT shows a 1.7 cm homogeneous mass with attenuation of 78 HU on nephrographic phase image. Bosniak Category II hyperdense cyst versus solid, enhancing renal neoplasm. (**B**) Fifteen-minute-delayed scan revealed no significant de-enhancement with attenuation measurement of 81 HU. *Abbreviations*: CT, computed tomography; HU, Hounsfield unit.

This group included nine proven renal cell carcinomas, two metastases, a nonlipomatous hamartoma, and five other lesions that showed enhancement when pre and postcontrast images were compared. Seven of the group of nine masses not showing de-enhancement had no evidence of enhancement where precontrast scans were available for comparison. This group also showed stability on short-term follow-up.

A potential pitfall in the analysis of delayed imaging to detect wash-out or de-enhancement of contrast is the lack of an adequate bolus of contrast on the initial contrast-enhanced scan, preventing peak parenchymal opacification. The degree of de-enhancement in that case may not be sufficient to distinguish a benign hyperdense lesion from a hypovascular solid mass. Also, it should be noted that de-enhancement is a feature of all solid lesions, not just renal cell carcinoma. Other solid lesions, both benign and malignant, such as lipid poor hamartomas, oncocytomas, metastases, and lymphoma, would be expected to show this imaging characteristic, as noted in the above series.

Suh et al. evaluated portal venous phase contrast-enhanced CT to determine what CT features might distinguish renal cell carcinomas from high attenuation renal cysts when only contrast-enhanced images were available (24). They investigated 57 renal cell carcinomas and 37 high attenuation cysts in 90 patients. The renal cell carcinomas were significantly larger in size, were greater in heterogeneity, and had higher attenuation than the hyperdense cysts. All lesions in their series measuring more than 110 HU were cancers. With regression analysis, they suggested that a threshold of 70 HU might be used to distinguish a cyst from neoplasm, but this is at odds with several previous reports of hemorrhagic cysts with attenuation measurements exceeding 70 HU. Although their study suggests that these features can be helpful in suggesting the presence of malignancy rather than a high attenuation cyst when unenhanced CT images have not been obtained, this information should not serve as a substitute for a dedicated, high quality, multiphasic CT examination, which, as previously mentioned, should include preliminary noncontrast images.

IS THE BOSNIAK CLASSIFICATION USEFUL?

It was established by Aronson et al., in a small study in 1991, that the Bosniak classification system was a useful management tool (25). In an investigation of 16 proven lesions, they found that all Category II lesions were benign and all Category IV lesions were malignant. Of the seven indeterminate cystic lesions in Category III, four (57%) were malignant.

There were a few subsequent series that retrospectively investigated the utility of this system and yielded varying results. A report by Wilson et al. in 1996 offered analyses of 22 resected renal cysts and concluded that the system was not helpful because 4 of 5 masses assigned to Category II were found to be malignant (26). This study has been criticized for its small number of Category II and III cases, inadequate CT evaluation (a dedicated renal CT examination was performed in only one of the four Category II malignant cystic masses), and the likelihood of inaccurate classification because so many Category I and II cysts underwent operation (27,28).

Another report in 1996 by Cloix et al. also cast doubt on the utility of the classification system in a study of 32 surgically proven lesions (29). They found two malignancies out of nine in the Category I/II group and 11 benign cysts out of 23 in the Category III/IV group. Thin section, dedicated renal CT had not been performed, however, on these patients.

In 1997, Siegel et al. evaluated 70 lesions in 46 patients and deemed the classification system useful but reported significant interobserver variation (30). Although the number of patients and lesions was larger than in earlier series, many simple cysts ($n = 22$) were included, and only 19 Category II/III lesions were included. One of 8 Category II lesions was malignant and 3 of 49 Category IV lesions were benign. Only 55% to 60% of the lesions were investigated by pre/postcontrast CT and/or thin section CT, and attenuation numbers were available in fewer than half the patients so that objective evidence of enhancement was lacking. All three readers agreed on the assignment of a category in only 41 masses (59%). Not unexpectedly, the largest interobserver variation found in that study was in distinguishing the most difficult categories, II and III. Although different levels of expertise might have been one factor, it is likely that suboptimal CT technique again also played a role in compromised performance.

A 1999 French series of cystic renal tumors that incorporated multimodality imaging found that the Bosniak classification system worked as expected. All Category I and II lesions were benign, all Category IV lesions were malignant, and Category III included benign and malignant masses (31). A Japanese series of 35 patients, reported in 2000, showed all 11 masses in Category I were benign, one of two Category II masses was malignant, and all 10 of Category III masses were malignant as well as 12 in Category IV (32). Unfortunately, imaging parameters were not specified, and it is unknown whether a proper CT technique was used.

What many of these studies inadvertently point out is the critical importance of proper CT technique to provide a basis for evaluation. In a larger series pooled from two institutions published in 2000, Curry et al. reported on 82 masses in 77 patients (33). Emphasis was placed on selection criteria maximizing the number of lesions evaluated by state-of-the-art CT protocol. There were 11 Category II and 49 Category III masses for a total of 60 lesions in the most-difficult-to-categorize groups. Of these, 81% were evaluated by thin section, dedicated renal CT. The classification system accurately classified all 15 cystic masses in Categories I and II as benign and all 18 Category IV lesions as malignant. Of the Category III indeterminate cystic masses, 59% were malignant. An additional group of 34 lesions in 32 patients that were followed up for 3 months to 10 years remained stable. The confirmatory results of this study were attributed to adherence to adequate CT technique.

In 2003, Israel and Bosniak published their own follow-up CT series of Category IIF lesions (13). They conducted a retrospective analysis of 42 moderately complex cystic masses that were followed for two years or more or had pathologic correlation. There were three of the latter. Number and appearance of septa, wall thickness, parenchymal/mass interface, calcification, and attenuation characteristics were all analyzed. Average and median follow-up time was about five years.

Three lesions decreased, and two lesions increased in size. One of the latter showed decreased complexity despite growth. The other was a renal cell carcinoma that showed an increase in size from 2 to 4 cm with thicker and more nodular septa three years after the initial examination. Another lesion did not increase in size, but over 16 months it too developed more internal complexity (thicker septa) and proved to be a cystic neoplasm as well. Their finding of a malignancy rate of approximately 5% in Category IIF is low enough to justify the follow-up strategy, because cystic cancers can generally be safely followed until their malignant nature becomes more obvious without fear that these cancers will metastasize before surgery or radiofrequency ablation is performed. Cystic renal cancers are usually of low malignant potential and are unlikely to metastasize before more definitive follow-up imaging is obtained (3).

ROLE OF BIOPSY IN COMPLEX CYSTIC RENAL MASSES

The recommended treatment for complex cystic masses is either observation or surgery, which traditionally has meant nephrectomy, partial nephrectomy, enucleation, or, more recently, laparoscopic surgery. Increasingly, radiofrequency ablation and cryosurgery are becoming options in patients who are not standard operative candidates. In the United States, unequivocal imaging diagnosis of renal malignancy is usually followed by surgical intervention without other confirmation. Biopsy is rarely performed, being reserved for selected cases where the patient has a known primary nonrenal tumor or lymphoma and biopsy is necessary to direct appropriate therapy.

One recent paper, however, advocates the biopsy of Category III cystic renal masses to avoid unnecessary surgery in the cases that prove to be benign. Harisinghani et al. described the results of CT-guided biopsies of 28 Bosniak Category III lesions (34). Fine needle aspirations and core biopsies were obtained of the suspicious areas of the cyst wall, septa, or calcification in multiple passes. Seventeen (61%) of the lesions were malignant and 11 (39%) were benign. The benign cases were followed up for periods of one to two years (median 18 months).

This study was subject to criticism, however, for misclassification of at least some lesions and inadequate period of follow-up in the benign group to assure stability (35). The authors' claim of a negative predictive value of biopsy of 100% has not been achieved by other investigators. In another study that included 16 cystic renal masses, Rybicki et al. showed percutaneous biopsy was only 33% sensitive with a negative predictive value of 87% (36). The authors do not advocate biopsy in these cases because of these results. Pathologists agree that the sensitivity of percutaneous biopsy in diagnosing cystic renal cell carcinoma is very low, rendering a negative result highly unreliable, a fact that should be communicated to the clinician (37). To be confident that a tumor will not manifest aggressive behavior, pathologic analysis of the entire lesion is mandatory (3). Another criticism of biopsy of cystic lesions is that less tissue is obtained, and it is well known that sampling errors can occur due to tumor cellular heterogeneity even in core solid tumor specimens. A false negative rate of 20% and a false positive rate of 34% were reported by Goethuys et al. in intraoperatively obtained renal mass core biopsies (38).

In addition to continued uncertainty, any biopsy may sufficiently alter a lesion's imaging characteristics to make follow-up for stability (which may be required in the case of a negative biopsy result) more confusing. Finally, complications of renal biopsy, such as pneumothorax, bleeding, pseudoaneurysm, infection, and tumor spill, are rare, but cannot be disregarded (35,36). Given the low sensitivity of biopsy for cystic renal cell carcinoma and the lingering problem of false negatives, Category III cystic renal masses appropriately classified with proper CT technique should be evaluated surgically (35–37).

MANAGEMENT RECOMMENDATIONS

Category IIF characterization implies that the lesion in question is probably benign, but some uncertainty exists because of the complex features described above. Thus, Category IIF cysts should be followed to make sure that the lesion shows stability over time. The finding of two malignancies in 42 (5%) followed-up renal cystic masses in Bosniak's series should not be cause for alarm. As previously stated, cystic renal cell carcinomas are much less aggressive tumors than solid malignant renal neoplasms, obviating the need for urgent intervention (3,39,40). They have a better prognosis and less potential for metastasis, so that a period of watchful waiting in these cases is unlikely to compromise the patient's ultimate well-being.

Bosniak recommends the first follow-up be obtained by dedicated renal CT at six months and then annually thereafter for five years if the patient is older than 50 years of age. Even longer follow-up might be considered in younger patients because of lack of data on these patients. Because of concerns with radiation exposure,

(A)   **(B)**

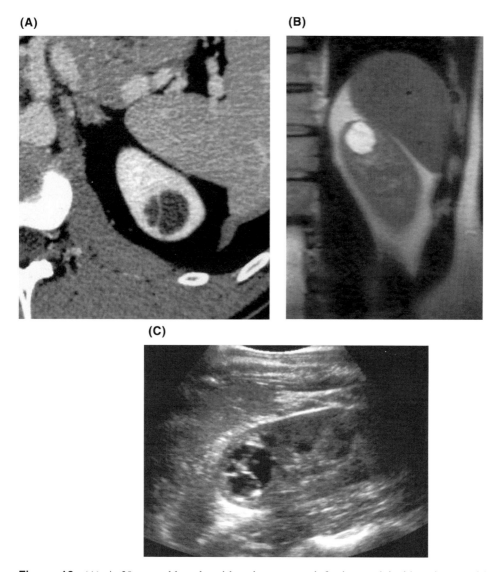

(C)

Figure 16 (**A**) A 30-year-old male with urinary tract infection and incidental cyst with slightly thickened septa. Bosniak Category IIF cyst. (**B**) Coronal T2-weighted MR scan shows minimal septation and slight wall irregularity. (**C**) Ultrasound examination shows more septa with associated nodular thickening appearing significantly more complex than the CT or MR. Lesion has remained stable for over a year of follow-up imaging. *Abbreviations*: CT, computed tomography; MR, magnetic resonance.

(A)   **(B)**

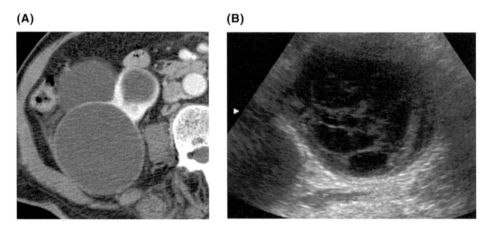

Figure 17 Bosniak Category IIF cyst. (**A**) An 87-year-old male with gross hematuria and aortic valvular disease. CT shows multiple simple cysts and one large homogeneous cyst with no internal enhancement and a uniformly thick wall. (**B**) The corresponding ultrasound examination performed the same day shows a striking internal architecture compared to the CT. *Abbreviation*: CT, computed tomography.

follow-up with MR might be considered for extended follow-up in these patients, as well as in those with renal insufficiency.

One pitfall in the substitution of MR for CT, however, is that while findings are often equivalent (Fig. 16), in some cases MR shows significantly greater internal complexity than does CT. Israel and Bosniak compared 71 cystic renal masses that were evaluated by CT and MR within one year of each other, with pathologic correlation in 23 cases (41). The findings were similar in 54 (76%) with the remaining 24% being discordant. MR showed more septa in 8 (11%), more wall/septal thickness in 5 (7%), and a single mass showed more of both. Four lesions whose enhancement was equivocal on CT showed no enhancement on MR with subtraction techniques. Overall, MR upgraded seven lesions, from Category II to IIF ($n = 2$), IIF to III ($n = 3$), and III to IV ($n = 2$). The most significant upgrade is from IIF to III because this change in categorization would mean that a lesion would be resected instead of being followed. One of the three IIF–III upgraded cases was a young patient with a large lesion that that proved to be a hemorrhagic cyst at operation. The other two patients were elderly. One refused surgery, and the lesion has remained stable after one year of observation. The other, who also refused surgery, has shown progression of findings highly suggestive of malignancy.

Ultrasound frequently shows far more internal complexity to cystic renal masses (Figs. 16 and 17) than CT and is most useful when it shows that a lesion is anechoic (Fig. 14). If a follow-up strategy is based on the CT findings, periodic sonographic examinations may be helpful to avoid the expense and radiation that dedicated renal CT entails. Replication of similar imaging planes can be difficult, however.

SUMMARY

By utilizing proper multiphasic CT protocols performed on single or multislice helical equipment, it is possible to accurately characterize most cystic renal masses exceeding 3 cm in size. Those that are smaller or have only mildly complex features can safely be followed. The truly indeterminate masses, Category III, are a relatively small subset of renal cysts and are best handled surgically. It cannot be expected that all or even most of these masses will be malignant, because benign inflammatory conditions and cystic nephromas are included in this group. As laparoscopic renal surgery becomes more available, the risks associated with resection will be reduced, lessening the impact of intervention. It should be remembered that the gross appearance of a lesion at visual inspection or imaging analysis is not reliably predictive of histology. Ultimately, the pathologist is the final judge regarding benign versus malignant nature of highly complex cystic masses.

REFERENCES

1. Kissane JM. Congenital malformations. In: Heptinstall RH, ed. Pathology of the Kidney. 2d ed. Boston: Little, Brown, and Company, 1974:69–119.
2. Witten DM, Myers GH, Utz DC. Renal cysts. In: Clinical Urography. 4th ed. Philadelphia: WB Saunders Company, 1977:1371–1466.
3. Eble JN, Bonsib SM. Extensively cystic renal neoplasms: cystic nephroma, cystic partially differentiated nephroblastoma, multilocular cystic renal cell carcinoma, and cystic hamartoma of renal pelvis. Semin Diagn Pathol 1998; 15:2–20.
4. Yuh BI, Cohan HR. Different phases of renal enhancement: role in detecting and characterizing renal masses during helical CT. AJR 1999; 173:747–755.
5. Birnbaum BA, Jacobs JE, Ramchandani P. Multiphasic renal CT: comparison of renal mass enhancement during the corticomedullary and nephrographic phases. Radiology 1996; 200:753–758.
6. Coulam CH, Sheafor DH, Leder RA, et al. Evaluation of pseudoenhancement of renal cysts during contrast-enhanced CT. AJR 2000; 174:493–498.
7. Bosniak MA. The current radiologic approach to renal cysts. Radiology 1986; 158:1–10.
8. Bosniak MA. Difficulties in classifying cystic lesions of the kidney. Urol Radiol 1991; 13:91–93.
9. Bosniak MA. Problems in the radiologic diagnosis of renal parenchymal tumors. Urol Clin North Am 1993; 20:217–230.
10. Bosniak MA. Diagnosis and management of patients with complicated cystic lesions of the kidney (commentary). AJR 1997; 169:819–821.
11. Bosniak MA. The use of the Bosniak classification system for renal cysts and cystic tumors. J Urol 1997; 157:1852–1853.
12. Israel GM, Bosniak MA. Calcification in cystic renal masses: is it important in diagnosis? Radiology 2003; 226:47–52.
13. Israel GM, Bosniak MA. Follow-up CT of moderately complex cystic lesions of the kidney (Bosniak category IIF). AJR 2003; 181:627–633.
14. Curry NS, Brock G, Metcalf JS, Sens MA. Hyperdense renal mass: unusual CT appearance of a benign renal cyst. Urol Radiol 1982; 4:33–35.
15. Fishman MC, Pollack HM, Arger PH, Banner MP. High protein content: another cause of CT hyperdense benign renal cyst. J Comput Assist Tomogr 1983; 7:1103–1106.
16. Sussman S, Cochran ST, Pagani JJ, et al. Hyperdense renal masses: a CT manifestation of hemorrhagic renal cysts. Radiology 1984; 150:207–211.
17. Dunnick NR, Korobkin M, Silverman PM, Foster WL. Computed tomography of high density renal cysts. J Comput Assist Tomogr 1984; 8:458–461.
18. Coleman BG, Arger PH, Mintz MC, Pollack HM, Banner MP. Hyperdense renal masses: a computed tomographic dilemma. AJR 1984; 143:291–294.
19. Zirinsky K, Auh YHB, Rubinstein WA, et al. CT of hyperdense renal cysts: sonographic correlation. AJR 1984; 143:151–156.

20. Sussman S, Cochran ST, Pagani JJ, et al. Hyperdense renal masses: a CT manifestation of hemorrhagic renal cysts. Radiology 1984; 150:207–211.

21. New PFJ, Aronow S. Attenuation measurements of whole blood and blood fractions in computed tomography. Radiology 1976; 121:645–640.

22. Dunnick NR, Korobkin M, Clark WM. CT demonstration of hyperdense renal carcinoma. J Comput Assist Tomogr 1984; 8:1023–1024.

23. Macari M, Bosniak MA. Delayed CT to evaluate renal masses discovered at contrast-enhanced CT: demonstration of vascularity with deenhancement. Radiology 1999; 213:674–680.

24. Suh M, Coakley FV, Qayyum A, et al. Distinction of renal cell carcinomas from high attenuation renal cysts at portal venous phase contrast-enhanced CT. Radiology 2003; 228:330–334.

25. Aronson S, Frazier HA, Baluch JD, Hartman DS, Christenson PJ. Cystic renal masses: usefulness of the Bosniak classification. Urol Radiol 1991; 13:83–90.

26. Wilson TE, Doelle EA, Cohan RH, Wojno K, Korobkin M. Cystic renal masses: a reevaluation of the usefulness of the Bosniak classification system. Acad Radiol 1996; 3:564–570.

27. Bosniak MA. Letter to the editor. Acad Radiol 1996; 3:981–984.

28. Curry NS. Atypical cystic renal masses. Abdom Imaging 1998; 23:230–236.

29. Cloix P, Martin X, Pangaud C, et al. Surgical management of complex renal cysts: a series of 32 cases. J Urol 1996; 156:28–30.

30. Siegel CL, McFarland EG, Brink JA, et al. CT of cystic renal masses: analysis of diagnostic performance and interobserver variation. AJR 1997; 169:813–818.

31. Levy P, Helenon O, Merran S, et al. Cystic tumors of the kidney in adults: radiohistopathologic correlations. J Radiol 1999; 80:121–133.

32. Koga S, Nishikido M, Inuzuka S, et al. An evaluation of Bosniak's radiological classification of cystic renal masses. BJU Int 2000; 86:607–609.

33. Curry NS, Cochran ST, Bissada NK. Cystic renal masses: accurate Bosniak classification requires adequate renal CT. AJR 2000; 175:339–342.

34. Harisinghani MG, Maher MM, Gervis DA, et al. Incidence of malignancy in complex cystic renal masses (Bosniak category III): should imaging-guided biopsy precede surgery? AJR 2003; 180:755–758.

35. Bosniak M. Letter to the editor. Should we biopsy complex cystic masses (Bosniak category III)? AJR 2003; 181:1425–1426.

36. Rybicki FJ, Shu KM, Cibas ES, et al. Percutaneous biopsy of renal masses: sensitivity and negative predictive value stratified by clinical setting and size of mass. AJR 2003; 180:1281–1287.

37. Renshaw AA, Granter SR, Cibas ES. Fine-needle aspiration of the adult kidney. Cancer 1997; 81:71–88.

38. Goethuys H, von Poppel H, Oyen R, Baert L. The case against fine-needle aspiration cytology for small solitary kidney tumors. Eur Urol 1996; 29:284–287.

39. Murad T, Komaiko W, Oyasu R, Bauer K. Multilocular cystic renal cell carcinoma. Am J Clin Pathol 1991; 95:633–637.

40. Bielsa O, Lloreta J, Gelabert-Mas A. Cystic renal cell carcinoma: pathologic features, survival and implications for treatment. Br J Urol 1998; 82:16–20.

41. Israel GM, Hindman N, Bosniak MA. Comparison of CT and MRI imaging by using the Bosniak classification system. Radiology 2004; 231:365–371.

5

CT Urography

Richard H. Cohan and Elaine M. Caoili
Department of Radiology, University of Michigan Health System, Ann Arbor, Michigan, U.S.A.

INTRODUCTION

Over the past few years, CT urography (CTU; CT: computed tomography) has emerged as a promising tool for imaging patients with suspected urinary tract disease, due to its ability to image all aspects of the urinary tract at the same time. CT is already known to be superior to excretory urography (EU) and ultrasonography for detecting and characterizing renal masses (1,2) and in detecting urolithiasis (3,4). The only potential problem with using CT for examination of the urinary tract has been its perceived limited accuracy in evaluating the renal collecting systems, ureters, and bladder. If CT could be performed in such a way as to assess these components of the urinary tract with at least similar accuracy to EU, CT would then be able to completely replace EU. A comprehensive CT evaluation of the urinary tract would offer the advantage of allowing information that has until now been acquired from many different imaging studies, including EU, ultrasound, and standard CT, to be obtained from only one study. This is a tremendous advantage. Multiexamination work-ups are inconvenient. They require much patient effort (including repeat trips to an imaging center and bowel preparation) and are expensive.

In this chapter, we will review the various strategies being employed for CTU. A brief discussion of CTU technique will follow. We will then review the initial reported experience with CTU detection of urinary tract pathology. Potential problems in CTU interpretation will be summarized. Published CTU radiation dose estimates will be discussed. Reported data on CTU cost-effectiveness will be mentioned as well. Finally, a few current controversies concerning the CTU technique will be addressed.

APPROACHES TO CTU

For a CT examination to allow for comprehensive urinary tract imaging, it must be able to adequately detect urinary tract calculi, renal masses, and renal collecting system, bladder, and ureteral abnormalities. Given the already widely acknowledged ability of CT to visualize renal masses and urolithiasis, recent modifications in

CT technique have centered around the creation of a protocol allowing for detailed evaluation of the renal collecting systems, ureters, and bladder.

There are several different philosophies concerning how to perform CTU. The approach that has existed the longest (but which is used by only a minority of investigators) involves combining precontrast and contrast-enhanced axial CT imaging with direct coronal imaging of the kidneys, ureters, and bladder, after injected contrast material have been excreted into the renal collecting systems (5). The coronal images were initially obtained with plain radiography. To do this the patient was removed from the CT scanner after the initial unenhanced and contrast-enhanced CT scans were obtained, and then conventional radiographs were taken at 10 to 15 minutes. Using this approach, a combined CT–excretory urogram was performed, with the latter portion of the study allowing for a detailed assessment of the urothelium.

Unfortunately, the radiographic images from these combined studies are not always of the best quality. This is because it is not always easy to ensure that once a patient is removed from a CT scanner, he or she will have prompt access to a radiography room. If there is too long a delay between the CT scanning and conventional X-ray acquisition, then the renal collecting system and ureteral distention and opacification will not be optimal at the time that the radiographs are obtained.

As a response to this potential timing difficulty, radiologists at the Mayo Clinic in Rochester, Minnesota, installed X-ray equipment in a CT scanning room (6). By doing this, they could obtain conventional radiographs at any time after CT images are acquired. This solution is probably not practical for most institutions, because such CT room modification is costly and the use of installed radiography equipment is restricted almost entirely to those patients referred for combined CT–EU. There is a significant cost of slowing down patient throughput in such a modified CT room. Obviously, regular CT examinations cannot be performed while the conventional abdominal radiographs are being obtained, processed, and reviewed.

As an alternative, investigators at the Mayo Clinic and others (7) explored the option of obtaining scan projection radiographs or digital scout radiographs instead of conventional radiographs after completion of the first two series of CT images (unenhanced scans evaluating patients for urolithiasis and enhanced scans evaluating patients for renal masses). This technique offers the advantage of requiring only a CT scanner rather than both a CT scanner and standard radiography equipment; however, it has an important limitation: the resolution of a digital scout radiograph is inferior to that of a conventional radiograph. Thus, the renal collecting systems, ureters, and bladder cannot be evaluated as accurately. In response to this problem, software has been developed that has been shown to significantly improve the quality of the scan projection radiograph (8). Using this software, so-called "enhanced" scan projection radiographs can be obtained.

At least two studies have compared the quality of standard and enhanced digital scout radiographs with that of standard film-screen radiographs (7,9). Both have determined that conventional radiography allows for superior imaging of the urinary tract compared with standard digital scout or scan projection radiography. In particular, intrarenal collecting system detail, interface, and bone image quality are significantly inferior on standard scan projection radiographs than on conventional radiographs. In contrast, enhanced scan projection radiographs appear to be similar to plain films at least in some aspects, such as in detecting urinary tract calculi (7).

Most researchers evaluating CTU have performed this study in a very different fashion (8,10–15). They have chosen, instead, to rely exclusively on the acquisition of an additional series of axial images obtained after renal excretion of injected contrast material has occurred. These excretory-phase axial images are used for a detailed evaluation of the renal collecting systems, ureters, and bladder (instead of relying on conventional radiography or CT scan projection radiography). Although there are a number of variations in the reported techniques for this excretory-phase image acquisition, all rely upon the same principle: a series of axial images are obtained using extremely thin sections (usually 2.5 mm thick or less) obtained at a delay far beyond that employed for standard abdominal and pelvic CT or renal mass CT. In CTU, the last set of images is obtained anywhere from 5 to 15 minutes after the initiation of the contrast material injection. Because most institutions utilizing this technique perform their scans on multidetector-row helical CT equipment, many refer to this technique as multidetector CTU or MDCTU. Although these images can also be obtained on single-detector helical scanners or even nonhelical scanners, they are much more quickly acquired and more easily processed when MDCTU is used.

At most centers where MDCTU is performed, thick-section three-dimensional (3-D) reconstructed images are also created. This is done, in part, because thick-section 3-D images more closely resemble the excretory urographic images with which radiologists and urologists are most familiar. To maximize postprocessed image quality when such reconstructions are obtained, the source axial images are usually reconstructed at overlapping intervals (usually with 50% overlap). It must be emphasized, however, that reliance solely on standard postprocessed 3-D images is not appropriate at the present time, because this will lead to many interpretative errors (most commonly false negative studies). The axial images have to be reviewed in addition to these 3-D images (although this can be done using another set of axial images reconstructed at contiguous rather than overlapping intervals).

In contrast, preliminary work has suggested that it may be possible to use thin-section (3 mm or less) 3-D or reformatted images instead of axial images to evaluate the renal collecting systems, ureters, and bladder without sacrificing sensitivity or specificity in diagnosing urinary tract pathology. In a recent study performed by Feng et al. (16), false negative and false positive diagnoses of urothelial cancer were identical for thin-section axial and thin-section coronal reformatted images (the latter actually being 2 mm thick 3-D images reconstructed in the coronal plane). The reformatted images offered the advantage of allowing reviewers to completely evaluate the urinary tract using a smaller number of images (about 100 rather than more than 500) in less time (three minutes rather than four minutes or longer).

Several preliminary studies have suggested that of the two CT-only urographic approaches, excretory-phase axial image acquisition is more sensitive (even when comparison is made with the enhanced scan projection radiographs). In one series that included 26 preselected patients with 97 urinary tract abnormalities detected on axial CT images, only 61 (63%) of these abnormalities could be prospectively identified on simultaneously obtained enhanced scan projection radiographs, 17 of which could not even be seen in retrospect (17). In this study, reviewers also subjectively graded urinary tract visualization to be inferior on digital scout radiographs, and they also rated the vast majority of detected abnormalities as more conspicuous on 3-D reconstructions than on the enhanced digital scouts. Other studies have also suggested that the accuracy in detecting urinary tract abnormalities is far superior if the MDCTU approach is utilized (8,12). It may be for this reason that some researchers who previously advocated the use of the digital scout radiograph have also begun to use axial CT image acquisition to assess the urinary tract.

RECOMMENDED CTU TECHNIQUE

At the present time, we recommend performing CTU by utilizing the MDCTU approach according to one of the two following techniques: the three-phase protocol or the split-bolus protocol. The two specific protocols that follow are those currently being employed at our institution. For both approaches, scanning begins with a renal stone CT, performed at contiguously reconstructed 5 mm thick axial images obtained from the upper poles of the kidneys to the symphysis pubis.

For the three-phase protocol, the patient is then injected with 150 mL of non-ionic contrast material (at a concentration of 300 mg I/mL and a rate of 3–4 mL/sec). Axial images are then acquired from the diaphragms through the lower poles of the kidneys (renal mass CT) using a delay of 100 seconds. Finally, at 720 seconds, thin-section (usually 1.25 mm on 16-row and 0.625 or 1.25 mm on 64-row multidetector scanners) excretory-phase images are obtained at 0.625 mm intervals from the tops of the kidneys to the symphysis pubis.

For the split-bolus protocol, after the renal stone CT images are obtained, the patient is injected with 75 mL of nonionic contrast material (at the same concentration used in the three-phase protocol), again at a rate of 3 to 4 mL/sec. After 600 seconds, an additional 100 mL of contrast material is administered intravenously at the same rate. Then at 720 seconds, thin-section (0.625 or 1.25 mm thick) images are obtained at 0.625 mm intervals from the diaphragms to the symphysis pubis.

For both the three-phase and the split-bolus protocols, the last thin-section excretory-phase series of images is then used as source images for 3-D reconstructions; however, axial images are also reconstructed at a thickness of 2.5 mm and at intervals of 1.25 mm. It is only these axial images that will be reviewed at the time that the study is interpreted. The initial source axial images are not utilized for image interpretation due to their much larger number.

Postprocessing, which is usually performed by a technologist, involves creating anteroposterior and bilateral 30° coronal oblique maximum-intensity projection and volume-rendered images. Coronal thin-section average-intensity projection images are also obtained (at 3 mm thickness and 3 mm reconstruction intervals). This technique creates, in all, several hundred images that must be reviewed. Such a review is best performed on a workstation.

INDICATIONS FOR MDCTU

Due to the radiation intensive nature of MDCTU (see section "Radiation"), some investigators (12) have suggested that this study be performed only on patients who are preidentified by subspecialists (such as urologists) as being at a high risk for having urinary tract pathology, especially transitional cell carcinoma. When these restrictions are enforced, MDCTU is generally performed on patients more than 40 years of age and patients with at least one of the following: a history of transitional cell carcinoma (and who are therefore likely to have recurrences or metachronous tumors), positive urine cytology, previous equivocal imaging studies (18), and persistent symptoms (e.g., ongoing hematuria). In this setting, there are some patients who might not qualify for MDCTU and who might still be referred to EU or standard abdominal and pelvic CT examinations instead. In contrast, others suggest performing MDCTU as a screening test on any patient who presents with hematuria (10,13,14). According to these authors, MDCTU is already in a position to replace EU completely. Regardless of the differing recommendations as to when MDCTU should be performed, all investigators are extremely enthusiastic about its potential. Even those advocating limited use have stated that with a few additional radiation-restricting modifications in CT hardware and changes in CT technique, MDCTU is poised to make EU obsolete in the very near future (12).

ASSESSING THE DIAGNOSTIC CAPABILITY OF CTU: PRELIMINARY RESULTS

Results from preliminary studies suggest that CTU can identify a wide range of urinary tract pathologies. In one of the earliest reports, Caoili et al. (12) reviewed 65 consecutive CT urograms performed in patients who were preidentified by urologists as being at high risk for urinary tract disease. CTU was able to detect 15 of 16 subsequently diagnosed uroepithelial neoplasms (of both the upper tracts and the bladder), as well as a number of additional benign abnormalities that were previously believed to be detectable only with EU or antegrade or retrograde pyelography, including renal tubular ectasia and papillary necrosis. In a follow-up review (19) that included these and an additional 305 patients undergoing CTU, 24 (89%) of 27 subsequently diagnosed upper-tract uroepithelial cancers and 42 (95%) of 44 subsequently diagnosed bladder cancers were detected, as well. Interestingly, whereas all 24 upper-tract cancers could be seen on axial images, only six were identifiable on 3-D reconstructed images. This underscores the limitations of the standard 3-D image review.

Anderson and Cowan reviewed their experience of a series of 130 CT urograms performed in patients with hematuria who had already had equivocal excretory urograms (18). Pathology was detected on 76 CT urograms, including 25 transitional cell carcinomas and 50 benign abnormalities. Yet another multi-institutional study reported by Lang et al. included 350 consecutive patients with microscopic hematuria who were referred for CTU (14). In this study 158 (93%) of 171 diagnosed abnormalities were correctly identified. In another report including 26 patients with painless macroscopic hematuria and/or known recurrent urinary cancer, CTU was also found to be very sensitive in identifying uroepithelial neoplasms (15).

CTU has also been utilized to evaluate patients after urinary diversion. In one study (20), CTU was able to detect 9 abnormalities in 24 patients following such surgery, including four ureteral strictures, and single cases of renal parenchymal scarring, bilateral renal collecting system and ureteral dilatation, vascular compression of a ureter, a calculus in a urinary reservoir, and tumor recurrence in the afferent limb of a neobladder.

Aside from these reviews, a number of anecdotal reports have appeared in which the CTU appearance of several other benign urinary tract abnormalities has been noted, including caliectasis, calyceal diverticula, parapelvic cysts, ureteritis cystica, benign ureteral strictures, blood clots, fibroepithelial polyps, mucus, ureteral endometriomas, ureteropelvic junction obstructions, partial and complete duplications, ureteroceles, pelvic kidneys, and horseshoe kidneys (8,10,21–24).

Only a few studies have actually directly compared the sensitivity of CTU in detecting pathology with that of EU (25) or retrograde pyelography (8). One found CTU to be more sensitive than EU in detecting renal collecting system, ureteral, and bladder pathology (25). O'Malley et al. obtained thin-section axial excretory-phase images in 91 patients within two hours of injection for a previously performed excretory urogram (25). Of 22 subsequently diagnosed abnormalities, CT correctly identified 18, while EU detected only 15. All four cases missed on CTU were bladder cancers. Additionally, there were two false positive CT urograms, but three false positive excretory urograms.

McCarthy and Cowan directly compared the sensitivity of CTU with retrograde pyelography in 106 high-risk patients (8) and found CTU to be superior in detecting both benign and malignant urinary tract pathologies with a sensitivity of 98% for the former versus 79% for the latter. In this series, all upper-tract uroepithelial neoplasms were visualized with CTU, while two upper-tract cancers were missed with retrograde pyelography.

CTU APPEARANCE OF URINARY TRACT PATHOLOGY

Renal Masses

As with conventional CT, CTU can easily detect cystic and solid renal masses. It is now well accepted that CT and magnetic resonance imaging are far more sensitive in detecting and accurate in characterizing renal masses than is EU (1,2). If solid renal masses are identified, accurate staging of these neoplasms (which are considered renal cell carcinomas until proved otherwise) can then be performed (Fig. 1).

Urolithiasis

Because CTU includes a series of noncontrast images, renal and ureteral calculi are usually easily identified, as is the case with renal stone CT. Studies have now clearly demonstrated that CT can identify many more renal and ureteral calculi than can EU (3,4). Calculi can occasionally be identified on contrast-enhanced excretory-phase axial and 3-D reconstructed images (as a filling defect or as an area of increased attenuation or double density, in the renal collecting systems or ureters), provided that images are viewed with wide windows (Fig. 2).

Upper-Tract Transitional Cell Carcinoma

Transitional cell carcinomas have a variety of CT urographic manifestations. They can appear as large masses that compress, distort, and obstruct the renal collecting system or ureteral lumen, thereby producing proximal renal collecting system or ureteral dilatation (Fig. 3). When these cancers are located in the intrarenal collecting system, the axial CT images can also be utilized to determine whether there has been renal parenchymal invasion (a feature of these tumors that affects their stage).

Some cancers are detected when they are still quite small (less than 5 mm in maximal diameter). Small cancers may produce tiny filling defects in the calices, infundibula, renal pelves, or ureters. These are best (and sometimes only) seen on MDCTU when the excretory-phase image review is performed using wide windowing. When only soft tissue windowing is utilized, such small tumors can be completely obscured by the very high attenuation of adjacent excreted contrast material (Fig. 4).

In addition, rather than producing focal masses or filling defects, some transitional cell carcinomas produce circumferential renal collecting system thickening or ureteral wall thickening that is also usually easily detectable on CTU. Whereas such wall thickening is often associated with irregular compression of the adjacent collecting system or ureteral lumen, less frequently, circumferential ureteral wall thickening does not produce any luminal narrowing or irregularity, an appearance not widely described previously (Figs. 5 and 6). Cancers causing wall thickening without luminal narrowing or irregularity are not detectable with EU or even with retrograde

(A)

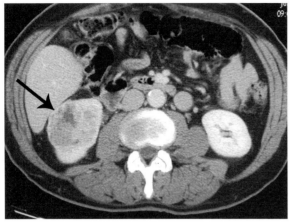

(B)

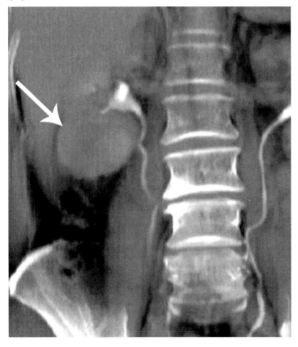

Figure 1 Renal cell carcinoma. (**A**) Contrast-enhanced nephrographic axial CT image demonstrates a large heterogeneous solid mass in the lower pole of the right kidney (*arrow*). (**B**) The mass is also well seen on the coronal, excretory-phase, average-intensity projection 3-D image (*arrow*). *Abbreviation*: CT, computed tomography.

pyelography, because these studies rely solely upon luminal abnormalities to identify urinary tract pathology. They do not image the ureteral wall.

On CTU, one cannot rely solely on 3-D reconstructions or thick-section coronal reformatted images for detecting transitional cell carcinomas. Axial images must be evaluated. The majority of transitional cell carcinomas (particularly those that are small or produce no luminal abnormality) are not seen if only these post-processed contrast-enhanced images are reviewed.

(A)

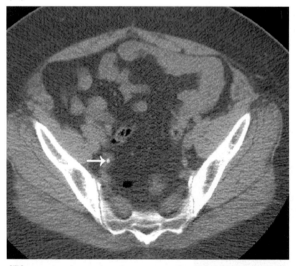

(B)

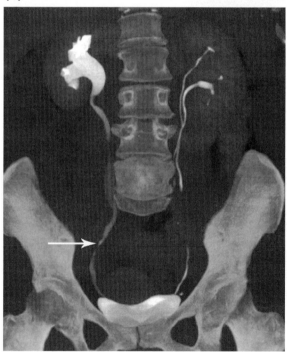

Figure 2 Ureteral calculus. (**A**) Noncontrast axial image demonstrates a small calculus in the distal right ureter surrounded by a rim of soft tissue attenuation (soft tissue rim sign) (*arrow*). (**B**) The calculus is also identified on the coronal excretory-phase, maximum-intensity projection image as a small, higher attenuation focus within the contrast-enhanced ureter (*arrow*). Note that there is mild dilatation of the more proximal portions of the ureter and of the renal collecting system, despite the fact that excretion was not significantly delayed.

(A)

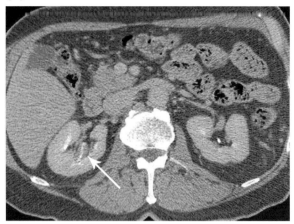

(B)

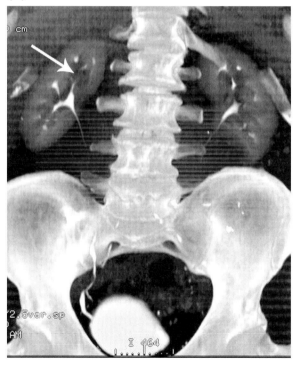

Figure 3 Transitional cell carcinoma. (**A**) A mass in the upper pole of the right kidney surrounds and grossly thickens the wall of the contrast-containing right upper pole infundibulum on this excretory-phase axial image (*arrow*). (**B**) Although the mass itself is not seen, irregular narrowing of the infundibulum is suggested on the coronal excretory-phase, volume-rendered 3-D reconstruction (*arrow*). *Source*: From Ref. 22.

Renal Collecting System and Ureteral Inflammation

Ureteral inflammation may also cause circumferential ureteral wall thickening with or without luminal narrowing and irregularity. Such thickening is indistinguishable from the thickening caused by infiltrative transitional cell carcinoma. Sources of

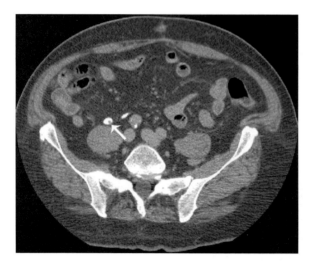

Figure 4 Tiny transitional cell carcinoma. A small (3–4 mm) soft tissue attenuation urothelial malignancy projects into the contrast-containing lumen of the mid-right ureter on this excretory-phase axial image (*arrow*).

ureteral inflammation that have been observed to cause wall thickening on MDCTU include in-dwelling double-J ureteral stents, infectious ureteritis, retroperitoneal fibrosis, and amyloidosis.

Upper-Tract Blood Clot

Blood clots are easily visualized on CTU. On noncontrast scans they may or may not be of characteristically high attenuation (60–80 Hounsfield Units). They do not demonstrate any enhancement after contrast material administration. They conform to the shape of the renal collecting system and ureter and may be completely surrounded by contrast material (because they have no mural attachment) on excretory-phase images (Fig. 7). As has been observed using EU, intraluminal blood clots also change in morphology over time and can actually lyse and resolve (if there is no rebleeding) due to the natural presence of urokinase in the urine.

Other Upper-Tract Filling Defects

Thus far, there are no reported cases of fungus balls imaged with CTU. In comparison, intracollecting system mucus has been imaged. These filling defects may have attenuation values similar to those of tumors and blood clots. Like blood clots, they are completely intraluminal.

Renal Tubular Ectasia

As with EU, renal tubular ectasia produces easily visualized linear areas of high attenuation in the renal pyramids on CTU. These dilated collecting tubules (which may be associated with nephrocalcinosis that can be visualized on noncontrast CT images) are best seen on wide-window images. Renal tubular ectasia may be completely missed if only standard soft tissue windowing is employed (Fig. 8).

(A)

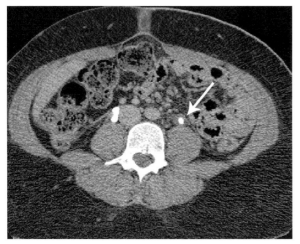

(B)

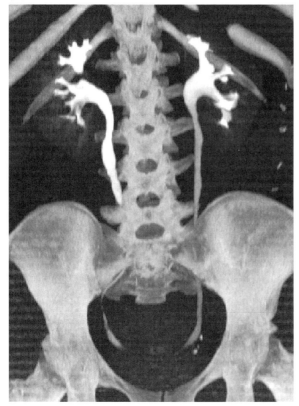

Figure 5 Infiltrative transitional cell carcinoma. (**A**) There is marked circumferential ureteral wall thickening (*arrow*) in the mid-left ureter produced by an extensive transitional cell carcinoma. Note that the ureteral lumen is not obstructed or narrowed and its contour appears smooth. (**B**) In fact, the ureter appears normal both in diameter and in contour on the coronal excretory-phase, volume-rendered reconstruction. It is likely that no abnormality would have been detected on EU as well. *Abbreviation*: EU, excretory urography.

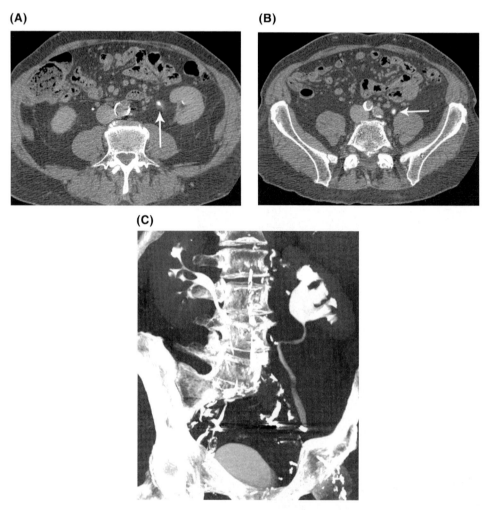

Figure 6 Transitional cell carcinoma. (**A**) Nearly circumferential left ureteral wall thickening is noted at the level of the lower pole of the left kidney (*arrow*). (**B**) The wall thickening continues all the way caudal to the pelvic inlet (*arrow*). (**C**) Left posterior oblique coronal volume-rendered reconstruction shows that the left ureter is normal in caliber throughout. The diffuse nature of this extensive transitional cell carcinoma cannot be identified. The extent of the cancer would have not been accurately identified on EU. In fact, the cancer would likely have been missed altogether. *Abbreviation*: EU, excretory urography.

Papillary Necrosis

Papillary necrosis can also be easily detected with CTU. As on EU, it can have a variety of appearances. There may be small linear or rounded collections of contrast material in the renal pyramids (Fig. 9), contrast material surrounding the necrotic papillae, or merely caliectasis. All of these changes represent permanent and irreversible damage to the renal papillae.

    Lang et al. have suggested that CT can be utilized to find changes related to renal medullary vascular insufficiency that can be reversed with appropriate therapy (termed by the authors as a type of medullary and papillary necrosis) (26). In this report, 39 of 57 patients were felt to have developed medullary and papillary necrosis as a result

(A)

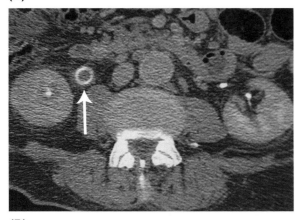

(B)

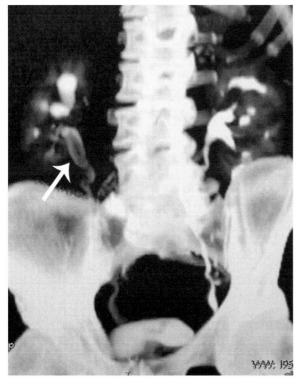

Figure 7 Blood clot. (**A**) A large blood clot fills and expands the right ureteral lumen on an excretory-phase axial image in this patient with a right renal transitional cell carcinoma. Note that the blood clot is surrounded by a rim of contrast material–containing urine (*arrow*). (**B**) Right posterior oblique coronal volume-rendered reconstruction also easily demonstrates the blood clot, which conforms to the shape of the dilated proximal right ureter (*arrow*).

of bacterial infection. The medullary and papillary necrosis produced small (usually less than 5 mm maximal diameter) areas of decreased enhancement in the renal medulla in these patients. Of the 39 patients, 28 then received antibiotic treatment, and follow-up CT demonstrated resolution of the abnormalities in more than half (16 patients).

(A)

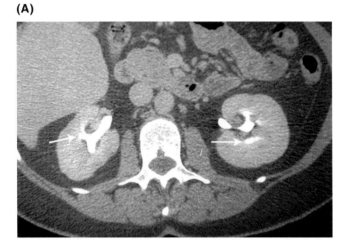

(B)

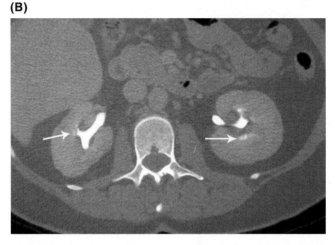

Figure 8 Renal tubular ectasia. (**A**) Areas of very high attenuation are noted within or adjacent to the calices in this excretory-phase axial image, when viewed using standard soft tissue windowing (*arrows*). (**B**) When the same image is viewed using wide windowing, discrete linear collections of contrast material can now be identified in the renal pyramids (*arrows*), establishing the diagnosis of renal tubular ectasia. This diagnosis would not have been made had the image been evaluated only at soft tissue windows.

Caliceal Diverticula

Caliceal diverticula appear as water attenuation lesions on precontrast and, often, on early enhanced images but usually fill in with contrast material on the excretory-phase images. Three-dimensional reconstructed or reformatted images can be obtained to assist the radiologist or urologist in preprocedural planning if intervention is anticipated (usually with percutaneous nephrostomy or retrograde catheterization followed by ablation) due to the presence of stones and/or infection within the diverticulum (Fig. 10). These additional images may allow the interventional radiologist or urologist to better visualize the relationship of the caliceal diverticulum to the adjacent renal collecting system.

(A)

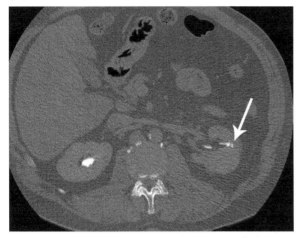

(B)

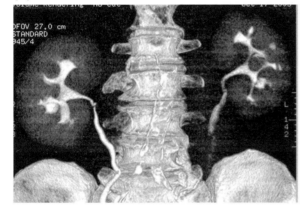

Figure 9 Papillary necrosis. (**A**) A tiny extracaliceal collection of contrast material is noted (*arrow*) in the lateral aspect of the mid–left kidney on this excretory-phase axial image. (**B**) This area of papillary necrosis is also easily identified on a coronal volume-rendered 3-D reconstructed image.

Pyeloureteritis Cystica

The tiny impressions from the submucosal ureteral cysts that occur in pyeloureteritis cystica are best (and often only) seen on CT urographic studies when wide-window images are reviewed. As with renal tubular ectasia, changes of pyeloureteritis cystica may be obscured on standard soft tissue windows. Given the characteristically large number of cysts, their mural location, and the similar size of these cysts to one another, a specific diagnosis of this entity can frequently be made (Fig. 11).

Bladder Cancer

As with upper-tract cancers, bladder cancers can produce large masslike areas of bladder wall thickening, in which case the diagnosis is strongly suggested (Fig. 12).

(A)

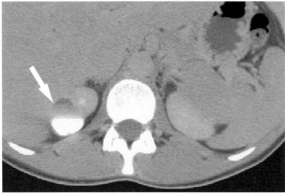

(B)

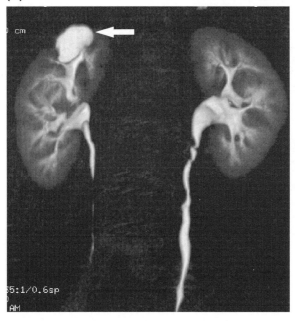

Figure 10 Caliceal diverticulum. (**A**) Excretory-phase axial image demonstrates a urine-contrast level in a mass in the upper pole of the right kidney (*arrow*). This mass had uniform water attenuation on the precontrast images. Based upon these findings, a diagnosis of caliceal diverticulum can be made. (**B**) This large caliceal diverticulum is also easily seen on the coronal volume-rendered 3-D reconstruction (*arrow*).

Bladder cancers may also produce small mural nodules. These can be detected by CTU even when quite small (again, often best and occasionally only seen with wide-window image viewing) (Fig. 13).

In some patients, bladder neoplasms merely produce linear areas of wall thickening that are detectable by CTU. Although bladder cancers usually produce focal bladder abnormalities and cystitis usually produces diffuse wall thickening, there is overlap. Each type of thickening can be caused by either benign or malignant disease. In the report by Caoili et al. (12), eight of ten patients with focal bladder wall

(A) **(B)**

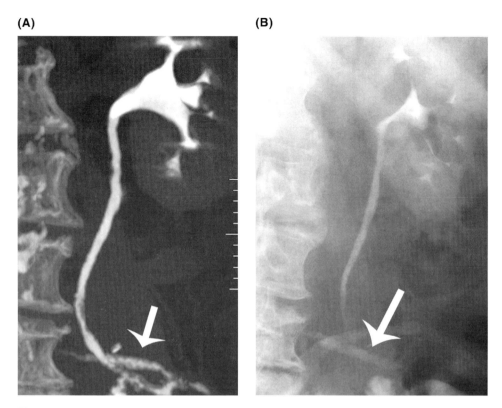

Figure 11 Ureteritis cystica. (**A**) Multiple tiny mural filling defects are easily seen in the distal right ureter (*arrow*), which is crossing over into the left lower quadrant on this coronal volume-rendered image in a patient with a left-sided ileal loop urinary diversion. Similar findings are present in the mid and distal portions of the left ureter. (**B**) These findings are less apparent (*arrow*) on this left posterior oblique abdominal radiograph taken during an excretory urogram, which preceded the CT by several months. *Abbreviation*: CT, computed tomography.

thickening had bladder cancer, while bladder cancer was the cause of wall thickening in only one of ten patients when such thickening was symmetric and diffuse.

Bladder Hematoma

Although bladder hematomas can have an appearance similar to that of bladder neoplasms (Fig. 14), they can occasionally be identified correctly when they have characteristic high attenuation (60–80 Hounsfield Units) on precontrast scans. Sometimes, the cause of hemorrhage (which is often a bladder neoplasm, cystitis, or upper-tract bleeding) can also be identified.

Cystitis

As mentioned above, cystitis frequently causes uniform diffuse bladder wall thickening (Fig. 15). In many instances, cystitis can be suggested on CTU (when such thickening is visualized); however, false negative studies are occasionally encountered (because urothelial inflammation need not produce detectable wall thickening).

(A)

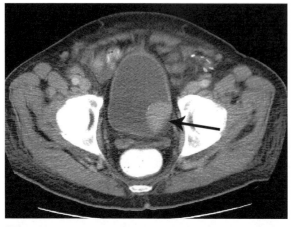

(B)

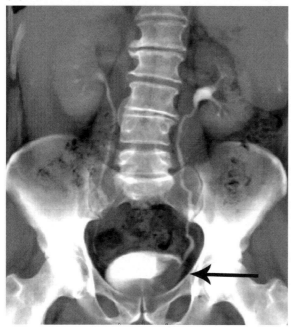

Figure 12 Large bladder cancer. (**A**) Nephrographic-phase axial image shows a large enhancing mass in the left posterolateral aspect of the urinary bladder (*arrow*). Mild diffuse bladder wall thickening is noted elsewhere. (**B**) The mass is also easily seen on the coronal average-intensity projection-reconstructed image (*arrow*).

PITFALLS IN IMAGE INTERPRETATION

Several problems can be encountered when performing and interpreting CT urograms. Knowledge of these potential pitfalls is important so that studies can be performed with the optimal technique and erroneous interpretations minimized.

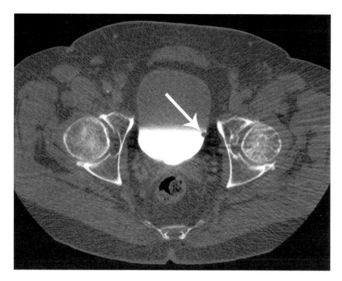

Figure 13   Tiny bladder cancer. A 3 mm diameter bladder cancer projects into the contrast-containing lumen of the urinary bladder (*arrow*), producing a small filling defect. This could not be seen on any of the 3-D reconstructed images.

Potential Technical Problems

A variety of criteria must be satisfied for CTU to be of excellent quality. Patients must be able to cooperate. Specifically, they must be able to hold still and to hold their breath briefly. As newer generation multidetector scanners have appeared, scan times have continued to diminish, such that with the newest 64-row scanners, thin-section images can be obtained through the entire abdomen and pelvis in only about 10 seconds. This has eliminated the need for prolonged breath-hold scanning.

Patients should also not be exceedingly obese and should not have a large amount of metallic material located adjacent to any portion of the urinary tract, because these situations can result in the production of extensive artifacts. A number of other high attenuation structures can also interfere with the interpretation of 3-D reconstructions. Overlying calcification (such as gallstones) can be mistaken for renal or ureteral calculi on 3-D images. If patients are mistakenly asked to ingest oral contrast material (which should not be administered to patients undergoing CTU), it may also interfere with the assessment of the urinary tract on subsequently created 3-D images.

Nonopacification

Nonopacification of some or all portions of the urinary tract can be seen in several instances. The most commonly encountered problem during CTU relates to incomplete opacification of one or more segments of nonobstructed peristalsing ureters on the excretory-phase images, a problem also seen with EU (11,13,27). Although, in many patients, the entirety of both ureters is opacified, it is not uncommon for at least a short segment of one or both ureters (usually the distal portion of a ureter) to be collapsed at the time of image acquisition due to ureteral peristalsis (Fig. 16). This has been encountered with all CTU techniques, although the

(A)

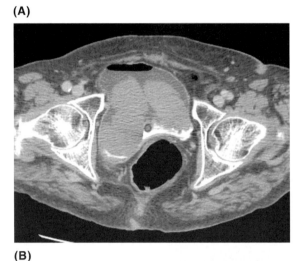

(B)

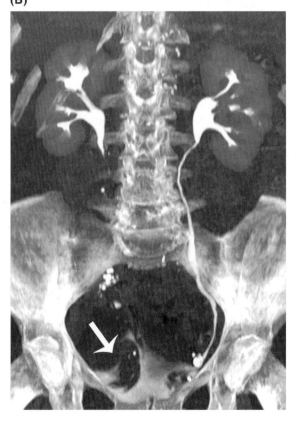

Figure 14 Bladder blot clot. (**A**) Large soft tissue attenuation masses fill the bladder lumen in this axial image of a patient whose bladder also contains a Foley catheter and air. The intraluminal blood clot is easily seen because it is well delineated by the surrounding low-attenuation unenhanced urine along its anterior, medial, and lateral borders and by a small amount of contrast-containing urine along its posterior border. (**B**) The blood clot is also identified on the excretory-phase, volume-rendered, reconstruction (*arrow*); however, it is much more difficult (if not impossible) to determine whether the abnormality is extrinsic, mural, or intraluminal on this image.

(A)

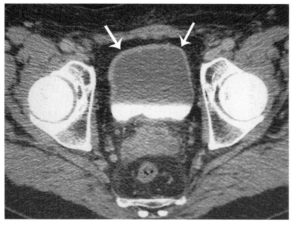

(B)

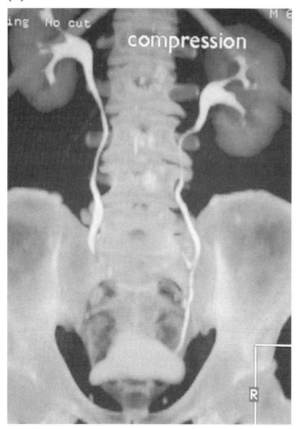

Figure 15 Cystitis. (**A**) Mild circumferential bladder wall thickening (*arrows*) is identified in this patient, who was later diagnosed as having cystitis. When bladder wall thickening is diffuse, it is most commonly due to inflammation rather than neoplasm. Conversely, focal bladder wall thickening is often due to cancer. (**B**) As with EU, the excretory-phase, coronal, volume-rendered 3-D image allows only for visualization of the bladder lumen, so that bladder wall thickening is not suspected. The bladder base is elevated due to prostatic enlargement. *Abbreviation*: EU, excretory urography.

(A)   (B)

(C)

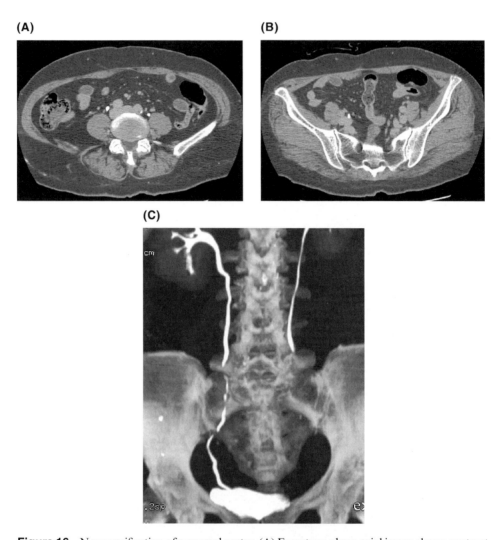

Figure 16 Nonopacification of a normal ureter. (**A**) Excretory-phase axial image shows contrast material in both ureters. No ureteral wall thickening or luminal filling defects are identified. (**B**) Several centimeters more caudally, the right ureter is again noted to be opacified; however, the left ureter no longer contains any contrast material, due to peristalsis. (**C**) Coronal, excretory-phase, volume rendered image reveals that a large portion of the left ureter was not opacified during image acquisition. The authors' solution to this problem is to read such a study as "negative," with the understanding that on rare occasions, tiny, nonobstructing ureteral lesions could be missed.

frequency with which nonopacification occurs does appear to vary. In a study by Inampudi et al. (27), portions of the proximal, middle, and distal ureters were not opacified on excretory-phase CTU images obtained at 300 seconds in 5%, 19%, and 33% of patients, respectively; however, by 450 seconds, the percentage of nonopacified ureters in each of these three locations was generally lower (at least more distally), at 8%, 16%, and 24% (27).

It is difficult or even impossible to assess nondilated, nonopacified ureteral segments for intrinsic pathology. Still, the likelihood of any pathology being present in such segments is low. Therefore, we recommend that these segments be considered normal, even though, in rare instances, abnormalities will be missed. Of more than

1000 CTUs performed at our institution thus far, we are aware of only one instance in which a ureteral polyp was not prospectively identified because it was located in a nonopacified segment of a normal caliber ureter.

Nonopacification can also be a problem in patients with urinary tract obstruction. When obstruction is present, excretion into the renal collecting systems and ureters may be delayed, and there may be minimal or no contrast material in the renal collecting systems, ureters, or bladder at the time of excretory-phase image acquisition. Fortunately, pelvicaliectasis and ureterectasis are usually present, and the water-attenuating urine can serve as a negative contrast agent within which urinary tract abnormalities (including the cause of obstruction) are often easily identified (Fig. 17).

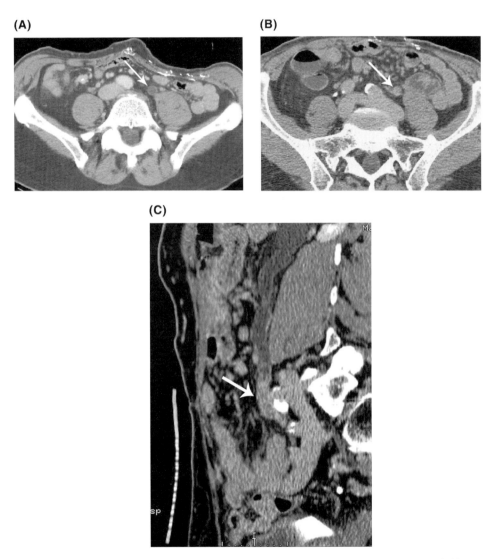

Figure 17 Nonopacification of an obstructed ureter. (**A**) Nephrographic-phase axial image reveals a markedly distended urine-containing left ureter (*arrow*). (**B**) The ureter becomes filled with soft tissue attenuation material more caudally (*arrow*), indicating the presence of a large mass, subsequently confirmed to be a transitional cell carcinoma. (**C**) The ureteral carcinoma is also well seen (*arrow*) on this sagittally reformatted image.

Finally, partial nonopacification can occur after there has been excretion into any dilated/distended portions of the renal collecting system, ureter, or bladder, due to the nondependent layering of unopacified urine above the heavier high-attenuation urine containing the excreted contrast material. This is most commonly encountered in the bladder if the patient has not been asked to move (by turning over or by walking around) after excreted contrast material begins to enter the bladder. In a motionless patient, the excreted contrast–containing urine layers dependently, or posteriorly, in the bladder of a supine patient, whereas unopacified urine layers nondependently, or anteriorly. Uroepithelial abnormalities, including neoplasms, are more likely to be missed if they are located in the nonopacified areas in the bladder or in dilated renal collecting systems or ureters. We have encountered one patient in whom a large transitional cell carcinoma in the anterior aspect of the bladder was not prospectively identified for this reason.

Normal Variants That Can Mimic Abnormalities

Two findings that are of no clinical significance can occasionally present interpretive problems because they can mimic important renal collecting system or ureteral pathology. When the ureter is tortuous, areas of redundancy/kinking may lead to confusion when only axial images are reviewed. Apparent filling defects may be suggested in places where the ureter loops back upon itself, leading to false positive diagnoses of ureteral lesions, including transitional cell carcinoma. False positive diagnoses due to ureteral kinking can usually be avoided by recognizing that the ureter has a tortuous course. Postprocessing can also be helpful. The anatomy is frequently most easily understood by reviewing 3-D coronal- or sagittal-plane reformatted images (Fig. 18).

Another occasionally confusing anatomic variant is due to prominent but normal renal papillae. Prominent papillae may bulge quite strikingly into the calices, producing pronounced concave impressions that can be mistaken for small uroepithelial neoplasms. Here, careful review of axial images usually facilitates differentiation of these normal papillae from pathology. Pronounced papillary impressions are usually multiple, similar to one another, and bilaterally symmetric (Fig. 19).

RADIATION

The biggest potential problem with CTU performed using excretory-phase axial image acquisition is the incremental radiation that patients receive with multiphase CT. The amount of radiation to which patients are exposed is directly related to the mA and kVp, as well as to the number of phases acquired. Radiation dose can be estimated in a variety of ways. The amount of radiation emitted from the scanner during image acquisition that is absorbed by the patient can be calculated [previously in rad and more recently in grays (with 100 rad equaling 1 Gy)]. It is more accurate, however, to use the equivalent or effective patient radiation dose, which takes into account the toxicity of any absorbed dose of radiation. The equivalent effective dose was previously measured in rem, but is now measured in Sieverts [with 1 rad of absorbed radiation equaling 1 rem, and 1 Gy of absorbed radiation equaling 1 Sv)].

Herts estimated that CT exposes a patient to an estimated surface radiation dose of 2 rem [or 20 millisievert (mSv)] for each series of acquired images (21). According to this data, the absorbed surface radiation dose from standard

(A)

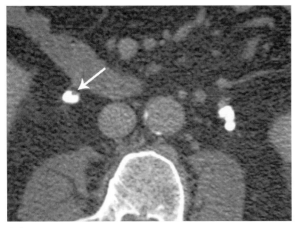

(B)

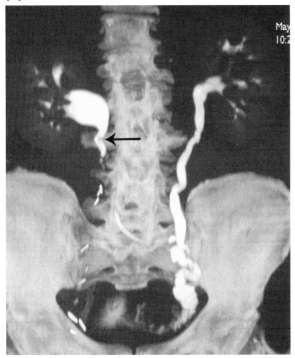

Figure 18 Ureteral kink. (**A**) Excretory-phase axial image demonstrates a tiny filling defect along the anteromedial aspect of the mid-right ureter (*arrow*). The left ureter also has an irregular contour. This is indicative of a small transitional cell carcinoma. (**B**) The coronal, excretory-phase, volume-rendered image reveals that the area of the filling defect (*arrow*), which was seen on this and other images, was merely the result of partial volume averaging in the region of a ureteral kink. Several kinks are also identified in the left ureter.

three-phase CTU protocols would be 6 rem (or 60 mSv). This is fairly similar to the radiation exposure these authors approximated for their 10 to 14 film excretory urograms of 5 to 7 rem (50–70 mSv). In another report, McTavish et al. estimated skin and total absorbed radiation doses resulting from their three-phase MDCTU

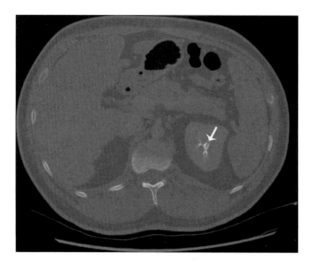

Figure 19 Prominent papillae. Excretory-phase axial image shows a prominent, concave impression on a left upper pole calyx due to a normal renal papilla (*arrow*). Note that a similar impression is also present on the more posteriorly located calyx. Nearly all of the other calices in both kidneys (seen on other axial images) showed the same appearance. The multiplicity of this finding and similarity of appearance across many calices indicate that this does not represent a true filling defect.

protocol to be 74.1 and 22.6 milligray (mGy) (13), as opposed to calculated doses of 81.2 and 11.4 mGy for EU. More recently, Nawful et al. estimated that the mean patient skin dose of their three-phase MDCTU protocol when calculated from phantom data and when measured with thermoluminescent dosimeter strips was 55 and 56 mGy, respectively (28). In this study, the mean effective dose for MDCTU was estimated to be 14.8 mSv, compared with 9.7 mSv for EU. Thus, the total effective dose resulting from three-phase MDCTU was estimated to exceed that of EU by a factor of at least 1.5 (28). Not surprisingly, Caoili et al. (12) calculated the total effective radiation dose for their four-phase protocol to be higher than that observed by McTavish et al. (13) and Nawful et al. (28). These authors estimated that an average-sized male studied using four-phase MDCTU (including two different excretory-phase image acquisitions, rather than one) received an effective total radiation dose of 25 to 35 mSv (12). This greatly exceeded the 5 to 10 mSv effective total dose for the 10 to 12 film EU that was routinely performed at the same institution.

Given the increased dose of three- or four-phase MDCTU (as assessed by the investigators referenced above), as previously mentioned, we and some others (17) have been reluctant to expand CTU indications to include all patients presenting with microscopic or gross hematuria. Instead, we have thus far reserved MDCTU for a selected group of patients in whom a high risk of urinary tract malignancy is believed to exist. This generally includes elderly patients with previously known urinary tract neoplasms, positive urine cytology, or persistent gross hematuria. Only rarely have we agreed to perform MDCTU in younger patients (usually those with intractable symptoms). As previously discussed, our restrictions can be contrasted with the policies of others (10,13,14), who, even now, advocate using MDCTU in any patient presenting with hematuria.

It must be remembered, however, that prior to the emergence of CTU, many patients with persistent, unexplained hematuria would have undergone imaging with

EU first, followed by CT if the EU did not identify any etiology. Thus, for many patients it is more appropriate to compare MDCTU radiation dose with that of EU and standard abdominal and pelvic CT combined. In such instances, the doses of these two imaging approaches are nearly comparable. Even when the data obtained in Caoili et al.'s series (utilizing four-phase MDCTU) are utilized (12), MDCTU exposed patients to only about 1.5 times as much radiation as EU and standard single-phase CT combined.

It must also be remembered that the probable carcinogenic risks of increased radiation from CTU must be balanced against the risks of not performing CTU and potentially missing malignant urinary tract pathology at an early stage when such pathology is more likely to be effectively treated.

There is one increasingly popular technical modification that allows for radiation dose from CTU to be reduced: the previously mentioned split-bolus technique. This technique, based upon a concept described by Chow and Sommer (10) but now utilized by many others (18,29), involves administering an initial intravenous bolus of contrast material. After a delay (allowing for excretion of the initial bolus into the renal collecting systems and ureters), additional contrast material is injected. Finally, a single series of thin-section contrast-enhanced scans is obtained after a further delay, allowing for the second bolus of contrast material to have enhanced the renal parenchyma homogeneously, while the first bolus has already been excreted into the renal collecting systems. In this fashion, nephrographic and excretory-phase images can be acquired simultaneously. As described in section "Recommended CTU Technique", MDCTU can, therefore, be performed using only two series of images (one precontrast and one postcontrast).

Several authors have reported good success with the split-bolus technique (10,18), although there are a few potential drawbacks: use of a smaller volume of contrast material to opacify and distend the renal collecting systems and proximal ureters (the initial bolus), as well as a smaller volume of contrast material to enhance the renal parenchyma and remainder of the abdominal visceral organs (the second bolus). Additionally, it has been observed that, on occasion, excreted contrast material in the renal collecting systems and renal pelvis can create artifacts, which may interfere with the evaluation of the renal parenchyma (30). Although, in our experience, such artifact is rarely severe enough to interfere with one's ability to detect a renal mass, it can limit the accuracy of any subsequent measurements of regions of interest that are obtained of a detected lesion.

Although using the split-bolus technique eliminates one of the usual minimum of three CT series acquisitions, the savings in radiation is not as great as might initially be expected. At our institution, for example, employing the split-bolus approach allows us to avoid the second, nephrographic-phase only, acquisition, which is the least radiation-intense component of our MDCTU examination. This is because our nephrographic phase scans are performed only as far caudal as the lower poles of the kidneys (rather than to the symphysis pubis). They also utilize relatively thick sections (5 mm rather than 0.625 or 1.25 mm), permitting scan acquisition to be obtained with lower mAs than that used for the excretory-phase series. For these reasons, we estimate that using the split-bolus technique reduces MDCTU radiation to the point that the examination would expose patients to only about 1.2 times (rather than 1.5 times) that to which the patient is exposed for a 10 to 15 film excretory urogram.

It is also possible to reduce some of the technical parameters while performing CTU image acquisition (irrespective of whether two or three total series are obtained). mA can be reduced considerably on the initial precontrast series without interfering substantially with the ability to detect stones. A number of studies have demonstrated that radiation reduction can be accomplished during renal stone CT, by lowering mA settings, without sacrificing diagnostic accuracy (31,32).

Finally, additional CT modifications (dose modulation) may allow for further dose reductions (by allowing for reductions in mA and kV depending upon which body part is being imaged and which organs are closest to the X-ray beam as it enters the patient). Work in this area is still very preliminary.

COST EFFECTIVENESS

MDCTU generates a much higher patient charge than does EU. When performing MDCTU, most institutions charge for a CT of the abdomen and pelvis both without and with intravenous contrast material and then may also add an extra charge for image postprocessing. The charge for this examination is several times that of EU. Of course, the charges for a particular study do not necessarily reflect reimbursement for that study or the actual cost of performing that study. Differences in these other two areas are much less pronounced. However, by performing MDCTU instead of EU, it is likely that many possible follow-up imaging tests would no longer be needed. One study found that when EU was performed first in patients with hematuria, additional imaging was frequently obtained (33). In comparison, when MDCTU was performed first, additional studies were eventually performed only 10% of the time. Obviously, if performing MDCTU first eliminates the need for other studies that would have been obtained after an initial EU, the overall health care cost differential for an individual may ultimately be considerably smaller than the price difference between MDCTU and EU.

OTHER VARIATIONS IN UTILIZED CTU TECHNIQUES

Although all MDCTU involves acquisition of thin-section axial excretory-phase images through the kidneys, ureters, and bladder, many variations in the technique are being used.

Timing Delay for Excretory-Phase Imaging

As has been previously mentioned, there is wide variation in the time at which the excretory-phase images are obtained [generally from 5 minutes (10,12) to 12–15 minutes (34–36)]. As already described, one group has found that when the shortest delays are used, the number of nonopacified distal ureteral segments is greatest (27).

Compression, Saline Hydration, and Furosemide

There is also variation in use of a variety of other maneuvers designed to improve renal collecting system and ureteral distention and opacification. Because abdominal compression has long been successfully used during EU, a number of researchers have advocated its use during CTU (10,12,37–39). During MDCTU, compression is often applied at the time of contrast material injection. Compression excretory-phase images are then obtained through the kidneys, followed by compression release and acquisition of a second series of excretory-phase images performed, at the least, through the middle and distal portions of the ureters.

Although a few studies have suggested that the use of compression is beneficial (27,37,39), only one actually directly compared compression CT images with noncompression CT images (27). The others instead compared compression-CT opacification with opacification obtained during EU performed on the same patients (37,39). In the study that utilized only CT images (27), compression produced only a slight but significant improvement in distention of the renal calices, infundibula, pelves, and proximal ureters when compared with postcompression-release images through these structures; however, there was no significant improvement between compression images and images obtained in a group of patients in whom no compression was ever applied. Further, this study was not designed to determine whether the slight advantage of abdominal compression would improve detection of upper-tract pathology. In fact, a more recent series from the same group has suggested that sensitivity in detecting urinary tract abnormalities is not improved on excretory-phase CT images performed with abdominal compression (40).

As an alternative to using compression for increasing renal collecting system and ureteral distention, several investigators have chosen to hydrate patients orally or with a 100 mL (29) or 250 mL (13,16,27,28) intravenous bolus of normal (0.9%) saline administered immediately prior to or following contrast material injection. Thus far, only use of the larger intravenous volumes appears to be beneficial to any extent. One study found distal ureteral opacification to be significantly improved when patients received precontrast material injection hydration with 250 mL of saline (compared to a control group) (13). However, there were no opacification advantages in other portions of the urinary tract. Another study found that patients hydrated with 250 mL of saline (administered between contrast material injection and excretory-phase scan acquisition) demonstrated small but significant improvements in upper urinary tract opacification, compared with patients who did not receive saline (27). In comparison, another study did not find hydration with 100 mL of saline to be of any benefit (29).

Finally, it has been suggested that using a small dose of an intravenous diuretic improves urinary tract visualization to the greatest extent. Two groups administered 10 mg of intravenous furosemide three to five minutes before contrast material administration for CTU (11,41). One group found that using furosemide during CTU resulted in near-complete or complete opacification of all 32 imaged renal collecting systems and of 30 imaged ureters, as well as in a more accurate depiction of the pelvicaliceal system (in comparison with CTUs performed with saline hydration) (11). Another group noted that lower and distal ureteral opacification was significantly better in 26 patients who received intravenous furosemide and saline hydration compared with lower and distal ureteral opacification in 35 patients who received saline hydration alone (41). Interestingly, in this study, there was no significant difference in opacification between the patients who received furosemide and saline hydration and another group of 26 patients who received furosemide alone (without saline hydration).

The use of furosemide has a few potential drawbacks. At most institutions, a physician is responsible for administration of this agent (and must specifically order that this agent be administered to every patient referred for CTU, as well as be directly available whenever a CTU examination is being performed with furosemide). Also, patients become extremely uncomfortable soon after furosemide administration (due to rapid bladder distention) and they may need to get off the scanner quickly to go to the bathroom before all image acquisition has been completed.

SUMMARY

CTU is rapidly gaining widespread acceptance as the imaging study of choice for complete evaluation of the urinary tract. While it has already replaced EU for renal stone and renal mass imaging, many investigators also now perform CTU instead of EU for evaluation of the renal collecting systems, ureters, and bladder. Reliance entirely upon axial image acquisitions, most efficiently performed with CTU, appears to result in the highest sensitivity in the detection of abnormalities (rather than combining axial image acquisition with plain radiography or standard or enhanced scan projection radiography). Even subtle renal collecting system abnormalities and ureteral abnormalities can be detected with CTU, with a sensitivity that appears to equal or perhaps even exceed that of retrograde pyelography and EU. As can be seen, many of these abnormalities have characteristic CTU appearances. Although occasional false diagnoses do occur, awareness of potential pitfalls, such as ureteral kinks and prominent renal papillae, can help minimize interpretive errors. The only major concern about performing CTU exclusively rather than EU is the increased radiation dose of CTU; however, ongoing modifications in CTU technique and in CT hardware and software may soon eliminate this problem. Although slightly different CTU protocols are being utilized at different institutions, all CTU imaging relies upon the same principle: the acquisition of very thin–section excretory-phase axial images. Further, with the passage of time, differences in opinion about technique have decreased considerably. In summary, it can now be stated with a relatively high degree of certainty that rapidly growing experience with an increasingly standardized CTU approach has made it increasingly clear that CTU will very likely make the EU obsolete in the very near future.

REFERENCES

1. Warshauer DM, McCarthy SM, Street L, et al. Detection of renal masses: sensitivities and specificities of excretory urography/linear tomography, US, and CT. Radiology 1988; 169:363–365.
2. Jamis-Dow CA, Choyke PL, Jennings SB, et al. Small (< 3-cm) renal masses: detection with CT versus US and pathologic correlation. Radiology 1996; 198:785–788.
3. Smith RC, Verga M, McCarthy S, Rosenfield AT. Diagnosis of acute flank pain: value of unenhanced CT. Am J Roentgenol 1996; 166:97–101.
4. Levine JA, Neitlich J, Verga M, Dalrymple N, Smith RC. Ureteral calculi in patients with flank pain: correlation of plain radiography with unenhanced CT. Radiology 1997; 204:27–31.
5. Perlman ES, Rosenfield AT, Wexler JS, Glickman MG. CT urography in the evaluation of urinary tract disease. J Comput Assist Tomogr 1996; 20:620–626.
6. McCollough CH, Bruesewitz MR, Vrtiska TJ, et al. Image quality and dose comparison among screen-film, computed and CT scanned projection radiography: applications to CT urography. Radiology 2001; 221:395–403.
7. Kawashima A, LeRoy AJ, King BF, et al. Comparison of CT scanned projection radiographs (SPR) utilizing enhanced algorithms with original CT scan SPR and conventional screen-film radiographs (FSR) in detecting urolithiasis and with respect to image quality. Radiology 2002; 225(P):236.
8. McCarthy CL, Cowan NC. Multidetector CT urography (MD-CTU) for urothelial imaging. Radiology 2002; 225(P):237.

9. Coll DM, Sosa RE, Smith RC. CT urography for evaluation of the urothelial system: are plain films still necessary? Radiology 2002; 225(P):237.

10. Chow LC, Sommer FG. Multidetector CT urography with abdominal compression and three-dimensional reconstruction. Am J Roentgenol 2001; 177:849–855.

11. Nolte-Ernsting CC, Wildberger JE, Borchers H, Schmitz-Rode T, Gunther RW. Multi-slice CT urography after diuretic injection: initial results. Rofo Fortschr Geb Rontgenstr Neuen Bildgeb Verfahr 2001; 173:176–180.

12. Caoili EM, Cohan RH, Korobkin M, et al. Urinary tract abnormalities: initial experience with multi-detector row CT urography. Radiology 2002; 222:353–360.

13. McTavish JD, Jinzaki M, Zou KH, Nawfel RD, Silverman SG. Multi-detector row CT urography: comparison of strategies for depicting the normal urinary collecting system. Radiology 2002; 225:783–790.

14. Lang EK, Macchia RJ, Thomas R, et al. Computerized tomography tailored for the assessment of microscopic hematuria. J Urol 2002; 167:547–554.

15. Mueller-Lisse UG, Mueller-Lisse UL, Hinterberger J, Schneede P, Reiser MF. Tri-phasic MDCT in the diagnosis of urothelial cancer. Eur Radiol 2003; 13(S1):146–147.

16. Feng FY, Caoili EM, Cohan RH, et al. Coronal vs standard axial image review CT urography. Presented at the 30th Annual Meeting of the Society of Uroradiology, San Antonio, Texas, February 27, 2005.

17. Inampudi P, Caoili EM, Cohan RH, Ellis JH. Urinary tract visibility and abnormality detection on multidetector CT urography: comparison of 3D reformats and enhanced scouts. Presented at the 104th Annual Meeting of the American Roentgen Ray Society, Miami Beach, Florida, May 2–7, 2004.

18. Anderson KE, Cowan NC. Multidetector CT urography (MDCTU) for the investigation of hematuria. Presented at the 89th Scientific Assembly of the Radiological Society of North America, Chicago, Illinois, December 3, 2003.

19. Caoili EM, Inampudi P, Cohan RH, et al. MDCTU of upper tract uroepithelial malignancy. Am J Roentgenol 2005; 184:1873–1881.

20. Sudakoff GS, Guralnick M, Langenstroer P, et al. CT urography of urinary diversions with enhanced CT digital radiography: preliminary experience. Am J Roentgenol 2005; 184:131–138.

21. Herts BR. The current status of CT urography (2002). Critical Rev Comput Tomogr 2002; 43:219–241.

22. Caoili EM, Cohan RH, Inampudi P, et al. MDCT urography of upper tract urothelial neoplasma. Am J Roentgenol 2005; 184:1873–1881.

23. Joffe SA, Servaes S, Okon S, Horowitz M. Multi-detector row CT urography in the evaluation of hematuria. Radiographics 2003; 23:1441–1456.

24. Kim JK, Cho KS. Pictorial review: CT urography and virtual endoscopy: promising imaging modalities for urinary tract evaluation. Br J Radiol 2003; 76:199–209.

25. O'Malley ME, Hahn PF, Yoder IC, et al. Comparison of excretory phase, helical computed tomography with intravenous urography in patients with painless hematuria. Clin Radiol 2003; 58:294–300.

26. Lang EK, Macchia RJ, Thomas R, et al. Detection of medullary and papillary necrosis at an early stage by multiphasic helical computerized tomography. J Urol 2003; 170:94–98.

27. Caoili EM, Inampudi P, Cohan RH, Ellis JH. Optimizing multi-detector CT urography: effect of compression saline administration, and prolonging acquisition delay. Radiology 2005; 236:116–123.

28. Nawful RD, Judy PF, Schleipman AR, Silverman SG. Patient radiation dose at CT urography and conventional urography. Radiology 2004; 232:126–132.

29. Maher MM, Jhaveri KS, Lucey BC, et al. Does the administration of saline flush during CT urography (CTU) improve ureteric distention and opacification? A prospective study. Radiology 2001; 221(P):500.

30. Sussman SK, Illescas FF, Opalacz JP, Yirga P, Foley LC. Renal streak artifact during contrast enhanced CT: comparison of high versus low osmolality contrast media. Abdom Imaging 1993; 18:180–185.

31. Meagher T, Sukumar VP, Collingwood J, et al. Low dose computed tomography in suspected acute renal colic. Clin Radiol 2001; 56:873–876.

32. Tublin ME, Murphy ME, Deling DM, Tessler FN, Kliewer MA. Conspicuity of renal calculi at unenhanced CT: effects of calculus composition and size and CT technique. Radiology 2002; 225:91–96.

33. Gupta KB, Silverman SG, McTavish JD, O'Leary M, Bernazzani J. The impact on diagnostic yield, practice patterns, and cost of using CT urography rather than intravenous urography in the evaluation of hematuria. Radiology 2001; 221(P):501.

34. Noroozian M, Cohan RH, Caoili EM. Multislice CT urography: state of the art. Br J Radiol 2004; 77:S74–S86.

35. Frauenfelder T, Boehm T, Michael M, Marincek S, Wildermuth S. The urinary collecting system: different *post-process*ing methods (MIP, SSD, VR) using multidetector-CT-datasets versus conventional intravenous urography. Eur Radiol 2003; 13(S1):147.

36. Girish G, Agarwal SK, Salim F, Brown PWG, Morcos SK. Single-phase multislice CT urography: initial experience. Eur Radiol 2003; 13(S1):147.

37. McNicholas MMJ, Raptopoulos VD, Schwartz RK, et al. Excretory phase CT urography for opacification of the urinary collecting system. Am J Roentgenol 1998; 170:1261–1267.

38. Caoili EM, Cohan RH, Korobkin M, et al. Effectiveness of abdominal compression during helical renal CT. Acad Radiol 2001; 8:1100–1106.

39. Heneghan JP, Kim DH, Leder RA, DeLong D, Nelson RC. Compression CT urography: a comparison with IVU in the opacification of the collecting system and ureters. J Comput Assist Tomogr 2001; 25:343–347.

40. Hilmes MA, Caoili EM, Cohan RH, et al. Evaluation of the ability of individual phases of multi-detector CT urography and different windowing to detect urinary tract pathology. Presented at the 29th Annual Scientific Meeting of the Society of Uroradiology, March 6, 2004.

41. Gan Y, Asbar S, Mortele K, et al. Multi-detector row CT urography: comparison of furosemide and saline as adjuncts to contrast media for depicting the normal urinary collecting system. Presented at the 30th Annual Meeting of the Society of Uroradiology, San Antonio, Texas, February 27, 2005.

6

Diagnostic Imaging for Nephron-Sparing Surgery

Brian R. Herts
Section of Abdominal Imaging, Division of Diagnostic Radiology and The Glickman Urological Institute, The Cleveland Clinic Foundation, Cleveland, Ohio, U.S.A.

Erick M. Remer and Joseph C. Veniero
Section of Abdominal Imaging, Division of Diagnostic Radiology, The Cleveland Clinic Foundation, Cleveland, Ohio, U.S.A.

INTRODUCTION

The traditional role of diagnostic imaging in patients with a renal mass is to detect and characterize the mass and to stage neoplastic disease. Both computed tomography (CT) and magnetic resonance imaging (MRI) detect and characterize renal masses with a high degree of accuracy, but CT is considered the gold standard for detection, diagnosis, and staging of renal cell carcinoma (1,2). CT is highly sensitive for the detection of solid renal masses (3–5) and is also used to characterize cystic renal lesions. Criteria such as those developed and modified by Bosniak have proved useful in stratifying the potential for malignancy in complex cystic renal masses (6–8). This risk stratification provides a framework for clinical management used by many urologists. MRI is also sensitive and specific for characterizing solid and cystic renal lesions. It has a higher soft tissue contrast resolution and is more sensitive to intravenous contrast enhancement than CT, but its spatial resolution and availability are less than that of CT, and thus MRI is often reserved for problem solving or for those patients who cannot receive iodinated contrast material for CT, e.g., patients with renal insufficiency or who have a history of prior severe adverse reaction.

The traditional surgical treatment for most patients with a renal neoplasm is total or radical nephrectomy, but nephron-sparing surgery (NSS) is an important treatment option for many patients (9–15). The traditional indications for NSS are renal neoplasms in those patients with a prior nephrectomy, bilateral renal tumors, underlying renal parenchymal disease, or other risk factors for renal insufficiency. The successful use of NSS in treating renal neoplasms in patients with the traditional indications has led to the expansion of its use to include some patients with a low-stage renal tumor and a normal contralateral kidney without any risk factor for renal

101

insufficiency. This includes many patients with incidentally detected renal neo-plasms, a presentation that has become much more common with the widespread use of cross-sectional imaging (16). NSS is most often performed using an open surgical partial nephrectomy, but laparoscopic partial nephrectomy (17–19) and ablative therapies (20–27) are now being used successfully as well.

NSS requires the surgeon to have an accurate understanding of the renal parench-ymal and vascular anatomy and the location of the tumor to preserve normal renal tissue and retain renal function (13,15). Therefore, urologists require more detailed information from diagnostic imaging, and the role of imaging has been expanded accordingly to provide additional information for both diagnosis and surgical planning. Imaging must now provide anatomic information that was not considered important previously for CT scan interpretation, including descriptions of the arterial anatomy, venous anatomy, and tumor location, and an assessment regarding the degree to which the tumor has extended into the parenchyma or central renal sinus. Imaging must also provide information on the proximity of the tumor to the vascular structures and the pelvocalyceal system, and identify the number and course of the ureters (9–12). Accu-rate surgical planning information helps to minimize perioperative and postoperative complications, such as urinary leak or renal infarct, and to maximize preserved renal parenchyma and renal function. Multidetector CT scanners and two-dimensional (2-D) and three-dimensional (3-D) visualization software provide this anatomic infor-mation rapidly and reliably, but CT and MRI protocols must be designed appropriately.

The role of imaging has also expanded into the operating room. Imaging is frequently used during NSS: intraoperative ultrasound is used to localize a tumor, identify and characterize any additional lesions, and demarcate surgical margins. This can be done either during open surgery with a high-frequency transducer placed directly on the surface of the kidney or laparoscopically by using specially designed laparoscopic ultrasound transducers. When ablative techniques are used, either laparoscopically or percutaneously, ultrasound or CT can be used to monitor the ablation. After surgery, MRI or CT is used to assess the success of an ablation and to follow the patient for complications, local recurrence, and metastatic disease.

This chapter discusses the use of CT and MRI as surgical planning tools spe-cifically for NSS, although many of these principles have been applied in several other areas of urologic surgery. We will discuss dedicated CT and MRI protocols and their importance for surgical planning, the use of 3-D renderings, and intrao-perative as well as percutaneous imaging guidance during both partial nephrectomy and ablative procedures.

CT

Preliminary Considerations

CT and MRI are both excellent modalities for preoperative imaging of renal tumors, and either can be used for surgical planning (1,2,28–32). CT is the study used most frequently because it is readily available, has superior spatial resolution, and unlike MRI, is able to detect calcifications. Success with 3-D real-time rendering using CT datasets has also contributed to preferential use of CT. CT examinations are per-formed before and after administering intravenous contrast agents but without oral contrast material because any positive enteric contrast media interferes with 3-D ren-derings. In our institution, patients with normal or mildly elevated serum creatinine levels (below 2.0 mg/dL) are given a full dose of a low-osmolar nonionic contrast agent. Patients with elevated serum creatinine levels between 2.0 and 2.5 mg/dL are hydrated intravenously with normal saline solution before the examination and are also instructed to drink fluids after the scan; however, at the present time, the use of iso-osmolar contrast agents is also recommended in these patients because of the reported reduction in nephrotoxicity during coronary angiography (33). Patients with creatinine levels of 2.5 mg/dL or higher are referred for MRI, which avoids the increased risk for nephrotoxicity in already compromised kidneys. Also, when renal function is poor, the optimal enhancement of normal parenchyma that is needed to best detect small tumors does not occur.

CT Protocol for Planning NSS

Three-phase CT protocols are the state of the art for imaging the kidneys and provide all the information necessary to plan for NSS (Fig. 1) (9–11). Scans should be performed on a multidetector helical scanner, which allows for the efficient use of intravenous contrast and facilitates the creation of thin-slice datasets for smooth 2-D and 3-D reformations. Technical parameters, such as kVp and mAs, should be kept consistent across the scan phases.

The first scan phase is a noncontrast CT of the abdomen, including the adrenal glands and both kidneys. The noncontrast CT is essential not only because it helps to plan for the contrast-enhanced portion of the study but also because it provides baseline attenuation values for any detected renal masses and also because it allows for the identification of any calcifications in the urinary tract or in renal lesions.

The second scan phase is a vascular phase CT scan (34). The timing for this phase can be determined either by scanning after a test bolus of 20 mL of contrast material has been injected, usually at a rate of 3 or 4 mL/sec or by using an automated bolus-tracking technique set to trigger from a threshold value, set from enhancement in the upper abdominal aorta. Additional time is needed to assure enhancement of the renal veins. An additional five seconds is usually sufficient to allow renal venous enhancement. In otherwise healthy patients, most vascular-phase CT scan delays are between 25 and 35 seconds after the initiation of the contrast material injection.

The third scan phase is obtained during the parenchymal phase of enhancement, obtained after a 120- to 150-second delay from the initiation of the bolus contrast injection (the longer delay times are used for older patients or patients with cardiac dysfunction). The parenchymal phase images are the most sensitive and specific for lesion detection and characterization, although the vascular phase images can also be useful when characterizing masses (1,3–5,28,29,34).

For each scan phase, thin sections, typically obtained at 3 mm, are reconstructed without image overlap for diagnostic interpretation and filming. Softcopy reading is recommended using either a picture archiving and communication system (PACS) workstation or the scanner console. In addition to the 3 mm slices for diagnostic interpretation, a separate reconstruction set of 1 mm thick slices with 20% overlap (reconstruction interval of 0.8 mm) is also created and used for multiplanar reformations and 3-D real-time volume-rendering reconstructions. Multiplanar reformatted (MPR) images are created through the abnormal kidney for interpretation and sent to the referring urologist. True sagittal and coronal oblique images oriented parallel to the long axis of the kidney are helpful for localization of the tumor within the kidney. Thin-section (3–5 mm thickness) coronal oblique thin-slab maximum intensity projection (MIP) images through the aorta and kidneys are helpful for delineating the renal vasculature. These thin-slab MIP images improve

(A)

(B)

(C)

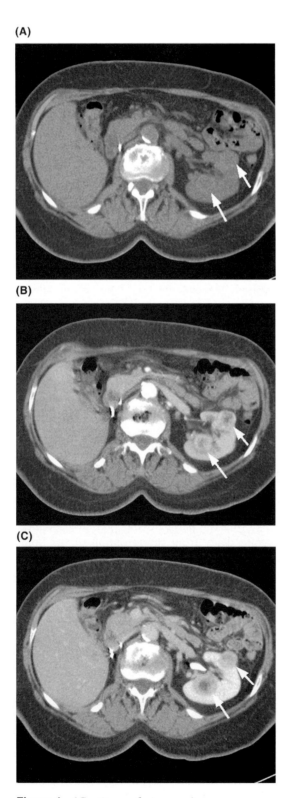

Figure 1 *(Caption on facing page)*

visualization of the renal vasculature and facilitate measurements of the distance to the first renal arterial branches and distances between renal arterial ostia in those patients with multiple renal arteries. MPR and MIP reformations are performed at the scanner console by the technologists using the thin-section (1 mm) dataset and then sent for image review along with the diagnostic axial images (Figs. 2 and 3).

MRI

General Considerations

As with CT evaluations, the preoperative evaluation for NSS with MRI also includes both pre- and post-contrast examinations (35). As with most body MRI examinations, the precontrast T1- and T2-weighted images are obtained to evaluate anatomy, to identify abnormalities, and to begin to characterize any identified renal or adrenal lesions (Fig. 4). Following intravenous gadolinium administration, postcontrast gradient-echo T1-weighted sequences are performed in multiple phases to define the enhancement characteristics of any detected lesions and to define the adjacent anatomy for surgical planning. Specifically the arterial, venous, and collecting system anatomy is again assessed.

The importance of patient preparation and general technique in body MRI cannot be understated. Anterior and posterior phased array surface coils should be used to increase the signal and must be positioned over the kidneys. Patient motion during image acquisition, including respiratory motion, leads to image artifacts, including blurring and ghosting in the phase-encoding direction. Eliminating this motion is an important factor in improving imaging quality in body MRI. In addition to eliminating image artifacts from respiratory motion, reproducible suspension of respiration is needed to take advantage of a variety of postprocessing techniques.

In general, motion compensation techniques can be used to eliminate these artifacts on precontrast scans. However, these techniques increase the acquisition time and could preclude the possibility of obtaining postcontrast scans confined to one specific phase of contrast enhancement, particularly the arterial phase. The most sensitive technique used to determine the presence of lesion enhancement is image subtraction. It requires reproducible breath-holding, because to perform accurate image subtraction, the datasets to be manipulated must be nearly perfectly registered in 3-D space. This is especially true for evaluating small lesions. Comparing imaging characteristics of lesions on different sequences requires their identification on similar or, even better, identical slices. Mathematically combining datasets requires near perfect anatomic registration.

In order to obtain motion-free imaging with a specific temporal resolution, the MRI sequences are kept as short as possible and patients are asked to breath-hold at end-expiration during image acquisition. Breath-holding is done during end-expiration because it is more reproducible. Patients tend to exhale to their functional residual capacity and stop, whereas there is significantly more variation in the

Figure 1 (*Figure on facing page*) Three-phase helical CT of the kidneys. (**A**) Noncontrast, (**B**) vascular phase, and (**C**) parenchymal phase axial images show two renal masses (*arrows*) in a 64-year-old male with a solitary left kidney. Note that the intrarenal mass is barely visible in (**A**), and best seen in (**C**). The parenchymal phase (**C**) is the most sensitive for lesion detection. *Abbreviation*: CT, computed tomography.

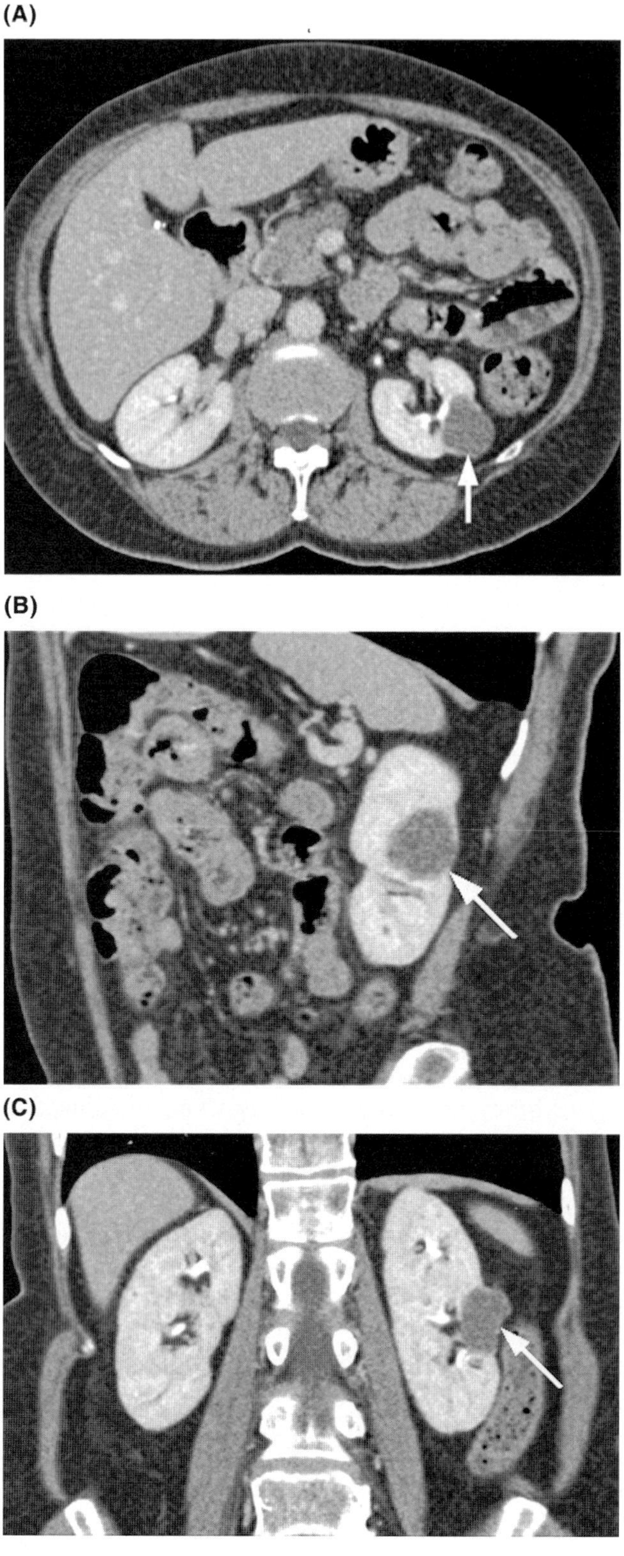

(A)

(B)

(C)

Figure 2 (*Caption on facing page*)

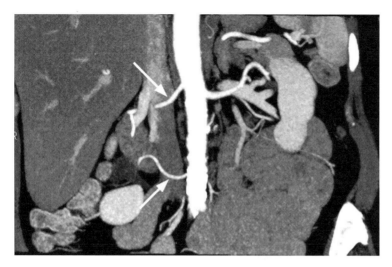

Figure 3 Thin-slab MIP reconstruction. This image, for surgical planning, is created from thin-section data obtained in the vascular phase. Coronal oblique MIP projection through the aorta shows two right renal arteries (*arrows*). *Abbreviation*: MIP, maximum intensity projection.

end-inspiratory lung volume when patients are asked to suspend respiration at end-inspiration. This can be a challenge for some patients, but in those who have difficulty suspending respiration at end-expiration, hyperventilation and supplemental oxygen can allow longer breath-holds, yielding much higher quality examinations. Using low-dose anxiolytic medication can allow for diagnostic studies to be obtained in anxious, nervous, or claustrophobic patients who would otherwise be unable to follow instructions.

When studies for surgical planning are performed, increasing the standard contrast material dose helps obtain better venous opacification. It may also be desirable to distend the calyces in order to better assess invasion in patients whose lesions approach the renal sinus. This can be accomplished with the administration of a small dose of intravenous furosemide. This is discussed in more detail in the following section.

MRI Protocol for Planning NSS

Localizer images are obtained to plan the diagnostic sequences. Typically, fast T1-weighted images are acquired in three planes. Then, T1-weighted in-phase and out-of-phase images are obtained using a 2-D fast gradient echo sequence without fat saturation. With a slice thickness of 5 to 6 mm, only about 20 slices are needed to cover the kidneys in a single breath-hold. On a 1.5 Tesla system, the out-of-phase time to echo (TE) is approximately 2 msec and the in-phase TE is approximately

Figure 2 (*Figure on facing page*) MPR reconstructions created for surgical planning. These images are created from thin-section data obtained in the parenchymal phase. (**A**) Standard axial image shows a hypodense left renal mass (*arrow*) in the lateral interpolar kidney. (**B**) Sagittal and (**C**) oblique coronal MPR images help to delineate the position of the tumor (*arrow*) with respect to the remaining normal renal parenchyma and are easy to create at the CT scanner console. *Abbreviations*: CT, computed tomography; MPR, multiplanar reformatted.

(A)

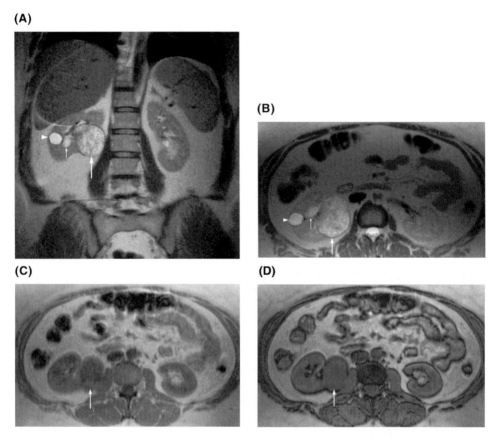

Figure 4 Precontrast T1- and T2-weighted MRI images. (**A**) Coronal and (**B**) axial precontrast T2-weighted images (half-Fourier single-shot turbo spin echo) show the heterogeneous mixed intensity of this exophytic renal cell carcinoma (*arrow*), a homogeneously hyperintense simple cortical cyst (*arrowhead*), and a distended collecting system in the right kidney (*small arrow*). (**C**) Axial in-phase and (**D**) out-of-phase precontrast T1-weighted images show the generally low precontrast T1-weighted signal of a renal cell carcinoma (*arrow*). *Abbreviation*: MRI, magnetic resonance imaging.

4 msec. If available, the use of a double echo technique to acquire both in-phase and out-of-phase images during a single breath-hold is advantageous for two reasons. First, it ensures precise registration of the in-phase and out-of-phase images, and second, it reduces the number of breath-holds the patient must perform. On this sequence, voxels containing both fat and water will have a degree of signal cancellation leading to signal intensity loss or signal dropout on the out-of-phase images when compared to the in-phase images. Thus, such tissue as lipid-rich adrenal adenomas and liver with fatty infiltration with intracellular or microscopic fat can be identified due to its signal dropout on the out-of-phase images (Fig. 5). A T1-weighted sequence with frequency-specific fat saturation is also employed to identify regions of bulk or macroscopic fat, as seen in angiomyolipoma. This is one of the same sequences used after contrast administration. Two goals are achieved by acquiring pre- and postcontrast data using the same sequence: first, the precontrast images identify bulk and macroscopic fat; and, second, postprocessing can be performed using the precontrast sequence as a mask for image subtraction.

(A)

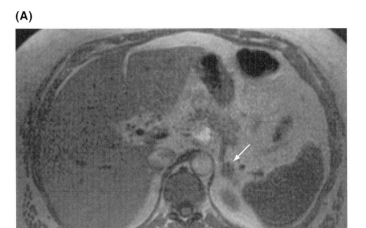

(B)

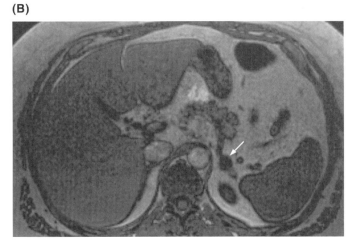

Figure 5 Axial (**A**) in-phase and (**B**) out-of-phase precontrast T1-weighted images of an incidental adrenal mass (*arrow*) in a patient with a renal tumor. There is signal drop-out on the out-of-phase image, indicating fat, and in this case, a lipid-rich adrenal adenoma.

Next, T2-weighted images are obtained to detect and evaluate areas of fluid, including cystic lesions and the renal collecting systems. Single-shot techniques are employed to obtain T2-weighted images in a single breath-hold and to image the entire region of interest with adequate resolution. Twenty slices can be obtained in approximately 20 seconds by utilizing a half-Fourier single-shot technique (HASTE). Thus, the kidneys and adrenal glands can be scanned using a slice thickness of 4 to 5 mm. If desired, axial imaging using the same technique can be performed with slice thickness and positioning corresponding to the in-phase and out-of-phase images.

A standard MRI contrast dose of 0.1 mmol/kg of gadolinium is adequate for most diagnostic studies and most MRI angiograms. However, as previously stated, it is helpful to increase the contrast dose when studies are performed for NSS surgical planning. A dose of 0.15 mmol/kg (1.5 times the standard dose, or, typically, 30 mL) is used to obtain better venous opacification for surgical planning studies. Contrast administration is ideally performed utilizing a power injector at a rate of 2 mL/sec followed by a saline flush at the same rate.

Because the intravenous contrast volume is small in MRI, there is typically only a 10-second window of ideal arterial opacification. Therefore, proper timing for scans acquired during the arterial phase of imaging is critical. More specifically, filling the data in the more "contrast-sensitive" center of k-space during optimal arterial opacification is necessary for best-quality imaging. A timing examination has been proven to be useful for obtaining images consistently during the arterial phase of contrast enhancement. The timing examination is performed by injecting a small amount of contrast (typically 1 mL) followed by a 20 mL saline flush and then obtaining images at fixed intervals (typically every 1–2 seconds) following the start of the injection. Usually, multiple images are obtained at the level of the kidneys for a period of 60 seconds, thereby defining the time course of contrast administration. Evaluation of these images allows for the easy determination of the delay needed to achieve peak arterial enhancement. In addition, evaluation of the enhancement of the renal parenchyma during this sequence provides a preliminary assessment of renal parenchymal perfusion.

Postcontrast imaging is obtained in multiple phases using T1-weighted gradient echo 3-D interpolated, fat saturated sequences. These sequences allow a slice thickness of 1.5 mm in the coronal plane and 2 mm in the axial plane. Since the resolution of each image is at or below the slice thickness, the voxels are nearly isotropic allowing for high quality multiplanar reconstructions in a manner similar to helical CT. Both arterial and venous phase imaging in the coronal plane are obtained using an angiographic sequence [such as fast low-angle shot (FLASH)]. This sequence tends to suppress background tissue signal in order to highlight vascular structures (36). Following this, anatomic imaging in the axial plane is obtained during the corticomedullary phase of renal enhancement using a more tissue-sensitive sequence [volume interpolated breath-hold examination (VIBE)] (37). Accurate assessment of the vasculature and accurate characterization of renal lesions are possible by combining these different techniques.

Coronal images are then obtained about 5 to 10 minutes after the initiation of the contrast material injection to obtain an MRI urogram. In patients whose lesions approach the renal sinus, it is desirable to distend the calyces in order to better determine whether the calyces are involved. Administering a small dose of intravenous furosemide during the timing examination will promote diuresis, distending the collecting system to achieve a better-quality MRI urogram. In patients who are not on chronic furosemide therapy, a dose of 10 mg given intravenously is almost always adequate. For patients who are on chronic therapy, dosage adjustments must be made.

IMAGE INTERPRETATION AND 3-D VOLUME-RENDERING

CT and MRI images are reviewed to evaluate each patient for a number of important features, including renal lesion size, lesion location, the number of renal arteries and veins, the presence or absence of renal vein tumor and inferior vena caval (IVC) tumor extension (and the degree of extension), enlargement of local, regional, and distant lymph nodes, and the presence or absence of local or regional metastatic disease. Tumor size and the presence of renal vein and IVC tumor thrombus and lymphadenopathy are all criteria used for staging. If the patient has a low-stage tumor and is an NSS surgical candidate, images are transferred to a dedicated 3-D imaging workstation for postprocessing typically using real-time volume-rendering techniques (38).

Surface-shaded display renderings have been used for NSS surgical planning but are limited by the need for intensive image editing, which is too time consuming for most radiologists. Volume-rendering typically requires little image editing and preserves the entire dataset (Figs. 6 and 7) (9,10,38,39).

(A)

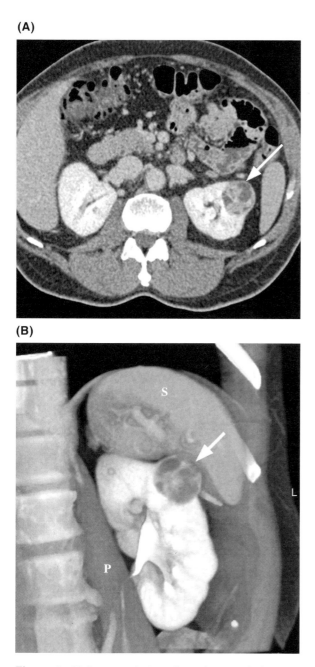

(B)

Figure 6 Volume-rendering of renal tumor before NSS. (**A**) Conventional axial image and (**B**) volume-rendered image; volume-rendering uses the entire dataset and projects a 3-D view of the renal tumor (*arrow*). The psoas muscle (P) and spleen (S) are seen and provide relational cues to interpreting the image. *Abbreviation*: NSS, nephron-sparing surgery.

(A)   **(B)**

(C)

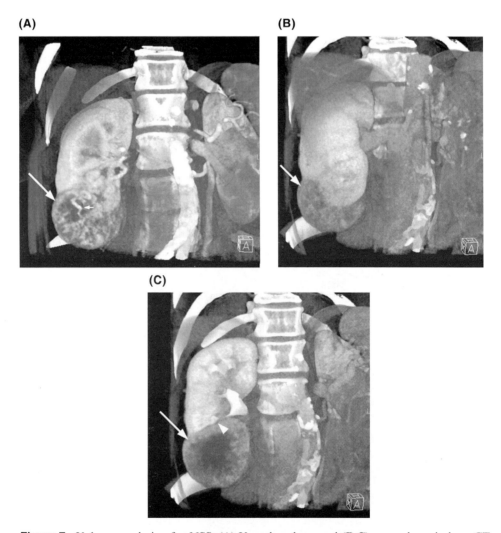

Figure 7 Volume-rendering for NSS. (**A**) Vascular phase and (**B,C**) parenchymal phase CT data volume-renderings show a right lower pole renal tumor (*arrows*). With the anterior plane of the image outside the kidney, the surface of the kidney is seen, and the component of the tumor exophytic from the kidney is identified in (**B**). By using a "clip plane" to image inside the kidney, a large arterial branch is seen within the tumor in (**A**) (*short arrow*), and the depth of extension of the tumor into the renal hilum is also seen in (**C**) (*arrowhead*). *Abbreviations*: NSS, nephron-sparing surgery; CT, computed tomography.

A CT technologist can create MPR and MIP images easily, but because of the quality of information needed for surgical planning, it is often most beneficial if the radiologist performs real-time 3-D volume-rendering on a dedicated 3-D work-station. Our current practice is to create one or two short MPEG-encoded (.avi) digi-tal movie files for each case illustrating the critical anatomy for surgical planning, but a set of static images, either digital or filmed, may also suffice. The scope of the information provided by the 3-D imaging was developed in conjunction with a urologist highly experienced in performing NSS. We recommend a thorough discus-sion between the radiologist and the referring urologist regarding their surgical approach and surgical planning needs.

Because the surgical technique necessitates control of the renal vasculature, the renal vasculature is rendered first using the images from the vascular scan phase. This portion of the rendering shows the size, origin, and course of all renal arteries and veins, major segmental arterial branches, the left adrenal vein, the gonadal vein, and any prominent lumbar veins (Figs. 8–11). Next, using the renal parenchymal phase, renderings are obtained to show the position of the kidney, location of the tumor, depth of extension, and relationship to the pelvocalyceal system (Fig. 12). The rendering process takes anywhere between 10 and 30 minutes, depending upon user experience and the complexity of the case.

Postcontrast 3-D MRI datasets are manipulated and displayed in the same manner as CT data, using a combination of the postcontrast image series. Image subtraction facilitates data analysis and display. Subtraction of the precontrast data

(A)

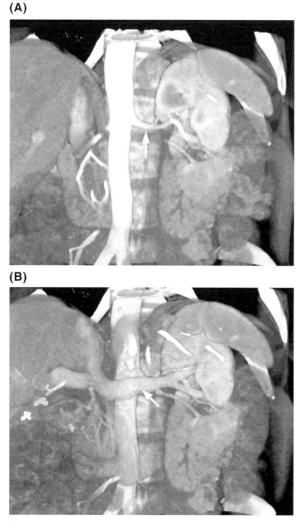

(B)

Figure 8 Conventional left renal vascular anatomy: Volume-rendered image of the left kidney during the vascular phase shows (**A**) single left artery (*arrow*) and (**B**) single left renal vein (*arrow*).

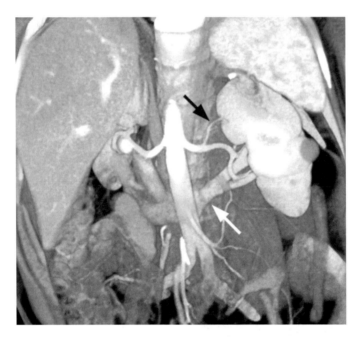

Figure 9 Anatomic left renal arterial and vein variants. An early apical polar branch is seen (*black arrow*) supplying the upper pole of the left kidney entering from the cortex. A retroaortic left renal vein (*arrow*) is also identified. Retroaortic left renal veins usually cross behind the aorta several centimeters below the level of the renal artery.

from the cortical phase data results in a dataset that can then be used to assess the true enhancement within renal lesions, facilitating characterization of the lesion (Fig. 13). A gadolinium-enhanced 3-D gradient echo magnetic resonance angiography (MRA) sequence provides inherent suppression of background signal and gives excellent volume-rendered views of the renal vasculature (Fig. 14). Subtraction of the precontrast data from the arterial phase data results in a dataset that has a high signal contrast within the arteries and a suppressed signal in the rest of the image, which can then be used to produce angiographic images, such as MIPs, with minimal additional editing needed (40). The venous phase–enhanced images are useful in determining whether there is any venous invasion (Fig. 15). Sequences acquired or reconstructed in the coronal or sagittal planes are often helpful to the urologist in defining lesion location/orientation within the kidney.

RADIOLOGICAL GUIDANCE DURING NSS

Another important role that imaging plays in surgical planning is in providing intraoperative guidance during open or laparoscopic ultrasound for partial nephrectomy and during laparoscopic and percutaneous ablative therapies.

Ultrasound Guidance for Partial Nephrectomy and Ablative Therapies

During intraoperative ultrasound, whether open or laparoscopic, dedicated intraoperative probes that yield high-resolution images are used (Fig. 16) (41). These

(A)

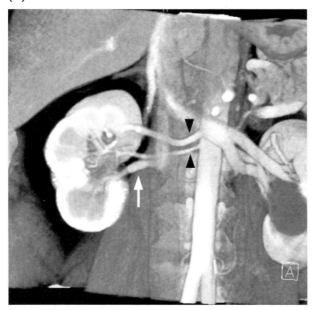

(B)

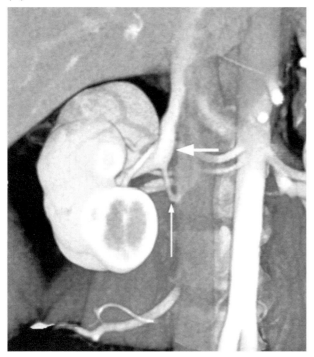

Figure 10 Anatomic right renal artery and vein variants. (**A**) Two right renal artery origins are seen (*arrowheads*) along with an accessory right renal vein (*arrow*). (**B**) The main right renal vein is seen (*arrow*) along with an unusual branch of the vein (*long thin arrow*) that results in a third renal vein entering into the inferior vena cava. The plane in image (**B**) is slightly more anterior than in image (**A**).

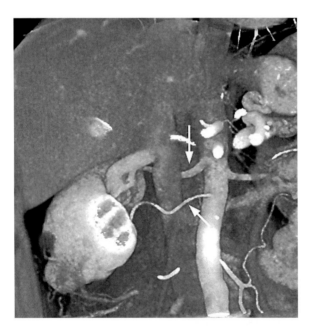

Figure 11 Accessory right renal artery. Vascular phase volume-rendering shows the main (*vertical arrow*) and an accessory right renal artery (*oblique arrow*). Right renal arteries that arise inferior off the aorta often course anterior to the IVC, as in this patient. *Abbreviation*: IVC, inferior vena cava.

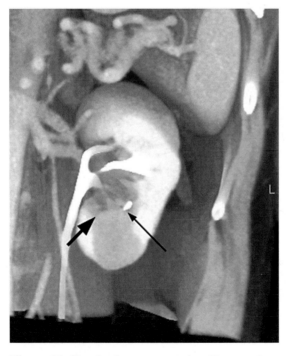

Figure 12 Depth of tumor extension. Tumors that extend into the renal hilum (*arrow*) will often abut larger vessels and the pelvocalyceal system (*thin arrow*). This is important for the urologist, who may opt for conservative surgery or be ready to anticipate repair of the collecting system and cauterize the vasculature.

(A)

(B)

(C)

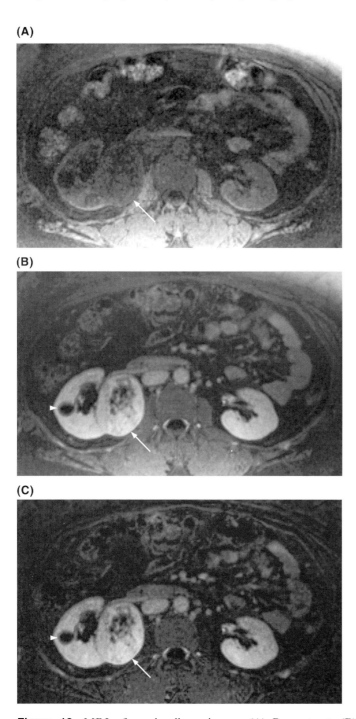

Figure 13 MRI of renal cell carcinoma. **(A)** Precontrast, **(B)** equilibrium postcontrast fat-saturated 3-D gradient echo T1-weighted (VIBE) images, and **(C)** subtraction image of a partially exophytic right renal mass (*arrow*). Tumor enhancement on the postcontrast image is confirmed on the subtraction image. This is most helpful when there is a high precontrast T1 signal in the investigated lesion such as that from internal hemorrhage. A laterally located renal cyst does not enhance and is black on the subtraction image (*arrowhead*). *Abbreviations*: MRI, magnetic resonance imaging; VIBE, volume interpolated breath-hold examination.

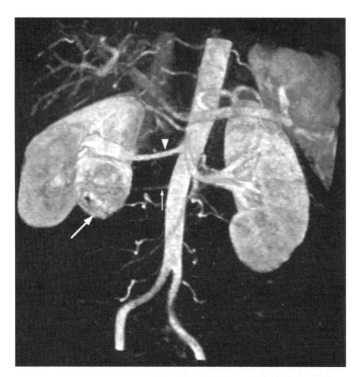

Figure 14 Volume-rendered arterial phase MRI for renal vasculature. Both the main right renal artery (*arrowhead*) and a small inferior accessory renal artery (*thin arrow*) are demonstrated on this volume-rendered angiogram. The partially exophytic tumor (*arrow*) is also seen. The arterial phase fat-saturated 3-D gradient echo T1-weighted (FLASH) data was used to create the image. *Abbreviation*: MRI, magnetic resonance imaging; FLASH, fast low-angle shot.

probes are smaller in size than conventional probes and are specifically shaped for the operative environment. The ultrasound transducer can be placed directly on the surface of the kidney during an open partial nephrectomy. The laparoscopic ultrasound transducer is constructed with the transducer elements on a flexible arm that fits through a 1 cm laparoscopic port. The transducer elements can typically be steered into different positions, although there are some limitations related to the locations of the access ports and the flexibility of the transducer. Doppler capability is helpful in facilitating the identification of vascular structures and their proximity to the surgical site.

During open partial nephrectomy, the urologist can palpate masses that extend to the renal surface. During these procedures, ultrasound is used to localize small intrarenal masses and to assess their proximity to the central sinus structures, the pyelocalyceal system, and vessels. The margins of the mass are demarcated on the renal surface using ultrasound, and then electrocautery is used to score the kidney surface. A search for additional lesions that may not have been identified on preoperative imaging is also performed.

During laparoscopic partial nephrectomy, unless a hand-assisted procedure is performed, the ability of ultrasound to localize a renal mass is invaluable because the tactile cues available during open surgery are not available. Most masses treated laparoscopically are small, and some may not be visible on the renal surface.

(A)

(B)

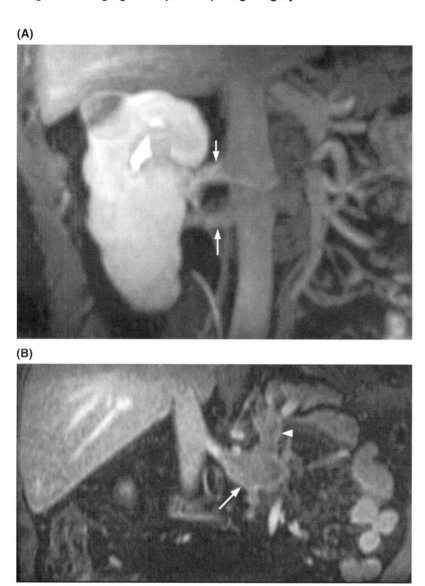

Figure 15   Renal vein evaluation by MRI. Oblique coronal thin MIP images show (**A**) two right renal veins (*arrows*) and (**B**) a left renal vein expanded by tumor thrombus (*arrow*) that does not extend to the IVC but is seen to extend into the left adrenal vein (*arrowhead*). The images are derived from the equilibrium phase postcontrast fat-saturated 3-D gradient echo T1-weighted (VIBE) data. *Abbreviations*: IVC, inferior vena cava; MRI, magnetic resonance imaging; MIP, maximum intensity projection; VIBE, volume interpolated breath-hold examination.

After identifying the mass by ultrasound, the surface of the kidney is scored using electrocautery as during the open procedure.

Laparoscopic ultrasound is also used to guide and monitor both cryoablation and radiofrequency ablation of renal masses. The position of the mass, as determined by preoperative CT or MRI with 3-D imaging, and any history of prior retroperitoneal or abdominal surgery are taken into consideration when deciding upon the laparoscopic approach. A retroperitoneal approach is commonly used for a

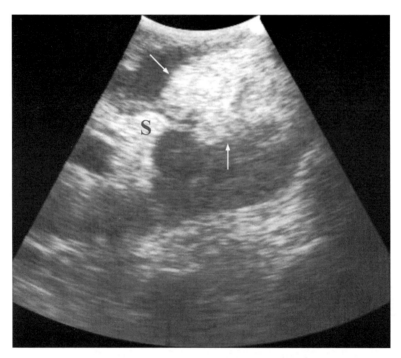

Figure 16 Intraoperative laparoscopic ultrasound shows an ovoid hyperechoic mass (*arrows*) that extends from the lower pole into hyperechoic fat of central renal sinus (S).

posteriorly or laterally located mass, whereas the transperitoneal approach is used for an anteriorly or anterolaterally located mass. Once the kidney is mobilized and fat excised for pathological analysis, the tumor and the remainder of the kidney are imaged with ultrasound. The mass is biopsied and then punctured with the ablative probe under ultrasound guidance. The probe is visualized as an echogenic line that casts an acoustic shadow.

During cryoablation, the critical steps are rapid freezing, slow thawing, and a repetition of the freeze–thaw cycle (42,43). The cryotherapy probe tip is advanced to the deep margin of the mass; the tip defines the deep margin of the ablation zone. Cryoablation, unlike radiofrequency ablation, creates a distinct margin of the ablated tissue on ultrasound. The deep margin of the tumor is most at risk for incomplete ablation (44). As cryoablation progresses, an iceball is seen as a hyperechoic arc with posterior shadowing (Fig. 17). Ultrasound findings correlate well with the actual size and location of the iceball at surgery. Scanning from the surface opposite the cryotherapy probe ensures shadowing does not obscure visualization of the deep margin and protects the probe from the cryoablation (45). Using multiple probe positions (i.e., rotating and translating the probe along the renal surface) may be necessary to

Figure 17 (*Figure on facing page*) Laparoscopic ultrasound monitoring of renal cryoablation. (**A**) Initial image shows the mass (*arrow*). (**B**) As cryotherapy begins, iceball formation is seen as a short hyperechoic arc (*arrow*). (**C**) As the iceball enlarges, the hyperechoic arc (*arrows*) increases in size and shows increasing shadowing.

(A)

(B)

(C)

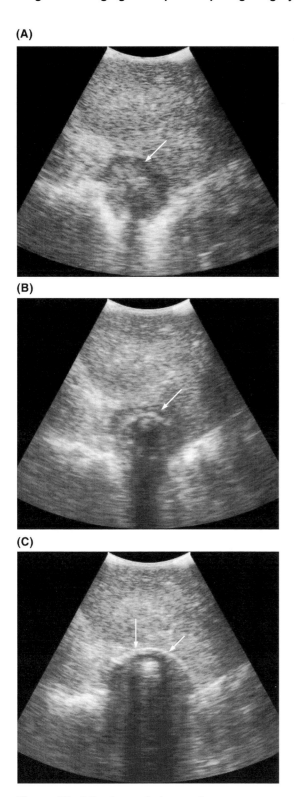

Figure 17 (*Caption on facing page*)

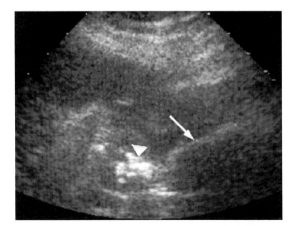

Figure 18 Percutaneous ultrasound guidance for renal radiofrequency ablation. The radio-frequency ablation electrode is seen as a linear echogenic structure (*arrow*). As the procedure continues, additional bright echoes (*arrowhead*) obscure the renal mass.

ensure complete ablation. Extension of the iceball more than 3 mm beyond the tumor margin ensures adequate freezing of the lesion resulting in desired cell death (20).

During radiofrequency ablation, an electrical current flows from the tip of a needle electrode into the surrounding tissue toward grounding pads that are placed on the patient's thighs. This leads to heat production and coagulative necrosis (21). The adequate treatment temperature is between 70°C and 100°C. When monitoring the ablation, increasingly bright echoes are visualized from the electrode tip on ultrasound due to microbubble formation (Fig. 18). This provides a rough estimate of the size of the treatment area (22). Larger lesions require the use of multiple overlapping treatment zones to achieve adequate coverage for complete ablation. However, the extent of coagulation cannot accurately be predicted and post-procedural imaging is necessary in order to assess the success of the ablation.

CT and MRI Guidance for Ablative Therapies

The principles described for ultrasound guidance for laparoscopically directed abla-tive therapies can also be used for percutaneous ablative therapies. A percutaneous approach may be used for accessible tumors: those that can be accessed without traversing the colon, small bowel, blood vessels, or lung. The percutaneous approach offers the added benefit of no postoperative recovery time. Most patients are dis-charged the same day.

CT and MRI are both used to guide percutaneous cryoablation and radiofre-quency ablation. The relative advantages of CT are its greater availability, ease of use, and the lack of need for specialized, MRI-compatible, nonferromagnetic equip-ment. The primary advantage of MRI is that it provides a more accurate determina-tion of the extent of the ablation during the procedure.

Of these two ablation techniques, there has been greater experience with radio-frequency ablation using CT guidance. In most hospitals, patients undergo deep sedation for CT-guided ablation procedures. After an initial preparatory scan, a skin site affording a safe and direct route to the mass is chosen. After skin cleansing and local anesthesia, the probe is advanced into the mass using CT fluoroscopy

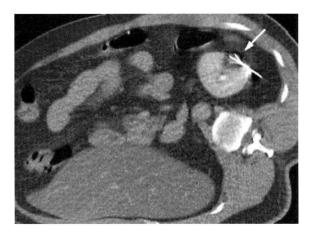

Figure 19 CT guidance of percutaneous RFA. An enhanced CT scan shows the RFA probe deployed in small peripheral renal cell carcinoma. *Abbreviations*: CT, computed tomography; RFA, radiofrequency ablation.

(Fig. 19) (23,24). The main role of CT during radiofrequency ablation is to direct the probe into the mass, because the location and amount of ablated tissue are not readily distinguished on unenhanced images. Postprocedural scans with intravenous contrast are necessary.

MRI has been used to guide cryoablation and radiofrequency ablation (25,26,46). It allows better evaluation than CT of the progress of ongoing ablation. MRI sequences afford a clear depiction of the ablation site, and temperature-sensitive sequences are available that can monitor ablation progress (47). In comparison to other modalities, MRI offers the advantage of better contrast resolution to discriminate between ablated and nonablated tissue. However, the specialized MRI scanners, expertise, and equipment needed are currently available in only a few centers.

POSTOPERATIVE IMAGING

At our institution, patients are seen four to six weeks after open partial nephrectomy for routine follow-up and have a physical examination, serum creatinine level check, and an excretory urogram (14). Imaging with CT or ultrasound is performed earlier on any patient who has clinical signs or symptoms of abscess, hematoma, urinary leak, or fistula. Generally, a CT scan with intravenous contrast should be performed, and if a urine leak is of concern, delayed images should be obtained.

Postoperative surveillance for recurrent disease should be tailored according to the initial pathological tumor stage (14). All patients are evaluated annually with a history, physical examination, and blood tests, including assessment of serum calcium, alkaline phosphatase, liver function, blood urea nitrogen (BUN), serum creatinine, and electrolytes. Patients with T1 tumors do not require early postoperative imaging because there is a low risk of recurrent malignancy (48,49). A yearly chest radiograph is recommended for patients with T2 or T3 tumors, because the lung is the most common site of metastasis. Low-dose chest CT may also be used. Patients with T2 tumors should have a CT examination every two years. Patients with T3 tumors have a higher risk of developing local recurrence, especially during the first two postoperative years, and they should have a CT examination every six months for two years, then at two-year intervals if there is no documented tumor recurrence.

The effectiveness of renal tumor ablation and laparoscopic partial nephrectomy has not yet been proven in long-term follow-up studies, and therefore imaging protocols following the procedure are not standardized, varying among institutions. In our opinion, conservative surveillance is appropriate. At our hospital, patients who have had laparoscopic partial nephrectomy undergo follow-up, with abdominal and pelvic CT and chest X-ray being taken at six months, at one year, and then at yearly intervals. Patients who have had cryoablation undergo postoperative MRI at one day, one month, six months, one year, and annually thereafter.

In most instances, contrast-enhanced CT is the test of choice to search for tumor recurrence in those patients with a normal serum creatinine (50). Contrast enhancement is important in detecting visceral organ metastases and local recurrence, but there is a risk of nephrotoxicity from iodinated CT contrast in those patients who have had NSS or those who have compromised renal function. Although MRI is not generally used as a screening examination, in patients with renal insufficiency it is a reasonable alternative to CT, because the gadolinium contrast used does not pose a risk to renal function.

Local tumor recurrences after NSS usually occur as masses at the resection site in the residual kidney (Fig. 20). Early on, postsurgical changes are significant for both laparoscopic partial nephrectomy and ablation and should not be confused

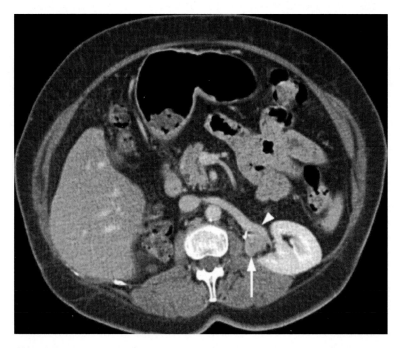

Figure 20 Recurrence at site of open partial nephrectomy. A 62-year-old woman had left open partial nephrectomy and right radical nephrectomy 2.5 years earlier. Contrast-enhanced CT shows a round soft tissue mass (*arrow*) abutting surgical clips and left renal vein (*arrowhead*). *Abbreviation*: CT, computed tomography.

(A)

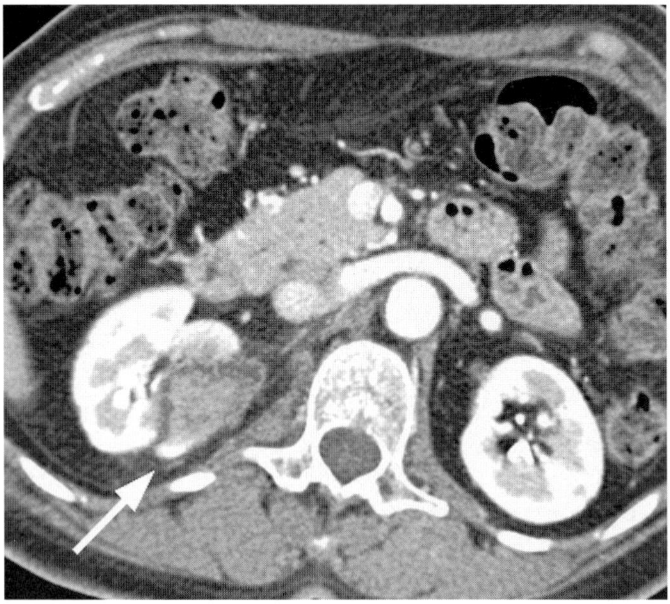

(B)

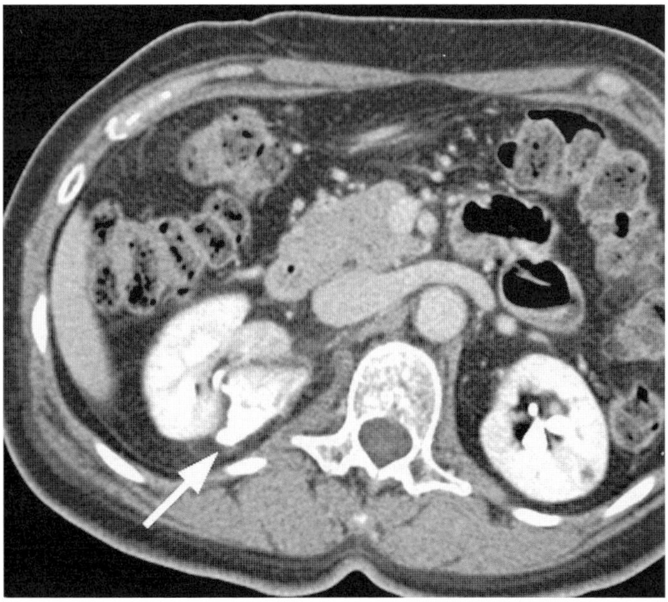

Figure 21 Postoperative urine leak following partial nephrectomy. If entry into the collecting system is not identified and repaired at surgery, urine leaks can result. (**A**) This patient has
a perinephric fluid collection (*arrow*) after partial nephrectomy that fills in with contrast on
(**B**) a delayed scan.

for residual disease. These postsurgical changes can include perinephric fluid, fat
necrosis, urine leak, scarring, or a defect at the operative site (Figs. 21 and 22).
Hemostatic agents, such as oxidized cellulose (Surgicel, Johnson & Johnson,
Arlington, Texas), may be present (51) and can mimic abscess formation (Fig. 23).

(A)

(B)

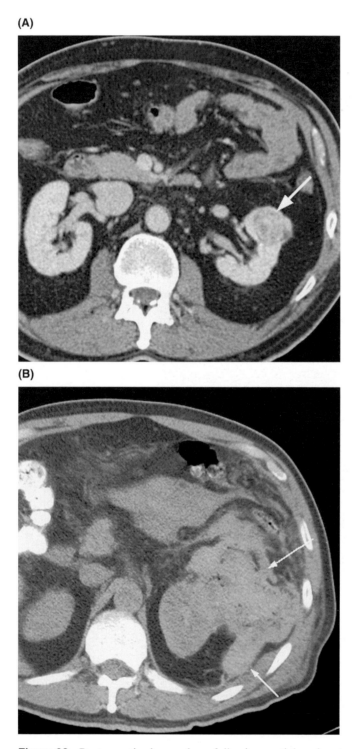

Figure 22 Postoperative hemorrhage following partial nephrectomy. The mass (*arrow*) in (**A**) was resected laparoscopically; the patient complained of left flank pain following the surgery and had a low hemoglobin. (**B**) Postoperative unenhanced CT scan shows a large perinephric hematoma (*thin arrows*). *Abbreviation*: CT, computed tomography.

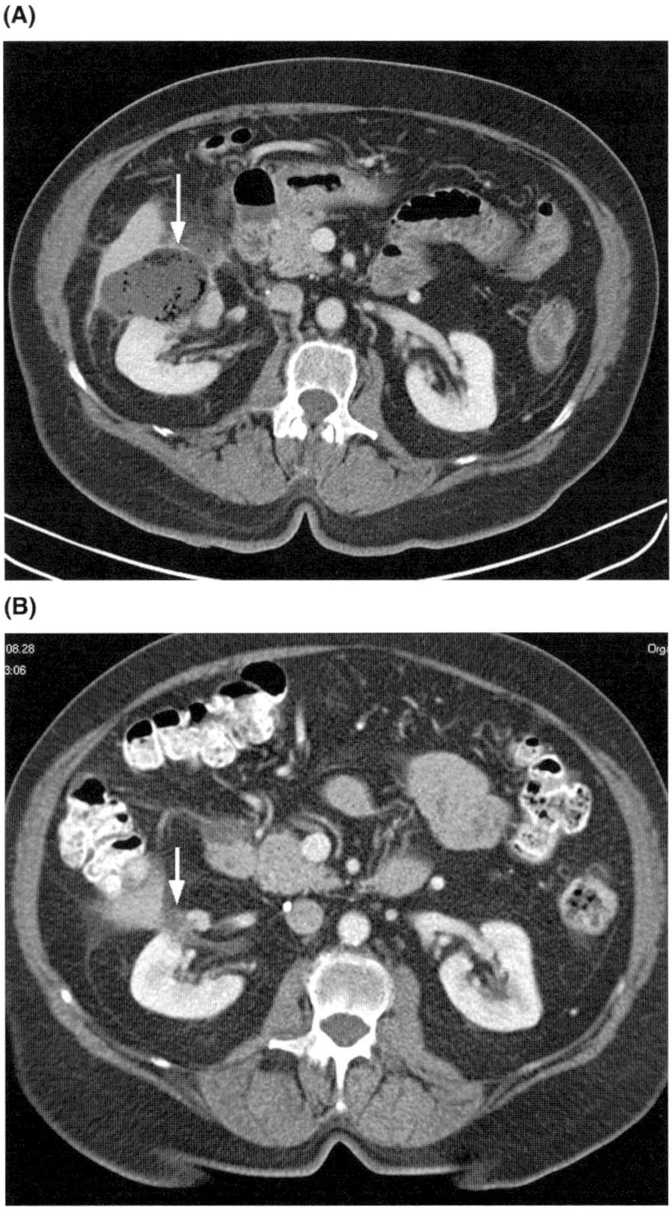

(A)

(B)

Figure 23 Oxidized cellulose (Surgicel) mimics abscess at laparoscopic partial nephrectomy site. This patient presented to the emergency department with flank pain after laparoscopic partial nephrectomy and had a normal white blood cell count. (**A**) Contrast-enhanced CT demonstrates an ovoid collection with scattered gas foci at partial nephrectomy site (*arrow*). No intervention was performed. (**B**) CT six months later shows resolution of collection with minimal residual low attenuation (*arrow*). *Abbreviation*: CT, computed tomography.

After ablation, the mass progressively decreases in size over time (52,53) and eventually presents only as cortical defect (Fig. 24). Incomplete ablation is seen as a residual enhancement at the site of the mass. In our experience, enhancement or a mass-like contour change suggests recurrent disease (54).

(A)

(B)

(C)

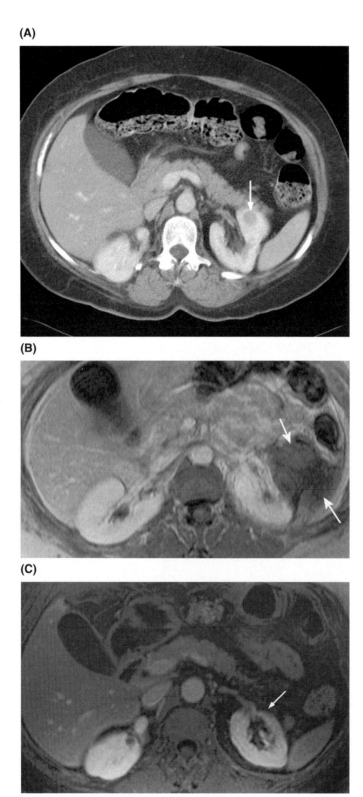

Figure 24   (*Caption on facing page*)

Figure 24 (*Figure on facing page*) Normal findings after cryoablation of renal cell carcinoma. (**A**) CT scan before cryoablation shows a small anterior mid-left renal cell carcinoma (*arrow*). (**B**) One month after cryoablation, gadolinium-enhanced T1-weighted 2-D gradient echo MRI shows no enhancement in the kidney at the cryoablation site. Low–signal intensity perinephric changes (*arrows*) merge imperceptibly with the ablated renal parenchyma. (**C**) 4.5 years after ablation, gadolinium-enhanced T1-weighted 3-D gradient echo MRI shows only cortical loss at the site of tumor ablation (*arrow*). *Abbreviations*: CT, computed tomography; MRI, magnetic resonance imaging.

Metastatic disease can occur in regional lymph nodes or in distant sites. Lung, mediastinal, bone, liver, contralateral kidney, adrenal gland, and brain metastases are common, but metastatic disease of the small bowel and peritoneal cavity can also occur (55). In this event, imaging reverts to the role of monitoring treatment for metastatic disease.

CONCLUSION

In summary, radiological imaging plays an increasingly important role in the diagnosis and treatment of renal cell carcinoma. Imaging is no longer used solely for the detection and characterization of renal tumors. It is now critical for surgical planning and for monitoring of patients during and after the new, less-invasive surgical and ablative therapies that have been recently developed.

REFERENCES

1. Zagoria RJ, Dyer RB. The small renal mass: detection, characterization, and management. Abdom Imaging 1998; 23:256–265.
2. Bosniak MA. The small (less than or equal to 3.0 cm) renal parenchymal tumor: detection, diagnosis, and controversies. Radiology 1991; 179:307–317.
3. Birnbaum BA, Jacobs JE, Ramchandani P. Multiphasic renal CT: comparison of renal mass enhancement during the corticomedullary and nephrographic phases. Radiology 1996; 200:753–758.
4. Szolar DH, Kammerhuber F, Altziebler S, et al. Multiphasic helical CT of the kidney: increased conspicuity for detection and characterization of small (<3-cm) renal masses. Radiology 1997; 202:211–217.
5. Cohan RH, Sherman LS, Korobkin M, Bass JC, Francis IR. Renal masses: assessment of corticomedullary-phase and nephrographic-phase CT scans. Radiology 1995; 196: 445–451.
6. Bosniak MA. The current radiological approach to renal cysts. Radiology 1986; 158:1–10.
7. Bosniak MA. Diagnosis and management of complicated cystic lesions of the kidneys. Am J Roentgen 1997; 169:819–821.
8. Israel GM, Bosniak MA. Follow-up CT of moderately complex cystic lesions of the kidney (Bosniak category IIF). AJR 2003; 181:627–633.
9. Coll DM, Uzzo RG, Herts BR, Davros WJ, Wirth SL, Novick AC. 3-dimensional volume rendered computerized tomography for preoperative evaluation and intraoperative treatment of patients undergoing nephron sparing surgery. J Urol 1999; 161:1097–1102.
10. Coll DM, Herts BR, Davros WJ, Uzzo RG, Novick AC. Preoperative use of 3D volume rendering to demonstrate renal tumors and renal anatomy. Radiographics 2000; 20: 431–438.

11. Wunderlich H, Reichelt O, Schubert R, Zermann DH, Schubert J. Preoperative simulation of partial nephrectomy with three-dimensional computed tomography. BJU Int 2000; 86:777–781.

12. Chernoff DM, Silverman SG, Kikinis R, et al. Three-dimensional imaging and display of renal tumors using spiral CT: a potential aid to partial nephrectomy. Urology 1994; 43:125–129.

13. Novick AC. Current surgical approaches, nephron-sparing surgery, and the role of surgery in the integrated immunologic approach to renal-cell carcinoma. Semin Oncol 1995; 22:29–33.

14. Novick AC. Nephron-sparing surgery for renal cell carcinoma. Ann Rev Med 2002; 53: 393–407.

15. Butler BP, Novick AC, Miller DP, Campbell SA, Licht MR. Management of small unilateral renal cell carcinomas: radical versus nephron-sparing surgery. Urology 1995; 45:34–40; discussion 40–41.

16. Smith SJ, Bosniak MA, Megibow AJ, Hulnick DH, Horii SC, Raghavendra BN. Renal cell carcinoma: earlier discovery and increased detection. Radiology 1989; 170:699–703.

17. Gill IS. Minimally invasive nephron-sparing surgery. Urol Clin North Am 2003; 30: 551–579.

18. Gill IS, Matin SF, Desai MM, et al. Comparative analysis of laparoscopic versus open partial nephrectomy for renal tumors in 200 patients. J Urol 2003; 170:64–68.

19. Gill IS, Desai MM, Kaouk JH, et al. Laparoscopic partial nephrectomy for renal tumor: duplicating open surgical techniques. J Urol 2002; 167:469–477.

20. Campbell SC, Krishnamurthi V, Chow G, Hale J, Myles J, Novick AC. Renal cryosurgery: experimental evaluation of treatment parameters. Urology 1998; 52:29–33; discussion 33–34.

21. Wood BJ, Ramkaransingh JR, Fojo T, Walther MM, Libutti SK. Percutaneous tumor ablation with radiofrequency. Cancer 2002; 94:443–451.

22. Pavlovich CP, Walther MM, Choyke PL, et al. Percutaneous radio frequency ablation of small renal tumors: initial results. J Urol 2002; 167:10–15.

23. Daly B, Krebs TL, Wong-You-Cheong JJ, Wang SS. Percutaneous abdominal and pelvic interventional procedures using CT fluoroscopy guidance. Am J Roentgenol 1999; 173:637–644.

24. Silverman SG, Tuncali K, Adams DF, Nawfel RD, Zou KH, Judy PF. CT fluoroscopy-guided abdominal interventions: techniques, results, and radiation exposure. Radiology 1999; 212:673–681.

25. Shingleton WB, Sewell PE Jr. Percutaneous renal tumor cryoablation with magnetic resonance imaging guidance. J Urol 2001; 165:773–776.

26. Lewin JS, Connell CF, Duerk JL, et al. Interactive MRI-guided radiofrequency interstitial thermal ablation of abdominal tumors: clinical trial for evaluation of safety and feasibility. J Magn Reson Imaging 1998; 8:40–47.

27. Murphy DP, Gill IS. Energy-based renal tumor ablation: a review. Semin Urol Oncol 2001; 19:133–140.

28. Curry NS, Bissada NK. Radiologic evaluation of small and indeterminant renal masses. Urol Clin North Am 1997; 24:493–505.

29. Davidson AJ, Hartman DS, Choyke PL, Wagner BJ. Radiologic assessment of renal masses: implications for patient care. Radiology 1997; 202:297–305.

30. Warshauer DM, McCarthy SM, Street L, et al. Detection of renal masses: sensitivities and specificities of excretory urography/linear tomography, US, and CT. Radiology 1988; 169:363–365.

31. Jamis-Dow CA, Choyke PL, Jennings SB, Linehan WM, Thakore KN, Walther MM. Small (≤3-cm) renal masses: detection with CT versus US and pathologic correlation. Radiology 1996; 198:785–788.

32. Silverman SG, Lee BY, Seltzer SE, Bloom DA, Corless CL, Adams DF. Small ($\leq$3 cm) renal masses: correlation of spiral CT features and pathologic findings. Am J Roentgenol 1994; 163:597–605.

33. Aspelin P, Aubry P, Fransson SG, et al. Nephrotoxic effects in high-risk patients undergoing angiography. N Engl J Med 2003; 348:491–499.

34. Herts BR, Coll DM, Lieber ML, Streem SB, Novick AC. Triphasic helical CT of the kidneys: contribution of vascular phase scanning in patients before urologic surgery. Am J Roentgenol 1999; 173:1273–1277.

35. Pretorius ES, Siegelman ES, Ramchandani P, Cangiano T, Banner MP. Renal neoplasms amenable to partial nephrectomy: MR imaging. Radiology 1999; 212:28–34.

36. Lee VS, Rofsky NM, Krinsky GA, Stemerman DH, Weinreb JC. Single-dose breath-hold gadolinium-enhanced three-dimensional MR angiography of the renal arteries. Radiology 1999; 211:69–78.

37. Rofsky NM, Lee VS, Laub G, et al. Abdominal MR imaging with a volumetric interpolated breath-hold examination. Radiology 1999; 212:876–884.

38. Johnson PT, Heath DG, Bliss DF, Cabral B, Fishman EK. Three-dimensional CT: real-time interactive volume rendering. Am J Roentgenol 1996; 167:581–583.

39. Calhoun PS, Kuszyk BS, Heath DG, Carley JC, Fishman EK. Three-dimensional volume rendering of spiral CT data: theory and method. Radiographics 1999; 19:745–764.

40. Lee VS, Flyer MA, Weinreb JC, Krinsky GA, Rofsky NM. Image subtraction in gadolinium-enhanced MR imaging. Am J Roentgenol 1996; 167:1427–1432.

41. Choyke PL, Daryanani K. Intraoperative ultrasound of the kidney. Ultrasound Q 2001; 17:245–253.

42. Gage AA, Baust J. Mechanisms of tissue injury in cryosurgery. Cryobiology 1998; 37:171–186.

43. Lee FT Jr, Mahvi DM, Chosy SG, et al. Hepatic cryosurgery with intraoperative 2US guidance. Radiology 1997; 202:624–632.

44. Gill IS, Novick AC, Soble JJ, et al. Laparoscopic renal cryoablation: initial clinical series. Urology 1998; 52:543–551.

45. Remer EM, Hale JC, O'Malley CM, Godec K, Gill IS. Sonographic guidance of laparoscopic renal cryoablation. Am J Roentgenol 2000; 174:1595–1596.

46. Merkle EM, Shonk JR, Duerk JL, Jacobs GH, Lewin JS. MR-guided RF thermal ablation of the kidney in a porcine model. AJR 1999; 173:645–651.

47. Jolesz FA. Interventional and intraoperative MRI: a general overview of the field. J Magn Reson Imaging 1998; 8:3–7.

48. Hafez KS, Novick AC, Campbell SC. Patterns of tumor recurrence and guidelines for follow-up after nephron sparing surgery for sporadic renal cell carcinoma. J Urol 1997; 157:2067–2070.

49. Saidi JA, Newhouse JH, Sawczuk IS. Radiologic follow-up of patients with T1-3a,b,c or T4N+M0 renal cell carcinoma after radical nephrectomy. Urology 1998; 52:1000–1003.

50. Newhouse JH, Amis ES Jr, Bigongiari LR, et al. Follow-up of renal cell carcinoma. American College of Radiology. ACR Appropriateness Criteria. Radiology 2000; 215(suppl):761–764.

51. Oto A, Remer EM, O'Malley CM, Tkach JA, Gill IS. MR characteristics of oxidized cellulose (Surgicel). Am J Roentgenol 1999; 172:1481–1484.

52. Gill IS, Novick AC, Meraney AM, et al. Laparoscopic renal cryoablation in 32 patients. Urology 2000; 56:748–753.

53. Remer EM, Weinberg EJ, Oto A, O'Malley CM, Gill IS. MR imaging of the kidneys after laparoscopic cryoablation. Am J Roentgenol 2000; 174:635–640.

54. Brady PS, Remer EM, Gill IS. MRI after renal cryoablation: findings at 1–2 year follow-up. Radiology 2000; 217(P):581.

55. Scatarige JC, Sheth S, Corl FM, Fishman EK. Patterns of recurrence in renal cell carcinoma: manifestations on helical CT. Am J Roentgenol 2001; 177:653–658.

7

Imaging of the Renal Arteries: Current Status

Graham J. Munneke and Uday Patel
Radiology Department, St. George's Hospital, London, U.K.

INTRODUCTION

Renal artery stenosis (RAS) has long been recognized as a potentially reversible cause of hypertension (1). It is also an important cause of renal impairment, especially in the elderly. However, there is also a further large reservoir of asymptomatic or unrecognized RAS. For example, postmortem studies have found various degrees of renal artery narrowing in previously normotensive patients (2). Thus some cases of RAS are clinically unimportant in the patient's lifetime, because it does not always produce a detrimental effect. The contemporary dilemma is the diagnosis of all cases of significant RAS without the misdiagnosis of clinically unimportant arterial stenosis. This demands a test of high specificity and of equally high sensitivity, a demand common with many other screening or quasi-screening scenarios. Furthermore, an ideal test should not only have a high diagnostic accuracy but also should be able to grade the stenosis. The "gold" or reference standard for the diagnosis of RAS is the renal arteriogram (Fig. 1), ideally with the measurement of the intra-arterial pressure gradient across the stenosis to grade its physiological significance. There is a lack of consensus about what percentage of reduction in lumen size identifies a clinically important RAS. Previous studies have used different thresholds of between 50% and 70%. In flow models, tube narrowing of greater than 70% cross-sectional area (or approximately 50% of the lumen diameter) will compromise flow and a further reduction in the diameter will lead to a corresponding exponential reduction in perfusion. At present there is no ideal cost-effective noninvasive "screening" investigation for RAS, and this chapter explores the ability and limitations of the various available modalities.

RAS

Prevalence

The true prevalence of RAS (all grades) is not known, but in an unselected hypertensive population, the prevalence of RAS runs between 1% and 5% (3–5). With such a low prevalence, screening for RAS may result in an unacceptably high false positive

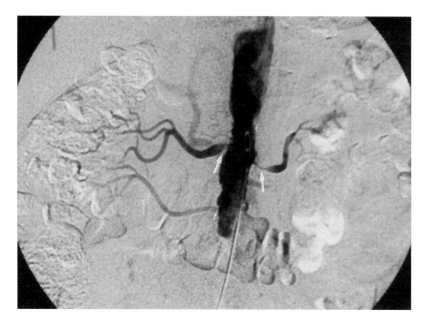

Figure 1 Bilateral RAS. AP aortogram with the pigtail flush catheter positioned just above the level of the renal arteries. There are two right renal arteries and a single left renal artery. All have severe ostial stenoses (*arrows*). Notice that the left kidney is small; it was found to be very poorly functioning on renography. *Abbreviations*: RAS, renal artery stenosis; AP, anteroposterior.

rate. Performance would be improved by increasing the pretest probability of RAS by identifying a high-risk group to make "screening," or more accurately, case finding a cost-effective proposition. Those with vascular disease in other territories have a higher incidence of RAS. Harding et al. (6) found RAS in 30% of patients undergoing cardiac catheterization, and the relationship with peripheral vascular disease is even stronger, with studies quoting RAS rates of between 38% and 49% (7,8). The athero-sclerotic patient who is also hypertensive has an even higher pretest probability of RAS, and the probability is further increased in those with severe hypertension. In the cooperative study (9) of renovascular hypertension, investigators compared 339 patients with essential hypertension with 175 patients with renovascular hypertension in order to identify the clinical findings most strongly associated with renovascular hypertension. Renovascular hypertension was characterized by advanced age, hypertension of short duration or accelerated hypertension, retinopathy, and the coexistence of cardiovascular, peripheral vascular, or cerebrovascular disease. Thus, clinical markers can allow more selective investigation of patients for RAS, improving the cost-effectiveness of any "screening" investigation: these clinical markers are shown in Table 1 and the grading of RAS is listed in Table 2.

Anatomy

The renal arteries usually arise from the abdominal aorta at the level of the L1/L2 vertebral interspace (10). As such, they are immediately inferior to the origin of the superior mesenteric artery. In most people the right renal artery is lower than the left and takes a longer, more caudal route behind the inferior vena cava to the kidney. The left renal artery commonly originates posterolaterally and the right slightly

Table 1 Clinical Predictors of RAS

Young hypertensive patients
Presence of peripheral or coronary vascular disease
Accelerated or malignant hypertension
Hypertension resistant to treatment
Bruit heard on abdominal auscultation
Deterioration in longstanding, previously well-controlled hypertensives
Worsening renal function after the instigation of an ACE inhibitor
Renal impairment but minimal proteinuria
Flash pulmonary edema
Differential in kidney size >1.5 cm
Grade III or IV retinopathy

Abbreviations: RAS, renal artery stenosis; ACE, angiotensin-converting enzyme.

more anteriorly. The average arterial diameter is 6 mm (range 5–8 mm in females, 6–9 mm in males). The main artery splits into anterior and posterior divisions outside the renal hilum. The divisions give rise to four or five segmental arteries that in turn divide into interlobar, then arcuate, and finally interlobular arteries. The renal arteries are end arteries and receive approximately 20% of cardiac output. Accessory arteries are present in 20% to 25%, the commonest being to the lower pole. Their presence has no bearing on the likelihood of renal arterial disease, but they may make endovascular treatment more technically difficult.

Pathophysiology

The renal artery may be narrowed at the ostium or within the main, segmental, or accessory artery. Narrowing beyond 70% of its cross-sectional area due to atherosclerosis or other causes compromises arterial flow and leads to a reduction in renal artery pressure and renal perfusion. This, in turn, causes a reduction in the glomerular filtration rate (GFR). The kidney adapts to preserve GFR by maintaining intraglomerular pressure via the renin angiotensin system (11). Reduction in renal blood flow triggers the secretion of renin in two ways. Baroreceptors in the afferent arteriolar wall detect decreased stretching from reduced blood flow. They signal the juxtaglomerular cells to secrete renin. With decreases in GFR and tubular flow, increased proportions of sodium and chloride are resorbed. The lower amount of these solutes in the distal tubule is detected by the macula densa, which also stimulates the release of renin. Renin converts angiotensinogen to angiotensin I. This is then converted to angiotensin II by angiotensin-converting enzyme (ACE).

Table 2 Grading of RAS

Grade	Stenosis (%)	Comment
0	0	No stenosis
I	<50	No significant stenosis
II	50–70	Significant stenosis
III	70–99	Critical stenosis
IV	100	Occlusion

Abbreviation: RAS, renal artery stenosis.

Angiotensin II bolsters GFR by selectively constricting the efferent glomerular arteriolar system, increasing glomerular capillary hydrostatic pressure. However angiotensin II also increases systemic vascular tone and stimulates aldosterone release, leading to renovascular hypertension. It should be apparent that treating renovascular hypertension patients with drugs that inhibit ACE or antagonize the angiotensin receptor itself can lead to a sudden drop in GFR. The administration of these drugs also provides the basis of some of the functional tests for RAS.

Consequences of RAS and Importance of Detection

The common causes of RAS are given in Table 3. Most cases of significant RAS are due to atherosclerosis, but whatever the cause, it has three important clinical sequelae:

Table 3 RAS: Causes

Cause	Pathology	Frequency	Epidemiology	Notes
Atherosclerosis	Atherosclerotic intimal lesion	65%	M > F; > 50 years old	Affects proximal 2 cm of renal artery Progressive and may lead to occlusion Presents as hypertension Associated with renal failure Common in patients with peripheral and cardiovascular disease Affects smokers
FMD	Hyperplasia of varying amounts of fibrous and smooth muscle tissue in the arterial wall	30%	M:F = 1:3; young	Affects distal renal artery and branches Not usually progressive, does not occlude Presents as hypertension Does not usually cause renal dysfunction Six types The most common, medial fibroplasia, has typical "string of beads" appearance on angio (alternating stenotic and aneurysmal segments)
Takayasu's	Aortoarteritis	Rare	F > M; children; mainly seen in Southeast Asians	The renal artery is the most commonly affected aortic side branch Produces severe ostial stenosis
Other causes				Neurofibromatosis Irradiation Thromboembolic disease Arterial dissection Infrarenal AAA

Abbreviations: RAS, renal artery stenosis; FMD, fibromuscular dysplasia; AAA, abdominal aortic aneurysm.

hypertension, renal failure, and pulmonary edema. However it is difficult to be sure that the RAS is solely responsible for morbidity in these patients. For example hypertension may be due to essential hypertension, renal failure due to hypertensive or atheroembolic nephropathy, and pulmonary edema from left ventricular failure (12).

Hypertension

RAS has classically been associated with hypertension. In reality it is seen in very few patients with a mild-to-moderate elevation in blood pressure. Its importance lies in malignant or drug-resistant hypertension when RAS is present in up to one-third of patients (13). Although excellent reductions in blood pressure have been reported following revascularization in fibromuscular dysplasia (FMD), the same is not true for atherosclerotic RAS (14,15). This may be due to the frequent coexistence of essential hypertension in these patients. Many will also have some degree of parenchymal renal disease. In these cases the role of intervention is to improve blood pressure control rather than effect a cure.

Renal Impairment

In a study in 1989 (11,16), 6% of new patients entering a dialysis program had RAS as the primary cause of chronic renal failure. The percentage was more than double that in patients over 50 years of age and may be as much as 25% in the over-60 age group (17). In these patients the mortality rate at two years is 50%; i.e., worse than many cancers. RAS detected in patients having coronary angiography had a significant bearing on prognosis: 65% four-year survival versus 86% survival in those with normal renal arteries (18). Zierler et al. (19) showed that in kidneys with 60% or greater stenosis, followed up on ultrasound, 19% lost 1 cm or more in length at one year. Guzman et al. (20) found 27% of similar patients lost an average of 19 mm in length when followed for a mean of 14 months. The diminished length reflects parenchymal loss due to fibrous replacement of glomeruli and tubules. This results in irreversible loss of function, but Watson et al. (21) found that this loss could be halted if the arteries were stented. Zierler's et al. prospective ultrasound study (19) has shown that the rate of stenosis progression can be up to 8% per year, most commonly from a less than 60% stenosis to a greater than 60% stenosis, and 10% will occlude within two years. In the setting of occlusion, the kidney may remain viable if sufficient collateral supply has developed, but nevertheless its function will be drastically compromised. Progression may in some cases be halted or even reversed with risk-factor modification and aggressive lipid-lowering therapy (22–24).

Renal function following technically successful angioplasty very rarely shows significant improvement (25); however, there are some reports of dialysis-dependent patients who regain function after revascularization (26). The aim of revascularization should be to prevent further decline in function. It is also useful to assess the status of the contralateral kidney, which may be at an earlier stage of the same process.

Pulmonary Edema

Pickering et al. (27) first reported bilateral RAS as a cause of congestive cardiac failure in 1988. It is thought to be due to a severe excess of angiotensin II and aldosterone, leading to hypertension, sodium retention, and fluid overload. Frequent associated left ventricular dysfunction from hypertension and coronary disease does not help matters. The association has been validated by the dramatic response to renal angioplasty. MacDowall et al. (28) looked at outpatients with New York Heart Association grade II–IV heart failure and found a 34% prevalence of RAS. Although there has been no study on the effect of revascularization in these patients on survival, it should in theory be beneficial because it would allow the use of ACE inhibitors.

DIAGNOSIS OF RAS

Ultrasound

Gray-Scale Ultrasound

Gray-scale ultrasound has little to contribute in the diagnosis of RAS except for the measurement of renal length and the exclusion of important morphological abnormalities.

Doppler Ultrasound

Since the development of color Doppler encoding, ultrasound has played an important role in imaging of the vascular system, including the renal arteries. Ultrasound has many advantages as a screening method. It is inexpensive, readily available, particularly noninvasive, and well tolerated by patients. Vascular sonography generally centers around the measurement of angle-corrected absolute arterial velocity, but historically, in the kidneys, direct velocity measurement has been difficult. Sonographic strategies for the detection of RAS broadly divide into the measurement of velocity and velocity change in the main artery and sampling of intrarenal arterial waveforms.

Direct Assessment of the Renal Arteries

An ultrasound examination of the entire renal artery is made, scanning the patient with the probe in an anterior or anterolateral position. Both color and power Doppler may be used to follow the course of the artery. The stenosis itself may be visualized on color Doppler imaging as a change in color due to turbulence (Fig. 2). Objective evidence is obtained by measurement of velocities on spectral Doppler— narrowing beyond the critical threshold ($>70\%$ reduction) results in a gradually increasing arterial velocity (the Bernoulli effect); the velocity gradient can help to grade the stenosis. Significant arterial stenosis produces an increase in the peak systolic velocity at or just distal to it (Fig. 3). Criteria for diagnosing a significant stenosis are presented in Table 4. The exception to this is in the near occlusive state when flow slows to a trickle. The artery is often tortuous, and scanning may be hampered by body habitus or interposed bowel gas, and in routine practice, complete and accurate interrogation is impossible in 10% to 50% (29).

Consequently, early reports on the use of this technique were somewhat less than promising, with quoted sensitivities as low as 0% (30). However technology and operator experience have moved on and current results are much better. Miralles et al. (31) reported that peak systolic velocity was the best ultrasound parameter for separating a less than 60% stenosis from a greater than 60% one. With a threshold of 198 cm/sec and a renal-to-aortic velocity ratio of 3.3, they obtained sensitivities of 87% and specificities of 91%. Other workers have reported sensitivities of 79% to 98% and specificities of 77% to 98% depending on the thresholds used (31–37). The results of these studies are shown in Table 5. Although accessory renal arteries

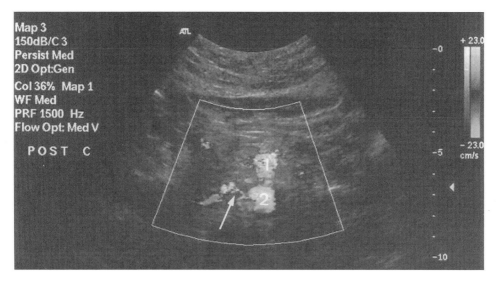

Figure 2 Right RAS in the same patient shown in Figure 1 on contrast-enhanced color Doppler ultrasound (*shown here in gray scale*). The renal artery is shown originating from the aorta in this transverse image. The superior mesenteric artery (1) is seen anterior to the aorta (2). The tight ostial RAS (*arrow*) can easily be appreciated on this image. Turbulent flow distal to the stenosis is seen as a markedly heterogeneous color display. *Abbreviation*: RAS, renal artery stenosis. *Source*: Courtesy of James Pilcher, St. George's Hospital, London.

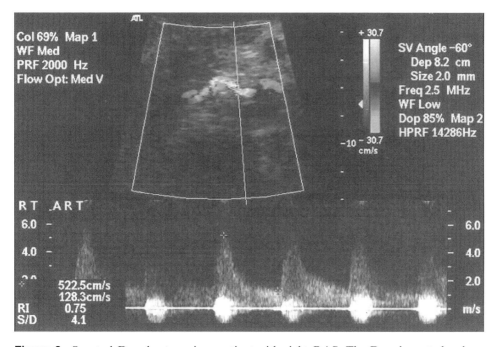

Figure 3 Spectral Doppler trace in a patient with right RAS. The Doppler gate has been placed at the site of stenosis. Measured velocities in excess of 5 m/sec indicate a high-grade stenosis in this case. *Abbreviation*: RAS, renal artery stenosis.

Table 4 Criteria for Diagnosis of Stenosis on Ultrasound

Peak systolic velocity at least 100–200 cm/sec
Ratio of renal artery to aortic peak systolic velocity > 3.5
Turbulent flow distal to the stenosis on color Doppler
No Doppler signal in the artery indicates occlusion

may be seen on ultrasound, their detection rate is universally very low in all series and much below the performance of other techniques (33,38).

Intrarenal Waveform Analysis

Due to the high rate of nondiagnostic scans with measurement of the renal artery velocity, considerable interest has been focused on the intrarenal arteries. These are much easier to scan, with waveform analysis being Doppler angle–independent. The results are thus far less operator dependent. The theory is that stenosis of the main renal artery will dampen the waveform of the downstream arteries, resulting in the so-called parvus-tardus effect ("parvus" meaning "small," and "tardus" meaning "slow" or "late"), with decreased peak velocity and a decreased slope of the systolic upstroke (Fig. 4) (39). Various parameters have been suggested to objectively measure this: prolonged systolic acceleration time (>0.07 seconds), decreased acceleration index (>4) (40), and resistive index (peak systolic velocity minus maximum end-diastolic velocity/peak systolic velocity). There are many reports of excellent results in the literature (41–43). Ripoles quoted a sensitivity of 89% and a specificity of 99% for the detection of RAS greater than 75%. However, others have shown that the tardus effect relates to vessel compliance (38), which changes with age and blood pressure, and has a poor correlation with stenosis (44). Most convincing is a study in which endovascular Doppler flow wires were placed in the patient's main and intrarenal arteries. Doppler traces obtained in this manner avoid the technical pitfalls of transabdominal ultrasound. The investigators found good correlation between main arterial peak systolic velocity and stenosis but no association with intrarenal parameters (45). Captopril can improve intrarenal Doppler ultrasound but not sufficiently (46).

Ultrasound Contrast Media

Because one of the main drawbacks of measuring renal artery peak systolic velocity is the inability to adequately image the artery in many subjects, efforts have been

Table 5 Performance of Doppler Ultrasound for the Detection of RAS Based on the Measurement of Main Renal Artery Velocity

Study	Number of patients	Doppler criteria (cm/sec)	Sensitivity (%)	Specificity (%)
Ref. 32	77	200	94	77
Ref. 33	45	200	79	93
Ref. 34	198	200	80	81
Ref. 31	78	198	87	91
Ref. 35	102	200	98	98
Ref. 36	41	180	95	90
Ref. 37	158	RAR	91	95

Abbreviations: RAS, renal artery stenosis; RAR, renal to aortic ratio.

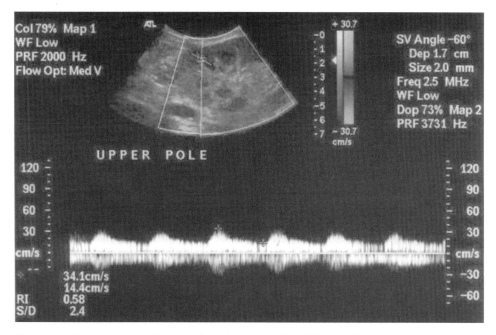

Figure 4 Intrarenal waveform analysis in a transplant kidney. The parvus-tardus effect is demonstrated with decreased peak velocity and a decreased slope of the systolic upstroke.

made to increase its visibility with the use of ultrasound contrast. These are micro-bubbles of air or other gas surrounded by a protective shell, allowing them to circulate around the vascular system several times. They provide a high-impedance interface, enhancing reflection of the ultrasound beam (47) and improving visibility (Fig. 5A,B). A study on a first-generation contrast (Levovist®, Schering-Plough, Berlin, Germany) showed that visualization of the renal artery could be significantly improved with contrast (75% of arteries demonstrated without enhancement compared to 90% with enhancement) (34). Other authors have reported accompanying improvements in sensitivity and specificity for the diagnosis of RAS with the use of ultrasound contrast and second harmonic imaging (48,49). A report that 97% of normal arteries could be visualized with newer contrast agents would suggest that a normal scan could effectively exclude stenosis (50). However, current agents still have a limited life, and long-lasting agents are keenly awaited, as are further refinements in ultrasound technology.

In conclusion, measurements of peak systolic velocity in the main renal artery and renal-to-aortic velocity ratios are the most accurate ultrasound methods for recognition of RAS. Waveform analysis is less accurate, but in the significant proportion of patients in whom the renal artery cannot be fully visualized, ultrasound contrast may help. Even then, sonographic evaluation has been lately overshadowed by the technical leaps in computed tomography (CT) and magnetic resonance imaging (MRI), and its routine use is limited to a few specialized centers.

Captopril Renography

Radionuclide imaging is an example of a functional rather than a structural imaging method. It provides information on the hemodynamic effect of a stenosis.

(A)

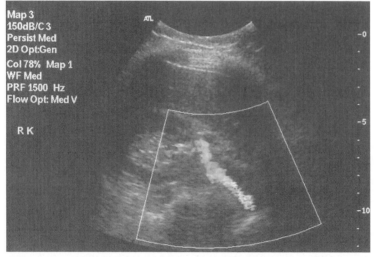

(B)

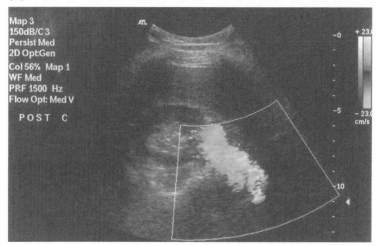

Figure 5 Contrast-enhanced ultrasound. (**A**) Unenhanced color Doppler image (*shown here in gray scale*) in the same patient shown in Figure 2. (**B**) Scan performed immediately after the administration of ultrasound contrast. Note the considerable increase in the color Doppler signal (*shown here in gray scale*). *Source*: Courtesy of James Pilcher, St George's Hospital, London.

As mentioned earlier, ACE inhibitors block the conversion of angiotensin I to angiotensin II. This results in a decreased filtration rate in patients with RAS. The detection of an increase in transit time of the tracer through the kidney, as a result of the change in GFR, is the basis of this test. Renography is performed with [99m]TC-MAG3, the preferred agent, or [99m]TC-DTPA. The test is performed before and an hour after the administration of an oral ACE inhibitor, usually 25 mg of captopril, on two consecutive days. Alternatively the post-captopril study may be performed first. If this is entirely normal, it obviates the need for a baseline study (51). Patients must not take ACE inhibitors for at least two days prior to the test. Sequential images are obtained for 30 minutes after the injection of the radiopharmaceutical and a time–activity curve generated. An increased time-to-peak of tracer in the kidney and an increased mean transit time suggest RAS (Fig. 6A, B). Changes may also be observed in the differential function. Obstruction of the kidney should be excluded before the test.

In patients with normal or near-normal renal function, sensitivities and specificities for detecting renovascular disease range from 65% to 96% and 62% to 100% (Table 6) (52–60). These studies mainly compare the functional results of scintigraphy with the structural gold standard (angiography). This may lead to unfair bias because hemodynamically insignificant stenosis will not be detected on the renogram. In a recent review of 10 studies with 291 patients on clinical improvement following revascularization as the standard, ACE inhibitor renography had a 92% positive predictive value (61). However, in those with abnormal renal function,

(A)

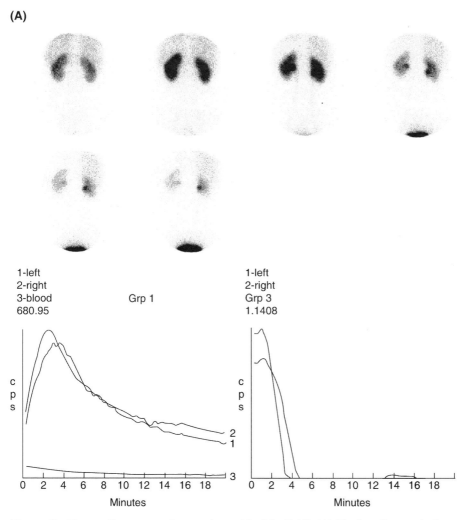

Figure 6 Captopril renogram in a patient with right RAS. (**A**) The baseline study (posterior images) shows normal uptake and excretion of tracer by both kidneys. (**B**) Post-captopril study. The left kidney continues to demonstrate normal uptake and transit of tracer (trace 1 on the left-hand graph). The right kidney has not peaked at 18 minutes and there is poor transit of tracer through the kidney (trace 2 on the left-hand graph). *Abbreviation*: RAS, renal artery stenosis. *Source*: Courtesy of Nigel Beharry, St. George's Hospital, London.

(B)

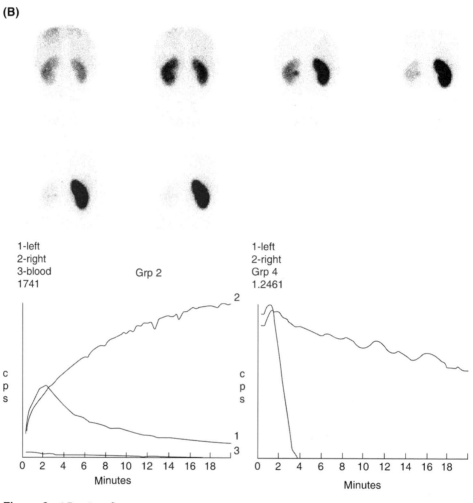

Figure 6 (*Continued*)

sensitivity fell drastically. Bilateral disease, urinary obstruction, dehydration, and chronic use of ACE inhibitors all decrease the sensitivity of the test (29). Finally, scintigraphy also provides valuable information about divided function and can ascertain whether a kidney is worth revascularizing.

Renal Arteriography

Not only is angiography considered the gold or reference standard for the diagnosis of RAS and the yardstick against which the other tests are measured, but it also allows treatment at the same sitting (Fig. 7A,B). The use of narrow-bore 3F catheters allow it to be performed as an outpatient procedure. However, it still carries the risks of arterial catheterization, namely groin hematoma, retroperitoneal hemorrhage, arterial pseudoaneurysm, and dissection. Angiography is performed via a common femoral artery (or brachial artery) puncture, with a pigtail flush catheter positioned just above the level of the renal arteries. This minimizes obscuration of the renal arteries from filling of mesenteric vessels. Left and right anterior oblique

Table 6 Results for Captopril Renography in the Detection of RAS

Study	Number of patients	Sensitivity (%)	Specificity (%)
Ref. 53	43	90	79
Ref. 54	45	72	73
Ref. 55	454	83	100
Ref. 56	20	65	–
Ref. 57	51	87	93
Ref. 58	55	94	95
Ref. 59	50	96	95
Ref. 60	94	91	62

Abbreviation: RAS, renal artery stenosis.

projections may be required to show the arterial ostia in profile. Oblique views should always be performed in patients with suspected FMD because the dilated segments tend to overlap the weblike stenoses (Fig. 8A,B) (62).

Selective catheterization may be required in these patients to demonstrate distal stenosis and allow pressure measurement. In patients with atherosclerotic disease, this is best avoided because of the risk of dissection and occlusion. However, if a significant stenosis is demonstrated, it is prudent to measure pressures across the lesion. Intra-arterial pressure measurement is regarded as the final reference standard for assessing the clinical significance of any arterial stenosis. This is achieved by passing a selective catheter past the stenosis and measuring paired pressures from beyond the stenosis and within the iliac artery (through the sheath). Alternatively, by steady withdrawal of the catheter, the gradient across the stenosis can be measured. As with change in lumen size, there is still a lack of consensus over the diagnostic thresholds used for intra-arterial pressure changes. An absolute change of between 7 and 34 mmHg or 10% to 15% of systolic pressure across the stenosis has been employed, either as a resting value or after vasodilatation. Bonn (63) summarized the data on this subject and concluded that further studies are necessary. The situation has not become any clearer since.

Angiography does have limitations in that eccentric plaques on the anterior or posterior wall of the artery may not be seen. Also ostial stenoses will be projected over the aorta and missed if the artery rises anteriorly (64). Likewise, an ostial stenosis may be missed on selective angiography if the catheter is placed distal to the stenosis. Three-dimensional arterial reconstruction has recently become available, but its value has not yet been defined. Further limitations include the potential for contrast medium–induced nephrotoxicity and the radiation dose rendered to the patient and radiologist.

The issue of contrast medium–induced nephrotoxicity may be addressed by the use of carbon dioxide (CO_2) angiography. In this technique CO_2 is injected intra-arterially in place of conventional iodinated contrast by means of a closed-system automated CO_2 injector (Fig. 7C). This avoids the potential for contamination with air possible during hand injection of CO_2 by syringe. CO_2 acts as a negative contrast by displacing rather than mixing with blood. It is highly soluble and is excreted via the lungs. Injection is safe but may provoke pain or nausea and vomiting in patients as it fills the mesenteric circulation. Its buoyancy as a gas may lead to underfilling of the renal arteries that travel posteriorly. This problem can be overcome by repeating the run with the patient obliqued to elevate the required side. Although the

(A)

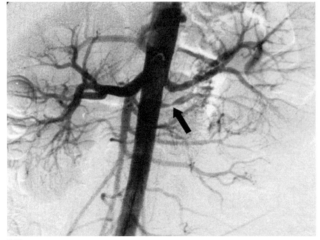

(B)

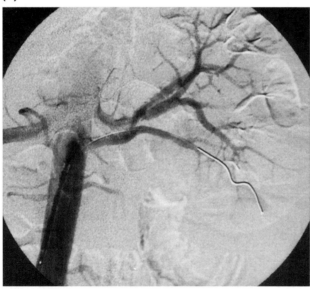

(C)

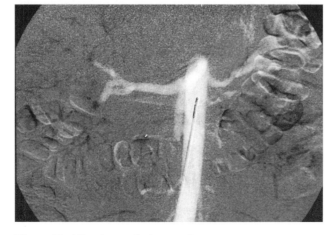

Figure 7   (*Caption on facing page*)

contrast opacification is not as good as with iodinated media, images are diagnostic in most cases (65). Opacification of the main artery and primary branches is good, but intrarenal branches and small accessory vessels may not be seen. Schreier et al. (66) reported 83% sensitivity and 99% specificity for CO_2 angiography in 100 patients. If CO_2 images do not allow confident diagnosis, they can be supplemented by a single iodinated run at an optimized obliquity as judged from the previous CO_2 images. CO_2 has several advantages over conventional contrast in that it has no nephrotoxic effect and may be used in patients allergic to contrast or those with brittle asthma. In addition, apart from the initial cost of the injector, the CO_2 itself is of negligible cost. Nevertheless, because of its inconvenience and significant minor morbidity, CO_2 angiography has a restricted place in renal artery imaging.

CT Angiography

The advent of helical and now multichannel CT has allowed CT to become a powerful tool for imaging the vascular system. The technique involves a thinly collimated helical scan through the renal vascular pedicle during a venous injection of iodinated contrast media. With each scanner generation, resolution has improved. Now we can image isotropically and reformat in any plane while maintaining image quality. Improved speeds now allow scanning of the aorta from diaphragm to iliac bifurcation within a single breath-hold. However, the imaging of renal arteries sets a difficult challenge for CT, because they run parallel or slightly oblique to the scanning plane and accessory vessels can have submillimeter dimensions. It has several advantages over conventional angiography. It is relatively noninvasive in that it does not require an arterial injection and so has consequent decreases in physician time, cost, in-patient hospital stay, patient discomfort, and complications. With improved technique it may also allow for a lower patient dose (67). CT angiography (CTA) may be used to plan the optimum projection for subsequent angiography and/or intervention (64).

Technique

For evaluation of the renal arteries, bowel contrast is not necessary; however, if this is desired, negative contrast with water should be used in preference to iodinated positive contrast. Precontrast, thick-section, low-dose scans should be obtained to localize the origins of the renal arteries and define the scanning volume. A scan from above the superior mesenteric artery to the aortic bifurcation will miss much less than 1% of accessory renal arteries (68). The thinnest slice collimation that allows adequate volume coverage within a single breath-hold should be selected. With single slice scanners, the volume to be scanned must be balanced against spatial resolution along the patient's (*z*) axis. This is obviously much less of a dilemma with multichannel scanners. Phantom studies have suggested that a maximum of 2 mm collimation is

Figure 7   (*Figure on facing page*) (**A**) LAO 20 view from the flush aortogram of a hypertensive patient. There are one right and two left renal arteries. A significant nonostial stenosis was present in the lower pole, accessory left renal artery (*arrow*). (**B**) This was resistant to conventional angioplasty but responded well to treatment with a 4 mm cutting balloon, followed by repeat dilatation with a 5 mm conventional balloon. The posttreatment appearance is shown with the guidewire still in the lower pole artery. (**C**) Pretreatment carbon dioxide angiogram in the same patient. Note that although the main renal arteries and large accessory artery are reasonably well opacified, the intrarenal vessels are not seen as a result of bolus fragmentation. *Abbreviation*: LAO, left anterior oblique.

(A)

(B)

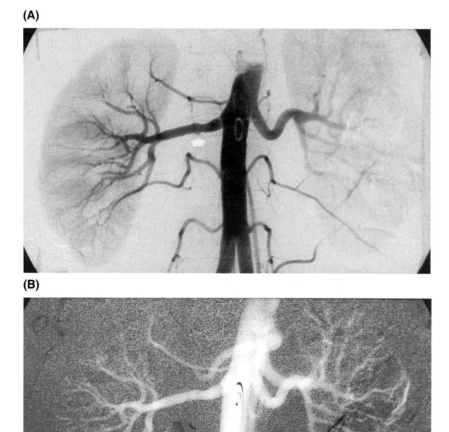

Figure 8 (**A**) Flush aortogram in a young hypertensive patient demonstrating minor aneurysmal beading (*arrow*) of the right main renal artery but no definite stenosis. The left renal artery was normal. (**B**) Carbon dioxide angiogram in the same patient. The aneurysmal segments are visible but less obvious. On selective catheterization and pressure measurement, there was a 30 mmHg gradient in the main artery. This was abolished following angioplasty. The appearances are consistent with FMD. *Abbreviation*: FMD, fibromuscular dysplasia.

required to accurately demonstrate RAS (69,70). With increasing pitch, the slice sensitivity profile is broadened, resulting in a larger effective slice thickness. However, if pitch is doubled, the volume scanned doubles, but the effective slice thickness only increases by 30% (68,71). Therefore, scans should be performed with high pitch and narrow collimation. Multichannel CT allows for much higher pitch factors. The patient should be coached in the breath-hold technique prior to the scan as respiratory artifacts can mimic a stenosis or aneurysm of the renal artery. Respiratory movement has less effect on the blood vessels caudal to the kidneys due to their being relatively fixed within the retroperitoneum. The data obtained with helical CT is converted into

Table 7 Multichannel CT of the Renal Articles

- No bowel preparation required
- Precontrast thick section localizer scan
- Scan from superior mesenteric artery to aortic bifurcation
- Dynamic bolus tracked injection of contrast
- Thinly collimated scan, for example, a slice thickness of 0.75 mm and table feed of 18 giving a pitch of 1.5

Abbreviation: CT, computed tomography.

axial slices by means of a linear interpolation algorithm. Currently, 180° interpolation is used because it decreases z-axis blur (62), allowing lower effective slice thickness. Contrast administration should maintain an enhancement plateau throughout the entire scanning period. This is best achieved by using bolus-triggering software. A region of interest is set in the aorta and sequential scans are performed at this level. When enhancement in the region reaches a predetermined threshold (usually 50–100 Hounsfield units), the scan is automatically triggered. With single slice scanners, 120 to 150 mL of contrast injected at 3 to 5 mL/sec is sufficient (68). As multichannel scanning is faster, the plateau phase can be shorter, and so less contrast is required. In addition, if the contrast bolus is chased with a 40 mL flush of saline, the plateau can be prolonged by up to eight seconds (68). Table 7 outlines an example of a scanning protocol for a 16-channel multislice CT.

Data Presentation

The volume of data gathered by helical scanning can be presented in a variety of ways, including traditional axial images, multiplanar reformats (MPRs) and curved reformats, maximum intensity projections (MIPs), and surface-shaded display (SSD). Axial images remain the mainstay of diagnosis and allow identification of nonvascular renal disease. They should be reviewed interactively on a workstation in a cine fashion, because the renal arteries may be tortuous and course through several images (72,73). Multiplanar reformatting is most useful for providing coronal images that allow appreciation of a cranio-caudally orientated stenosis that may not be obvious on axial imaging. Curved reformats are produced by tracing the course of the artery on source images followed by software straightening. They can accurately display the width of the vessel and help with grading of stenosis but are time consuming. MIP images first require editing of the data to remove overlying bony structures. Newer workstations may do this automatically. MIPs produce an angiogram-like image in which the relative attenuation values of structures are maintained, but their 3-D relationship is lost (Fig. 9). They are very sensitive for vascular calcification; unfortunately, overlying renal veins may obscure the artery. SSDs provide an attractive way of presenting findings to referring clinicians but are of limited diagnostic accuracy. In SSD, adjacent voxels above a predetermined threshold attenuation are modeled into a 3-D object (Fig. 10A,B). Apparent vessel size is very dependent on the chosen threshold for 3-D reconstruction. If the level is too low, artifacts from overlying enhancing structures will be present, too high and small vessels not seen, or stenosis overgraded (72). In single threshold reconstructions, contrast and calcified plaque cannot be separated, leading to underestimation of lumen narrowing. Both MIP and SSD perform poorly in demonstrating accessory arteries (72). Volume-rendering uses opacity curves instead of a single threshold

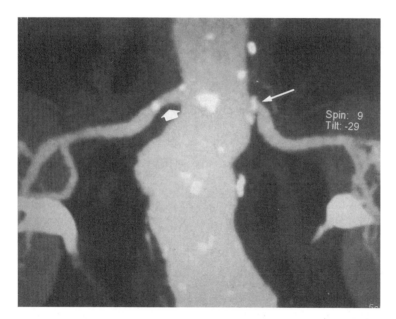

Figure 9 MIP image from a CTA in a patient with a 70% ostial stenosis of the left renal artery (*long arrow*) and a 50% nonostial stenosis of the right renal artery (*short arrow*). Note the associated small infrarenal aortic aneurysm. *Abbreviations*: CTA, computed tomography angiography; MIP, maximum intensity projection. *Source*: Courtesy of Joe Brookes, The Middlesex Hospital, London.

level. As such, the vessel lumen and calcified plaques remain separate. This rendering method can produce an angioscopic view from within the artery, allowing the arterial ostium to be viewed from the aortic lumen.

Results

The accuracy of CTA varies with the display technique utilized. Early work by Galanski et al. showed that review of the axial images with additional MPRs was superior to MIP or SSD (72). CTA was sensitive for detecting accessory renal arteries on axial images. MIP images were superior for the diagnosis of ostial stenosis. Rubin et al. found that MIP images were 92% sensitive and 83% specific for the detection of stenoses greater than or equal to 70%. SSD was only 59% sensitive and 82% specific. The accuracy for grading the stenosis was 80% for MIP but only 55% for SSD (74). A prospective comparison (75) of multislice CTA and contrast-enhanced magnetic resonance angiography (MRA) [with digital subtraction angiography (DSA) as the gold standard] showed no statistical difference between the two for evaluating aorto-iliac and renal arteries (sensitivity 92%, specificity 99%), but the authors commented that the CT images took significantly more time to read than MRA studies.

Nevertheless, many studies have shown CTA to be a highly effective method for the noninvasive diagnosis of RAS, with sensitivities of 88% to 100% and specificities of 87% to 99% (Table 8) (68,76–82) and in close agreement with DSA for grading of stenosis (80). A normal CTA virtually rules out significant RAS with a negative predictive value of 95% (83). A meta-analysis (51) found that CTA along with contrast MRA performed significantly better than ultrasound and captopril scintigraphy.

(A)

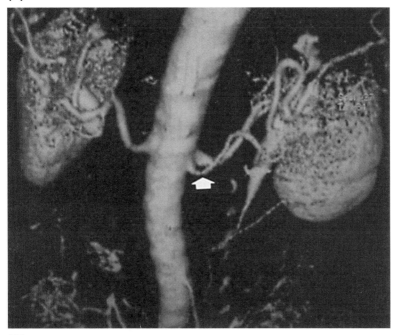

(B)

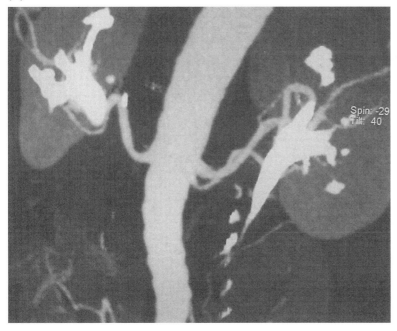

Figure 10 (**A**) SSD in a patient with one right and two left renal arteries. There is a nonostial stenosis of the lower of the left renal arteries (*arrow*). (**B**) Corresponding MIP image; note that the relative densities of the different structures are maintained here, whereas they are lost on the SSD. *Abbreviations*: SSD, surface-shaded display; MIP, maximum intensity projection. *Source*: Courtesy of Joe Brookes, The Middlesex Hospital, London.

Table 8 Performance of CT in the Detection of RAS

Study	Number of patients	Definition of significant stenosis (%)	Sensitivity (%)	Specificity (%)
Ref. 76	27	N/A	90	98
Ref. 77	50	50	94	95
Ref. 78	82	50	96	99
Ref. 79	25	50	94	87
Ref. 80	71	50	96	96
Ref. 81	50	50	88	98
Ref. 82	52	50	100	92

Abbreviations: CT, computed tomography; RAS, renal artery stenosis.

Furthermore, these results relate mainly to studies based on single slice technology. It can be expected that multichannel scanning will perform even better. One author (80) made the point that some false positive CTA results were in fact DSA false negatives—DSA is not infallible; e.g., the renal artery ostia may be obscured by the aorta especially with unusual (anterior) origins.

CT can also accurately define the site of stenosis and the degree of calcification, but it does have its limitations. If older scanners are used with wider collimation (3 mm), sensitivity drops appreciably (67–90%) (68,70,81,84,85). Calcification can obscure stenosis on MIP images (Fig. 11); in these cases, the axial images should be viewed. Even on these, "blooming" of calcium may overstate stenosis, but this effect can be decreased by viewing on bone windows (75). Arteries with high-grade stenosis may be discontinuous on CTA, mimicking occlusion. Contrast in the artery distal to the apparent occlusion favors stenosis over-occlusion.

Secondary signs of RAS are detectable on CT. For example post-stenotic dilatation and asymmetrical renal enhancement are specific but not sensitive for significant RAS (74). It is also possible to diagnose FMD on CTA. Beregi et al. (85) studied 20 patients, all with FMD, and found they could make the diagnosis in all of them with CTA—MIPs were more sensitive than review of axial images. Using both sets of images, the overall sensitivity for individual lesions was 87%. However some weblike FMD lesions are below the resolving power of even angiography, and so with its lower resolution, CTA cannot be recommended to exclude FMD; angiography with pressure measurement should remain the diagnostic method of choice.

Although diagnostically impressive and becoming more widely available, the radiation dose, potential for contrast nephrotoxicity, and its cost limit the use of CTA as a primary diagnostic or screening investigation. Patients with diabetes and renal impairment are at high risk for contrast-induced nephrotoxicity. These patients should be preferentially investigated with MRA. If this is not possible and CTA is required, they should receive prehydration with intravenous normal saline at a rate of 100 mL/hr, for at least six hours prior to the scan and continuing for 12 hours afterwards. The absolute minimum dose of nonionic contrast should be used.

MRA

Like CT, MRI has the capability to produce angiogram-like studies of the vascular system. It has the additional benefits of avoiding ionizing radiation and nephrotoxic contrast media. A 3-D volume of data is acquired and may be viewed in any plane

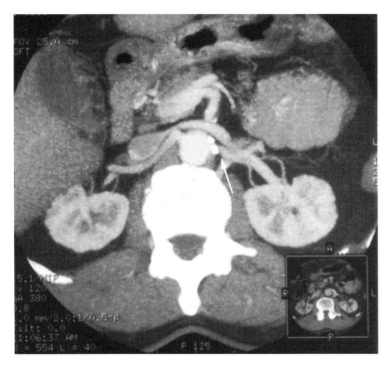

Figure 11 Axial MIP image from the CTA of a patient with bilateral RAS. The heavily calcified left renal artery ostium (*arrow*) partially obscures the stenosis. *Abbreviations*: CTA, computed tomography angiography; MIP, maximum intensity projection; RAS, renal artery stenosis. *Source*: Courtesy of Robert Morgan, St. George's Hospital, London.

from this single acquisition. Both renal ostia can thus be displayed to best advantage on a single study compared to perhaps multiple runs of conventional angiography. Two distinct methods of imaging are available: flow-enhanced and contrast-enhanced techniques.

Time-of-Flight and Phase Contrast Imaging

Both of these techniques rely on the effect of flow to provide a large differential in signal between flowing blood and stationary tissue. They are limited in that they can visualize only the proximal 3 to 3.5 cm of the renal artery; only around half of the accessory arteries are shown, and turbulence seen as signal loss may overgrade stenosis as occlusion (52). Published sensitivities and specificities for significant stenosis are 53% to 100% and 65% to 97% respectively (86–90). The advent of newer magnetic resonance (MR) systems with stronger, faster gradients have made gadolinium-enhanced scans possible and rendered these methods obsolete.

Contrast-Enhanced MRI

Many of the shortcomings of flow-enhanced imaging can be surmounted by the use of T1-weighted contrast-enhanced scanning (Table 9). Because the arterial contrast is not reliant on flowing blood, it avoids the artifacts that undermine other methods, namely spin dephasing and in-plane flow artifacts (91). Gadolinium, a paramagnetic contrast agent, is thought to be safe even in high doses in patients with abnormal renal function (92). However, there have been some reports of nephrotoxicity in

Table 9 Contrast Enhanced MR of the Renal Arteries

- High resolution T1-weighted gradient echo pulse sequence with a short TR and TE
- Phased array coil
- Field of view 30–36 cm to cover from the SMA to the aortic bifurcation
- 20–30 second breath hold
- Dynamic bolus tracked injection of contrast
- 2–3 mm sections acquired in the coronal plane from the anterior aortic wall backward

---

Abbreviations: MR, magnetic resonance; SMA, superior mesenteric artery; TR, time to repetition; TE, time to echo.

patients with diabetic nephropathy. Care should be taken when using it in these patients, but in general, the available data suggest that gadolinium is much safer than conventional contrast. Gadolinium is dynamically injected intravenously to enhance the signal from blood by shortening its T1 value. Images are acquired during a single breath-hold using a high-resolution 3-D T1-weighted gradient echo technique, pre- and postcontrast. Scanning should be performed in the coronal plane with 2 to 3 mm sections from the anterior border of the aorta back (91). The precontrast images can then be subtracted, thus improving the vessel-to-background contrast. Image quality is significantly increased by using a phased array coil. Images from the mesenteric vessels to the aortic bifurcation can be acquired in a 20 to 30 second breath-hold (93–95). As with CT, the timing of the scan is important. Too early, and there will be inadequate arterial enhancement; too late, and there will be excessive venous and soft tissue enhancement. The optimum start time can be determined by using a 2 mL contrast test bolus and performing sequential single slice imaging of the aorta to ascertain the transit time to the renal arteries. Alternatively, an automatic bolus-triggering software that starts the scan when the level of enhancement in the aorta reaches a threshold is now present on most MR systems. A dose of 0.2 mmol/kg of contrast is injected at a rate of 1.5 to 2 mL/sec. Additional precontrast T1 and T2 fast spin echo images may be obtained to assess the renal size and detect parenchymal disease, morphological anomalies, and adrenal pathology. Newer scanners read central k-space first, which encodes contrast, and fill peripheral, spatial k-space later. This allows the contrast data to be acquired early in the breath-hold when there is maximal enhancement. The data should be viewed on a workstation with multiplanar reconstruction capability. Coronal and axial MIP images may be generated from the 3-D volume, producing an angiographic image (Fig. 12). Multiplanar projection images are useful in analyzing the renal artery ostia, especially when there is superimposition of the renal vein. Recent experimental work has also explored the value of functional renal MRI. Binkert et al. (96) studied renal artery blood flow and renal volume with MR and found that it had a 91% sensitivity but only 67% specificity for the prediction of a clinical response to angioplasty. These methods await further validation, but they may extend the potential of MR in atherosclerotic renal disease (97).

Results

A recent meta-analysis (98) of contrast and noncontrast MRA showed the former to be significantly better. The investigators analyzed 25 studies comparing MRA blindly with catheter angiography. The contrast-MRA group included 499 patients with 993 renal arteries and 183 accessory arteries. Overall sensitivity was 97% and specificity 93%. The performance in the detection of accessory renal arteries was

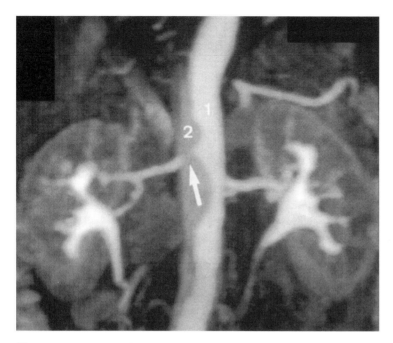

Figure 12 Coronal view from a contrast-enhanced MR angiogram in a patient with a type B aortic dissection. The renal arteries arise from the true lumen (1); the false lumen is marked (2). Note the associated stenosis of the right renal artery (*arrow*). *Abbreviation*: MR, magnetic resonance. *Source*: Courtesy of Joe Brookes, The Middlesex Hospital, London.

significantly better with contrast MRA than noncontrast MRA, with a detection rate of 82% compared with 49% (Fig. 13A,B). Most of the arteries missed on contrast MR either were very small or originated from unusual locations. In another meta-analysis, this time comparing different diagnostic tests for RAS, Boudewijn et al. (51) found CTA and enhanced MRA to be significantly better than the other tests. They calculated receiver-operating characteristic (ROC) curves for the different modalities and found areas under the curve of 0.99 for contrast MRA and CTA. This signifies that these tests can achieve a high sensitivity at low rates of false positivity. The results of other studies on contrast-enhanced MRA of the renal artery are shown in Table 10 (33,46,53,99–106). With regard to grading of stenosis, MRA has been found to have the same interobserver variability as conventional angiography (46,107). Like CTA, MRA can demonstrate secondary changes seen in RAS, i.e., post-stenotic dilatation (Fig. 14), reduction in size, asymmetrical enhancement, and concentration of contrast. Conversely, a study by Qanadli et al. (46) observed that with a normal MRA, RAS could be reliably excluded in 98% of patients.

Limitations and Pitfalls

Even with newer machines, visualization of vessels past the renal hilum is inconsistent. Therefore the evaluation of branch vessels is unsatisfactory when compared with DSA. However, technical advances are likely to provide better resolution in the future. Because FMD affects the distal artery and branches, it makes its exclusion with MRA difficult, and DSA with pressure measurement should remain the investigation of choice. Classical cases ("string of pearls") of FMD may be observed on MR (Fig. 15). MRA has a tendency to overestimate moderate stenosis. This is

(A)

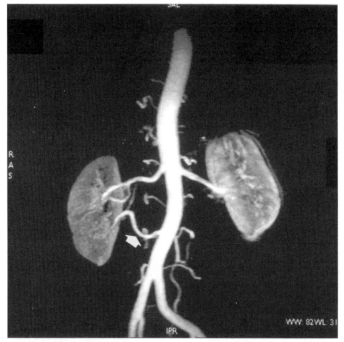

(B)

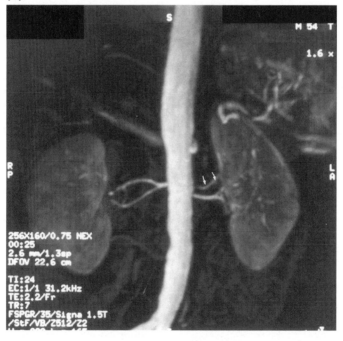

Figure 13 (**A**) Contrast-enhanced MR angiogram with subtraction of background image. A lower pole accessory renal artery is demonstrated on the right (*arrow*). (**B**) MR is increasingly being used in the preoperative work-up of living renal donors, providing vital information for the transplant surgeon. In this case there is early branching of the right renal artery and a left upper pole accessory artery (*arrows*). *Abbreviation*: MR, magnetic resonance.

Table 10 Performance of Contrast-Enhanced MRA in the Detection of RAS

Study	Number of patients	Definition of significant stenosis (%)	Sensitivity (%)	Specificity (%)
Ref. 99	39	50	100	100
Ref. 46	41	50	97	–
Ref. 100	26	50	96	93
Ref. 53	43	50	100	94
Ref. 33	45	50	100	93
Ref. 101	62	50	88	98
Ref. 102	44	50	97	92
Ref. 103	20	N/A	100	98
Ref. 104	55	50	94	96
Ref. 105	30	50	100	71
Ref. 106	32	N/A	100	89

Abbreviations: MRA, magnetic resonance angiography; RAS, renal artery stenosis.

due to signal loss from turbulent flow distal to the stenosis. MIPs may miss small accessory arteries because other structures may obscure them. The source images should be scrutinized for such vessels (104,108).

Transplant Artery Stenosis

Cadaveric transplant kidneys are joined to the recipient's external iliac artery via an end-to-side anastamosis. Living donor kidneys are joined to either the external iliac

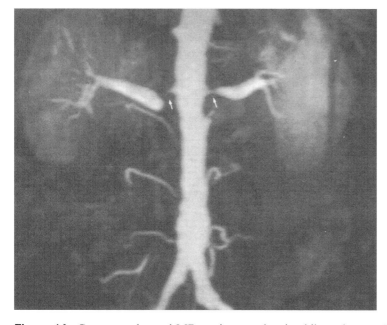

Figure 14 Contrast-enhanced MR angiogram showing bilateral severe RAS (*arrows*). Note the post-stenotic dilatation. *Abbreviations*: MR, magnetic resonance; RAS, renal artery stenosis. *Source*: Courtesy of Joe Brookes, The Middlesex Hospital, London.

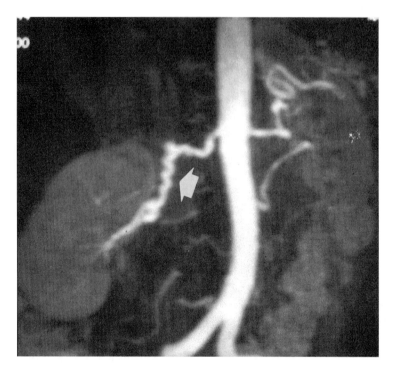

Figure 15 Contrast-enhanced MR angiogram showing the "string of pearls" (*arrow*) appearance of FMD in the right renal artery. *Abbreviations*: FMD, fibromuscular dysplasia; MR, magnetic resonance. *Source*: Courtesy of Joe Brookes, The Middlesex Hospital, London.

end-to-side or internal iliac end-to-end (109). Stenosis of the transplant artery is well recognized. Improved surgical techniques and immunosuppressive therapy have led to increased graft longevity. As a result, transplant artery stenosis is more of a clinical problem with an incidence of 1% to 15% (110,111), mostly within the first three years. Stenosis can occur in the recipient iliac artery, at the anastamosis, or distal to the anastamosis. Causes and predisposing factors include native vessel atherosclerosis, clamp injury, rejection, turbulence distal to the anastamosis, and surgical technique (109). Clinical pointers to stenosis include hypertension and worsening function in the absence of rejection or ureteric obstruction.

As with native renal arteries, a variety of noninvasive tests have been investigated to exclude stenosis. Contrast-enhanced MRA shows promise with sensitivities and specificities of up to 100% and 97% respectively (112). As before, its avoidance of radiation and nephrotoxic agents are particular strengths and its tendency to overgrade stenosis, a weakness. CTA should also provide an accurate assessment of the transplant artery but requires a large volume of contrast, and metallic surgical clips may cause streak artifact. Duplex ultrasound is the most commonly used screening method, with sensitivities of 87% to 94% and specificities of 86% to 100% (113–115) in experienced hands. Of the multiple Doppler indices, peak systolic velocity has been shown to be the most accurate (111). A peak systolic velocity of greater than 2.5 m/sec was 100% sensitive and 95% specific for the detection of stenosis greater than 50%. In our more recent experience, this threshold performs poorly in a low-risk or surveillance population (116), so we now use a threshold of 3.0 m/sec. However, vessel tortuosity can make scanning problematic, and inadequate angle correction may reap misleading results. Catheter angiography with pressure measurement may still be needed to exclude stenosis or differentiate it from vessel kinking (117). An ipsilateral approach is used if the transplant is joined end-to-side to the external iliac artery (Fig. 16A). End-to-end internal iliac anastamoses are easier to catheterize from the other side. Rotational angiography (118) with 3-D

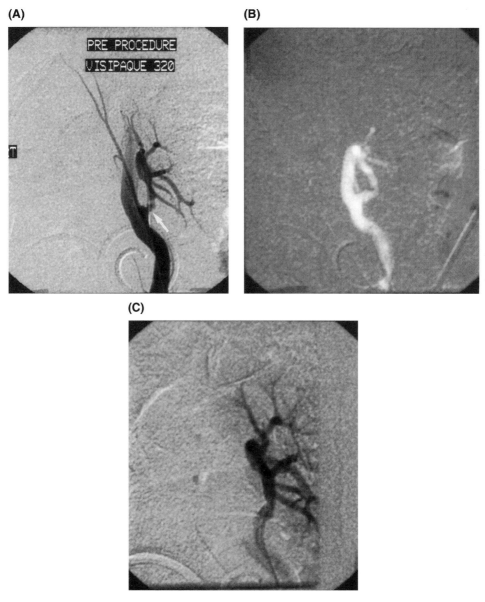

Figure 16 (**A**) Transplant angiogram, RAO 60 projection. The transplant artery is joined end-to-side to the external iliac artery. There is a significant proximal stenosis (*arrow*). (**B**) Carbon dioxide run at the same projection. Note the poor delineation of the peripheral vessels. (**C**) Gadolinium angiogram taken postdeployment of a 6 mm stent. Although the opacification is not as good as conventional contrast, the renal artery branches are well seen. *Abbreviation*: RAO, right anterior oblique.

reconstruction, or at least multiple projections, should be used to demonstrate the artery to advantage. The use of contrast agents carbon dioxide and gadolinium is limited by bolus fragmentation and poor visibility, respectively (Fig. 16B,C). As in the native renal artery, a pressure gradient should always be sought before intervention is performed.

Endovascular Therapy for RAS

Catheter-based treatments have revolutionized the management of occlusive renovascular disease. However, because many patients may have stenosis without clinical effect, treatment should be limited to hemodynamically significant stenoses in patients in the clinical scenarios mentioned earlier. Patients with significant truncal stenosis or FMD should be treated with angioplasty. Primary stenting is needed for ostial lesions because the elastic recoil of aortic plaques makes them resistant to angioplasty (Fig. 17). Factors suggestive of successful revascularization include: bilateral disease, preservation of renal mass, preserved function on nuclear scintigraphy, and minimal arteriolar sclerosis on biopsy (119). A meta-analysis by Rees (120) reported a 99% primary patency rate for stents in 1128 arteries (cf. 55% and 70% for percutaneous transluminal angioplasty of ostial and nonstial stenoses, respectively) and a secondary patency of 77% at a mean of 7.9 months.

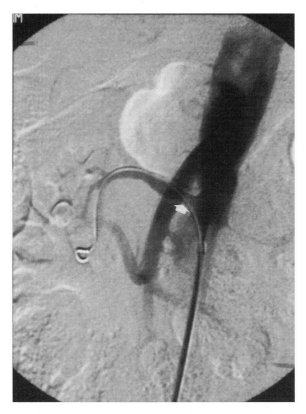

Figure 17 The same patient shown in Figure 1. Post-stent angiogram showing normal lumen dimensions following deployment of a 6 mm balloon expandable stent (*arrow*). The guidewire is still within the artery.

CONCLUSION

All of the efforts put into imaging the renal arteries will not be worthwhile if the treatments they subsequently direct do not bring improvements in patient outcome.

Although the results of endovascular therapy are technically impressive, at the time of writing, randomized controlled studies comparing pharmacological management with endovascular correction of RAS are keenly awaited. A meta-analysis of three small trials comparing angioplasty with best medical therapy alone has failed to give us a clear direction (14). The DRASTIC study (121) reported in early 2004 found that although there was a clear benefit from immediate angioplasty in patients with bilateral stenosis, it could be deferred in other patients unless they deteriorated clinically. Once again this study was small, with only 106 patients. Two other trials, STAR (122) and ASTRAL (123), are currently in progress in Europe. The largest of these, ASTRAL, will include 1000 patients (at the last report in late 2005, 600 patients had been enlisted). This trial should have the statistical power to conclusively prove or refute the value of treating RAS. They will use the objective end-points of renal preservation and hypertensive control, and the cost-effectiveness of the various investigations may be calculated. Only then will the case for early diagnosis or even screening or active case-finding become compelling. The main tools for diagnosis are likely to be MRA and CTA. However contrast-induced nephrotoxicity is a major source of concern in this group of patients.

To summarize, RAS is an important cause of hypertension and renal failure, especially in patients with arterial disease in other vascular territories. Narrowing of the artery beyond 70% of its cross-sectional area is generally accepted to represent a significant stenosis. However, RAS may be clinically silent. Its prevalence runs

Table 11 Benefits and Limitations of the Different Imaging Modalities

Modality	Advantages	Disadvantages
MRI	Reproducible No radiation/nephrotoxic contrast 3-D imaging shows arterial ostium to advantage	May overestimate stenosis Contraindicated for/not tolerated by some patients
CT	Reproducible 3-D Resolution improving all the time	Contrast and radiation dose
Ultrasound	Cost Availability Noninvasiveness	Accuracy may fall with inexperience of operator Less reproducible Misses accessory renal arteries High technical-failure rate
Nuclear medicine	May predict response to treatment Gives information on kidney function	Not as accurate as other methods
Angiography	Accurate Pressures can be measured May proceed directly to intervention	Cost Complications Contrast dose Ostial lesions may be projected over the aorta and missed

Abbreviations: MRI, magnetic resonance imaging; CT, computed tomography.

between 1% and 5% in an unselected hypertensive population. Clinical markers of RAS may be employed to allow a more selective investigation of patients. An overview of the strengths and weaknesses of the available imaging modalities is given in Table 11. At the moment MRA seems to be the best choice with its safety and accuracy. If MRA is not available or is contraindicated, a strong case can also be made for CTA. However in patients with renal impairment, contrast media–induced nephropathy is a major source for concern. In this group and others, contrast-enhanced Doppler ultrasound may be of assistance if there is local expertise in the technique.

REFERENCES

1. Goldblatt H, Lynch J, Hanzal RF, Summerville WW. The production of persistent elevation of systolic blood pressure by means of renal ischaemia. J Exp Med 1934; 59:347–378.
2. Schwartz CJ, White TA. Stenosis of the renal artery: an unselected necropsy study. BMJ 1964; 2:1415–1421.
3. Safian RD, Textor SC. Renal artery stenosis. N Engl J Med 2001; 344:431–442.
4. Derkx FH, Schalekamp MA. Renal artery stenosis and hypertension. Lancet 1994; 344:237–239.
5. Eardley KS, Lipkin GW. Atherosclerotic renal artery stenosis: is it worth diagnosing? J Hum Hypertens 1999; 13:217–220.
6. Harding MB, Smith LR, Himmelstein SI. Renal artery stenosis: prevalence and associated risk factors in patients undergoing routine cardiac catheterization. J Am Soc Nephrol 1992; 2:1608–1616.
7. Swartbol P, Thorvinger BO, Parsson H, Norgren L. Renal artery stenosis in patients with peripheral vascular disease and its correlation to hypertension. A retrospective study. Int Angiol 1992; 11:195–199.
8. Olin JW, Melia M, Young JR, Graor RA, Risius B. Prevalence of atherosclerotic renal artery stenosis in patients with atherosclerosis elsewhere. Am J Med 1988; (1N):46N–51N.
9. Maxwell MH, Bleifer KH, Franklin SS, Varady PD. Cooperative study of renovascular hypertension: demographic analysis of the study. JAMA 1972; 220:1195–1204.
10. Butler PF. Applied Radiological Anatomy. Cambridge: Cambridge University Press, 1999.
11. Scoble JE. Renal artery stenosis as a cause of renal impairment: implications for treatment of hypertension and congestive heart failure. J R Soc Med 1999; 92:505–510.
12. Main J. When should atheromatous renal artery stenosis be considered? Clin Med 2003; 3:520–525.
13. McLaughlin K, Jardine AG, Moss JG. ABC of arterial and venous disease. Renal artery stenosis. BMJ 2000; 320:1124–1127.
14. Ives NJ, Wheatley K, Stowe RL, Krijnen P. Continuing uncertainty about the value of percutaneous revascularisation in atherosclerotic renovascular disease: a meta-analysis of randomized trials. Nephrol Dial Transplant 2003; 18:298–304.
15. Ramsay LE, Waller PC. Blood pressure response to percutaneous transluminal angioplasty for renovascular hypertension: an overview of published series. BMJ 1990; 300: 569–572.
16. Scoble JE, Maher ER, Hamilton G, Dick R, Sweny P, Moorhead JF. Atherosclerotic renovascular disease causing renal impairment: case for treatment. Clin Nephrol 1989; 31:119–122.
17. Mailloux LU, Napolitano B, Belluci AG, Vernance M, Wilkes BM, Mossey RT. Renal vascular disease causing end-stage renal disease; incidence, clinical correlates and outcomes: a 20-year clinical experience. Am J Kidney Dis 1994; 24:622–629.

18. Conlon PJ, Athirakul K, Schwab SJ, Crowley J, Stack R, Albers S. Long term follow up of asymptomatic renal vascular disease. Am Soc Nephrol 1996; 7:1384.

19. Zierler RE, Bergelin RO, Isaacson JA, Strandness DE Jr. Natural history of athero-sclerotic renal artery stenosis. A prospective study with duplex ultrasonography. J Vasc Surg 1994; 19:250–258.

20. Guzman RP, Zierler RE, Isaacson JA, Bergelin RO, Strandness DE Jr. Renal atrophy and arterial stenosis: a prospective study with duplex ultrasound. Hypertension 1994; 23:346–350.

21. Watson PS, Hadjipetrou P, Cox SV, Piemonte TC, Eisenhauer AC. Effect of renal artery stenting on renal function and size in patients with atherosclerotic renovascular disease. Circulation 2000; 102:1671–1677.

22. Zocali C, Mallamaci F, Finochiaro P. Atherosclerotic renal artery stenosis: epidemi-ology, cardiovascular outcomes, and clinical prediction rules. J Am Nephrol 2002; 13: S179–S183.

23. Basta LL, Williams C, Kioschos JM, Spector AA. Regression of atherosclerotic stenos-ing lesions of the renal arteries and spontaneous cure of systemic hypertension through control of hyperlipidaemia. Am J Med 1976; 61:420–423.

24. Khong TK, Missouris CG, Belli AM, Macgregor GA. Regression of atherosclerotic renal artery stenosis with aggressive lipid lowering therapy. J Hum Hypertens 2001; 15:431–433.

25. Farmer CKT, Reidy J, Kalra PA, Cook GJR, Scoble JE. Individual kidney function before and after renal angioplasty. Lancet 1998; 352:288–289.

26. Stansby GP, Scoble JE, Hamilton G. Use of hepatic arterial circulation for renal revas-cularisation. Ann R Coll Surg Engl 1992; 7:260–264.

27. Pickering TG, Herman L, Devereux RB, et al. Recurrent pulmonary oedema in hyper-tension due to bilateral renal artery stenosis: treatment by angioplasty or surgical revas-cularisation. Lancet 1988; 2:551–552.

28. MacDowall P, Kalra PA, O'Donoghue DJ, Waldock S, Mamotora H, Brown K. Risk of morbidity from renovascular disease in elderly patients with congestive cardiac fail-ure. Lancet 1998; 352:13–16.

29. Soulez G, Oliva VL, Turpin S, Lambert R, Nicolet V, Therasse E. Imaging of renovas-cular hypertension: respective values of renal scintigraphy, renal Doppler US and MR angiography. Radiographics 2000; 20:1355–1368.

30. Dresberg AL, Paushter DM, Lammert GK, et al. Renal artery stenosis: evaluation with colour Doppler flow imaging. Radiology 1990; 177:749–753.

31. Miralles M, Cairols M, Cotillas J. Value of Doppler parameters in the diagnosis of renal artery stenosis. J Vasc Surg 1996; 23:428–435.

32. Chain S, Herrera RN, Mercau G, et al. Ultrasound Doppler technique and the renal arteries: diagnostic impact of the echo enhancer sh u 508a and a new renal hilar velo-cities index. Echocardiography 2004; 21:204.

33. De Cobelli F, Venturini M, Vanzulli A, et al. Renal artery stenosis: prospective compar-ison of color Doppler US and breath-hold, three-dimensional, dynamic, gadolinium-enhanced MR angiography. Radiology 2000; 214:373–380.

34. Claudon M, Rohban T. Levovist (SH U 508 A) in the diagnosis of renal artery stenosis: results of controlled multicentre study. Radiology 1997; 205:242.

35. Olin JW, Piemonte MR, Young JR, De Anna S, Grubb M, Childs MB. The utility of duplex ultrasound scanning of the renal arteries for diagnosing significant renal artery stenosis. Ann Int Med 1995; 122:833–838.

36. Hoffman U, Edwards JM, Carter S. Role of duplex scanning for the detection of ather-osclerotic renal artery disease. Kidney Int 1991; 39:1232–1239.

37. Kohler TR, Zierler RE, Martin RL. Noninvasive diagnosis of renal artery stenosis by ultrasonic duplex scanning. J Vasc Surg 1986; 4:450–456.

38. Bude RO, Rubin JM. Detection of renal artery stenosis with Doppler sonography: it is more complicated than originally thought (editorial). Radiology 1995; 196:612–613.

39. Lafortune M, Patriquin HB, Demeule E. Renal artery stenosis: slowed systole in the downstream circulation—experimental study in dogs. Radiology 1992; 184:475–478.
40. Handa N, Fukanga R, Uehara A. Echo-doppler velocimeter in the diagnosis of hypertensive patients: the renal artery Doppler technique. Ultrasound Med Biol 1986; 12:945–952.
41. Ripolles T, Aliaga R, Morote V, et al. Utility of intrarenal Doppler ultrasound in the diagnosis of renal artery stenosis. Eur J Radiol 2001; 40:54–63.
42. Stavros AT, Parker SH, Wayne FY. Segmental stenosis of the renal artery: pattern recognition of tardus and parvus abnormalities with duplex sonography. Radiology 1992; 184:487–492.
43. Patriquin HB, Lafortune M, Jequier JC. Stenosis of the renal artery: assessment of slowed systole in the downstream circulation with Doppler sonography. Radiology 1992; 184:479–485.
44. Kliewer MA, Tuple RH, Hertzberg BS. Doppler evaluation of renal artery stenosis: interobserver agreement in the interpretation of waveform morphology. Am J Roentgenol 1994; 162:1371–1376.
45. Van der Hulst VPM, Van Baalen J, Kool LS, et al. Renal artery stenosis: endovascular flow wire study for validation of Doppler US. Radiology 1996; 200:165–168.
46. Qanadli SD, Soulez G, Therasse E, et al. Detection of renal artery stenosis: prospective comparison of captopril-enhanced Doppler sonography, captopril-enhanced scintigraphy, and MR angiography. Am J Roentgenol 2001; 177:1123–1129.
47. Lencioni R, Pinto S, Napoli V, Bartolozzi C. Noninvasive assessment of renal artery stenosis: current imaging protocols and future directions in ultrasonography. J Comput Assist Tomogr 1999:S95–S100.
48. Calliada F, Bottinelli O, Campani R, Sala G, Corradi B, Draghi F. Optimization of color and spectral Doppler scanning of the renal arteries using a US contrast agent and second harmonic imaging. Radiology 1997; 205:241.
49. Lees WR. Echo-enhanced renal ultrasound imaging with Levovist SH U 508 A. Angiology 1996; 47:S31–S35.
50. Blebea J, Zickler R, Volteas N, et al. Duplex imaging of the renal arteries with contrast enhancement. Vasc Endovasc Surg 2003; 37:429–436.
51. Boudewijn G, Vasbinder C, Nelemans PJ, et al. Diagnostic tests for renal artery stenosis in patients suspected of having renovascular hypertension: a meta-analysis. Ann Int Med 2001; 135:401–411.
52. Grenier N, Trillaud H. Comparison of imaging methods for renal artery stenosis. BJU Int 2000; 86:S84–S94.
53. Bongers V, Bakker J, Beutler JJ, Beek FJ, De Klerk JM. Assessment of renal artery stenosis: comparison of captopril renography and gadolinium enhanced breath-hold MR angiography. Clin Radiol 2000; 55:346–353.
54. Gezici A, Ersay A, Antevska V, Heidental GK, Schreij G, Demirtas OC. Quantitative residual cortical activity measurement: appropriate test for renal artery stenosis? Urol Int 1999; 62:1–7.
55. Fommei E, Ghione S, Hilson AJW. Captopril radionuclide test in renovascular hypertension: European multicenter study. In: O'Reilly PH, Taylor A, Nally JV, eds. Radionuclides in Nephrourology. Blue Bell, PA: Field and Wood Medical Periodicals, Inc., 1994:33–37.
56. Jensen G, Moonen M, Aureli M. Reliability of ACE inhibitor-enhanced ^{99m} Tc-DTPA gamma camera renography in the detection of renovascular hypertension. Nucl Med Commun 1993; 14:169–175.
57. Dondi M, Fanti S, De Fabritiis A. Prognostic value of captopril renal scintigraphy in renovascular hypertension. J Nucl Med 1992; 33:2040–2044.
58. Mann SJ, Pickering TG, Tan S. Captopril renography in the diagnosis of renal artery stenosis: accuracy and limitations. Am J Med 1991; 90:30–40.

59. Erbsloh-Moller B, Dumas A, Roth D. Furosemide I-131-hippuran renography after angiotensin-converting enzyme inhibition for the diagnosis of renovascular hypertension. Am J Med 1991; 90:23–29.

60. Geyskes GG, de Bruyn AJG. Captopril renography and the effect of percutaneous transluminal angioplasty on blood pressure in 94 patients with renal artery stenosis. Am J Hypertens 1991; 4:S685–S689.

61. Taylor A. Renovascular hypertension: nuclear medicine techniques. Q J Nucl Med 2002; 46:268–282.

62. Rankin SC, Saunders AJS, Cook GJR, Scoble JE. Renovascular disease. Clin Rad 2000; 55:1–12.

63. Bonn J. Percutaneous vascular intervention—value of haemodynamic measurements. Radiology 1996; 201:18–20.

64. Verschuyl EJ, Kaatee R, Beek FJ. Renal artery origins: best angiographic projection angles. Radiology 1996; 199:637–640.

65. Beese RC, Bees NR, Belli AM. Renal angiography using carbon dioxide. Br J Radiol 2000; 73:3–6.

66. Schreier DZ, Weaver FA, Frankhouse J, et al. A prospective study of carbon dioxide—digital subtraction vs standard contrast arteriography in the evaluation of the renal arteries. Arch Surg 1996; 131:503–508.

67. Ruiz-Cruces R, Perez-Martinez M, Martin-Palanca A. Patient dose in radiologically guided interventional vascular procedures: conventional versus digital systems. Radiology 1997; 205:385–393.

68. Prokop M. Protocols and future directions in imaging of renal artery stenosis: CT angiography. J Comput Assist Tomogr 1999; 23:S101–S110.

69. Fielding JR, Silverman SG, Rubin GD. Helical CT of the urinary tract. Am J Roentgenol 1999; 172:1199–1206.

70. Brink JA, Lim JT, Wang G, Heiken JP, Deyoe LA, Vannier MW. Technical optimization of spiral CT for depiction of renal artery stenosis: in vitro analysis. Radiology 1995; 194:157–163.

71. Polacin A, Kalender WA, Marchal G. Evaluation of section sensitivity profiles and image noise in spiral CT. Radiology 1992; 185:29–35.

72. Galanski M, Prokop M, Chavan A, Schaefer CM, Jandeleit K, Nischelsky JE. Renal arterial stenoses: spiral CT angiography. Radiology 1993; 189:185–192.

73. Urban BA, Ratner LE, Fishman EK. Three-dimensional volume-rendered CT angiography of the renal arteries and veins: normal anatomy, variants, and clinical applications. Radiographics 2001; 21:373–386.

74. Rubin GD, Dake MD, Napel S. Spiral CT of renal artery stenosis: comparison of three-dimensional rendering techniques. Radiology 1994; 190:181–189.

75. Willmann JK, Wildermuth S, Pfammatter T, et al. Aortoiliac and renal arteries: prospective intraindividual comparison of contrast-enhanced three-dimensional MR angiography and multi-detector row CT angiography. Radiology 2003; 226: 798–811.

76. Hahn U, Konig CW, Miller S, et al. Multidetector CT angiography—is it a valuable screening tool to detect significant renal artery stenosis? Rofo Fortschr Geb Rontgenstr Neuen Bildgeb Verfahr 2001; 173:1086–1092.

77. Equine O, Beregi JP, Mounier-Vehier C, Gautier C, Desmoucelles F, Carre A. Importance of echo-doppler and helical angioscanner of the renal arteries in the management of renovascular diseases. Arch Mal Coeur Vaiss 1999; 92:1043–1045.

78. Wittenberg G, Kenn W, Tschammler A, Sandstede J, Hahn D. Spiral CT angiography of renal arteries: comparison with angiography. Eur Radiol 1999; 9:546–551.

79. Johnson PT, Halpern EJ, Kuszyk BS. Renal artery stenosis: CT angiography—comparison of real-time rendering and maximum intensity projection algorithms. Radiology 1999; 211:337–343.

80. Kaatee R, Beek FJ, De Lange EE, et al. Renal artery stenosis: detection and quantification with spiral CT angiography versus optimized digital subtraction angiography. Radiology 1997; 205:121–127.

81. Beregi JP, Elkohen M, Deklunder G, Artaud D, Coullet JM, Wattinee L. Helical CT angiography compared with arteriography in the detection of renal artery stenosis. Am J Roentgenol 1996; 167:495–501.

82. Galanski M, Prokop M, Chavan A, Schaefer C, Jandeleit K, Olbricht C. Leistungsfahigkeit der CT—Angiographie beim Nachweis von Nierenarterienstenosen. Rofo 1994; 161:519–525.

83. Fleischmann D. Multiple detector-row CT angiography of the renal and mesenteric vessels. Eur J Radiol 2003; 45:S79–S87.

84. Kim TS, Chung JW, Park JH, Kim SH, Yeon KM, Han MC. Renal artery evaluation: comparison of spiral CT angiography to intra-arterial DSA. J Vasc Interv Radiol 1998; 9:553–559.

85. Beregi JP, Louvegny S, Gautier C, et al. Fibromuscular dysplasia of the renal arteries: comparison of helical CT angiography and arteriography. Am J Roentgenol 1999; 172:27–34.

86. Debatin JF, Spritzer CE, Grist TM. Imaging of the renal arteries: value of MR angiography. Am J Roentgenol 1991; 157:981–990.

87. Richter CS, Krestin GP, Eichenberger AC, Schopke W, Fuchs WA. Assessment of renal artery stenosis by phase-contrast magnetic resonance angiography. Eur Radiol 1993; 3:493–498.

88. Loubeyre P, Revel D, Garcia P. Screening patients for renal artery stenosis: value of three-dimensional time-of-flight MR angiography. Am J Roentgenol 1995; 162:847–852.

89. Gedroyc WMW, Neerhut P, Negus R. Magnetic resonance angiography of renal artery stenosis. Clin Radiol 1995; 50:436–439.

90. Loubeyre P, Trolliet P, Cahen R, Grozel F, Labeeuw M, Tram Minh VA. MR angiography of renal artery stenosis: value of the combination of three-dimensional time-of-flight and three-dimemnsional phase-contrast MR angiography sequences. Am J Roentgenol 1996; 167:489–494.

91. Leung DA, Hagspiel KD, Angle JF, et al. MR angiography of the renal arteries. Radiol Clin N Am 2002; 40:847–865.

92. Prince MR, Arnoldus C, Frisoli JF. Nephrotoxicity of high-dose gadolinium compared to iodinated contrast. J Magn Reson Imaging 1996; 6:162–166.

93. Leung DA, McKinnon GC, Davis CP, Pfammater T, Krestin GP, Debatin JF. Breath-hold, contrast-enhanced, three-dimensional MR angiography. Radiology 1996; 200:569–571.

94. Prince MR, Narasimham DL, Stanley JC, Chenevert TL, Williams DM, Marx MV. Breath-hold gadolinium-enhanced MR angiography of the abdominal aorta and its major branches. Radiology 1995; 197:785–792.

95. Siegelman ES, Gilfeather M, Holland GA, Carpenter JP, Golden MA, Townsend RR. Breath-hold ultrafast three-dimensional gadolinium-enhanced MR angiography of the renovascular system. Am J Roentgenol 1997; 168:1035–1040.

96. Binkert CA, Debatin JF, Schneider E, et al. Can MR measurement of renal artery flow and renal volume predict the outcome of percutaneous transluminal renal angioplasty? Cardiovasc Intervent Radiol 2001; 24(4):233–239.

97. Grenier N, Basseau F, Ries M, Tyndal B, Joes R, Moonen C. Functional MRI of the kidney. Abdom Imaging 2003; 28:164–175.

98. Tan KT, Van Beek EJR, Brown PWG, Van Delden OM, Tüssen J, Ramsey LE. Magnetic resonance angiography for the diagnosis of renal artery stenosis: a meta-analysis. Clin Radiol 2002; 57; 617–624.

99. Masunaga H, Takehara Y, Isoda H, et al. Assessment of gadolinium-enhanced time-resolved three-dimensional MR angiography for evaluating renal artery stenosis. Am J Roentgenol 2001; 176(5):1213–1219.

100. Mittal TK, Evans C, Perkins T, Wood AM. Renal arteriography using gadolinium enhanced 3D MR angiography—clinical experience with the technique, its limitations and pitfalls. Br J Radiol 2001; 74:495–502.

101. Thornton J, O'Callaghan J, Walshe J, O'Brien E, Varghese JC, Lee MJ. Comparison of digital subtraction angiography with gadolinium enhanced magnetic resonance angiography in the diagnosis of renal artery strenosis. Eur Radiol 1999; 9: 930–934.

102. Bakker J, Beek FJA, Beutler JJ. Renal artery stenosis and accessory renal arteries: accuracy of detection and visualization with gadolinium enhanced breath-hold MR angiography. Radiology 1998; 207:497–504.

103. Telo R, Thompson KR, Witte D, Becker GJ, Tress BM. Standard dose Gd-DTPA dynamic MR of the renal arteries. JMRI 1998; 8:421–426.

104. De Cobelli F, Vanzulli A, Sironi S. Evaluation with breath-hold, three-dimensional, dynamic, gadolinium-enhanced versus three-dimensional, phase-contrast MR angiography. Radiology 1997; 205:689–695.

105. Rieumont MJ, Kaufmann JA, Geller SC. Evaluation of renal artery stenosis with dynamic gadolinium enhanced MR angiography. Am J Roentgenol 1997; 169:39–44.

106. Snidow JJ, Johnson MS, Harris VJ. Three dimensional gadolinium enhanced MR angiography for aortoiliac inflow assessment plus renal artery screening in a single breath hold. Radiology 1996; 198:725–732.

107. Gilfeather M, Yoon HC, Siegelman ES. Renal artery stenosis: evaluation with conventional angiography versus gadolinium-enhanced MR angiography. Radiology 1999; 210:367–372.

108. Holland GA, Dougherty L, Carpenter JP. Breath-hold ultrafast three-dimensional gadolinium-enhanced MR angiography of the aorta and the renal and other visceral abdominal arteries. Am J Roentgenol 1996; 166:971–981.

109. Sandhu K, Patel U. Renal transplantation dysfunction: the role of interventional radiology. Clin Radiol 2002; 57:772–783.

110. Rengel M, Gomes Da Silva G, Inchaustegui L. Renal artery stenosis after kidney transplantation: diagnostic and therapeutic approach. Kidney Int 1998; 54:S99–S106.

111. Baxter GM, Ireland H, Moss JG, et al. Colour Doppler ultrasound in renal transplant artery stenosis: which Doppler index? Clin Radiol 1995; 50:618–622.

112. Huber A, Heuck A, Scheidler J, et al. Contrast-enhanced MR angiography in patients after kidney transplantation. Eur Radiol 2001; 11:2488–2495.

113. Maia CR, Bittar AE, Goldani JC. Doppler ultrasonography for the detection of renal artery stenosis in transplanted kidneys. Hypertension 1992; 19:207–209.

114. Snider JF, Hunter DW, Muradian GP. Transplant renal artery stenosis: evaluation with duplex sonography. Radiology 1989; 172:1027–1030.

115. Baxter GM. Ultrasound of renal transplantation. Clin Radiol 2001; 56:802–818.

116. Patel U, Hughes N, Khaw KK. Doppler ultrasound for detection of renal transplant artery stenosis—threshold peak systolic velocity needs to be higher in a low-risk or surveillance population. Clin Radiol 2003; 58:772–777.

117. Chua GC, Snowden S, Patel U. Kinks of the transplant renal artery without accompanying intra-arterial pressure gradient do not require correction—five-year outcome study. Cardiovasc Intervent Radiol 2004; 27:643–650.

118. Seymour HR, Matson MB, Belli AMB, et al. Rotational digital subtraction angiography of the renal arteries: technique and evaluation in the study of native and transplant renal arteries. Br J Radiol 2001; 74:134–141.

119. Martin LG, Rundback JH, Sacks D, et al. Quality improvement guidelines for angiography, angioplasty and stent placement in the diagnosis and treatment of renal artery stenosis in adults. J Vasc Interv Radiol 2003; 14:S297–S310.

120. Rees CR. Stents for atherosclerotic renovascular disease. J Vasc Interv Radiol 1999; 10:689–705.

121. Krijnen P, van Jaarsveld BC, Deinum J, Steyerberg EW, Habbema JD. Which patients with hypertension and atherosclerotic renal artery stenosis benefit from immediate intervention? J Hum Hypertens 2004; 18:91–96.
122. Bax L, STAR study group. The benefit of stent placement and blood pressure and lipid lowering for the prevention of progression of renal dysfunction caused by atherosclerotic ostial stenosis of the renal artery. The STAR-study: rational and study design. J Nephrol 2003; 16:807–812.
123. Wheatley K. ASTRAL—the story so far. J Renovasc Dis 2003; 2:1–2.

8
MR Urography

Claus Nolte-Ernsting
Department of Diagnostic and Interventional Radiology, University Hospital Hamburg—Eppendorf, Hamburg, Germany

INTRODUCTION

During the past 10 years, magnetic resonance (MR) urography has evolved to become a serious clinical alternative to conventional intravenous urography (IVU) and computed tomography (CT) urography. The concept of MR urography has been promoted with the intention of providing typical urographic views without resorting to radiation exposure. MR urography features different techniques to image the upper urinary tract in a comprehensive way that is not achievable with conventional IVU. The MR urographic technique is based on unenhanced, heavily T2-weighted pulse sequences for obtaining static-fluid images of the urinary system without depending on the renal excretory function (1). MR urography can also be performed as a T1-weighted technique after renal excretion of an intravenously injected gadolinium chelate (2). A profound knowledge of the diverse principles and examination techniques make it easy to put MR urography into operation. Additionally, MR urography has proved to be of diagnostic value in numerous urinary tract disorders in adults and children. However, owing to the emerging problems of cost restraints in our health care systems, it is obvious that MR urography will mainly be regarded as a diagnostic tool of secondary preference after ultrasonography, IVU, and CT. Nevertheless, MR urography is certainly much better than being only a procedure of second or third choice. MR urography offers a number of first-choice applications and should not be limited to the use in patients who do not tolerate iodinated contrast agents. MR urography especially provides the option of being combined with other MR examination techniques in a single session, such as standard magnetic resonance imaging (MRI) of the abdomen, MR angiography, or MR nephrography. This kind of integrative approach of MRI in modern uroradiology may help avoid the need for multiple, separate diagnostic procedures, which in the sum are costly, time-consuming, and sometimes even invasive.

HARDWARE ATTRIBUTES AND PATIENT PREPARATION

Field strength is not a critical issue in MR urography, which is routinely carried out between 0.5 and 1.5 T. MR urography performed at 3 T is of marginal benefit in that the increased signal-to-noise ratio (SNR) facilitates the use of parallel imaging techniques such as sensitivity encoding (SENSE). Phased-array surface coils with abdominal coverage are routinely employed, preferably as multichannel coils allowing for parallel imaging.

In adult patients, no special preparation is necessary. Complete information about the whole examination procedure is a prerequisite. Data on the latest serum creatinine level should be available. Before starting, patients should be asked to empty their urinary bladder. A respiratory sensor should be fixed on the patient's abdomen to monitor the respiration curve and to check for the patient's cooperation during the acquisition of breath-hold pulse sequences. It is recommended that the patient be asked to suspend breathing for 20 to 30 seconds once or twice prior to the actual breath-hold imaging procedure in order to prepare for it (3).

To perform MR urography in babies, infants, and adolescents, several aspects of the examination procedure have to be accommodated to suit the requirements of the different age groups: patient preparation, use of sedation, patient positioning inside the magnet, selection of surface coil, adaptation of sequence parameters, dose of contrast material, etc. The MR examination should always be accomplished in close cooperation with the parents, who should be informed about the procedure and should generally be allowed to be present inside the magnet room during the examination. In babies and infants, medical sedation obviously provides for the best patient handling during the examination. Alternatively, several measures have been proposed that may help avoid medical sedation (4).

The examination may be scheduled around the usual sleeping time of an infant, who may be fed right before the examination to achieve a natural sedative effect. Babies are wrapped in a blanket and immobilized with sandbags on each side. Cotton wool plugs and headphones may be employed for noise protection. With these preparations, a prospective MR urographic study demonstrated that medical sedation was unnecessary in 62 of 65 examined children (4).

PRINCIPLES OF T2-WEIGHTED MR UROGRAPHY (STATIC-FLUID MR UROGRAPHY)

T2-weighted MR urography simply provides water images of the urinary tract by acquisition of heavily T2-weighted turbo spin-echo (TSE) sequence techniques. The water we intend to visualize is the urine itself, which may be regarded as an "intrinsic contrast medium." T2-weighted MR urography is well suited for imaging of obstructive urinary tract disorders, because the large amount of static fluid generates a good SNR (Fig. 1). Moreover, T2-weighted MR urography offers a diagnostic tool that is independent of the renal excretory function. Static-fluid MR urography may even provide excellent urographic views of hydronephroses associated with severe kidney malfunction (2,5–10).

Moderate or marked dilatation is often indicative of advanced-stage urinary tract obstruction. On the other hand, early-stage intrinsic or extrinsic tumor lesions often do not cause obstruction and are therefore not necessarily associated with an increase of static fluid. The value of T2-weighted MR urography for the visualization of the nondilated urinary system is limited (Fig. 1) (7,8,11–13). Thus, several authors evaluating T2-weighted MR urography recommend supplementary measures for increasing the fluid load of the nondilated collecting system, including the use of a compression device plus intravenous diuretics (6,14) or saline

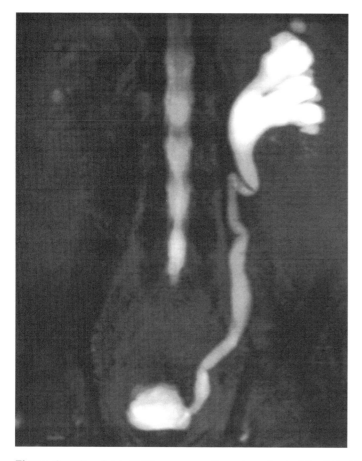

Figure 1   T2-weighted MR urogram of a male patient with a left-sided ureterohydronephrosis developed after prostatectomy. The large amount of static fluid on the left provides a good visualization of the dilated urinary tract on a heavily T2-weighted MR image. The unobstructed collecting system on the right remains invisible because of the lack of static fluid without application of a compression device. This MR urogram was obtained during a breath-hold of eight seconds by acquisition of a single-slice projection MR image with a thickness of 85 mm. *Abbreviation*: MR, magnetic resonance.

infusion plus intravenous diuretics; e.g., 0.3 mg furosemide per kg bodyweight combined with 20 mL saline infusion per kg (15). However, even the administration of an intravenous dose of 20 mg of furosemide cannot constantly ensure sufficient visualization of the nondilated urinary tract on T2-weighted MR urograms (11).

A second limitation of static-fluid MR urography is the inability of deriving functional information about the renal excretion and the urine flow through the collecting system and ureters (2,5,8,9).

The former objection that superimposed intestinal fluid collections may degrade the conspicuity of the urinary tract on T2-weighted MR urograms is nowadays less relevant because modern image postprocessing techniques, such as vector-of-interest editing, allow the elimination of fluid-filled bowel loops from MR urographic source images.

PULSE SEQUENCES FOR T2-WEIGHTED MR UROGRAPHY

Static-fluid MR urograms are performed using heavily T2-weighted TSE sequence techniques, such as rapid acquisition with relaxation enhancement (RARE) or half-Fourier acquisition single-shot turbo spin-echo (HASTE) (1,7,12,16,17). Initially, the RARE technique was employed to generate so-called nontomographic projection MR images of the urinary tract (1). Acquisition of a single-slice projection RARE image with a section thickness of 60 to 80 mm requires a short breath-hold of less than 10 seconds and provides a quick scout view of the pelvicalices and ureters in the coronal or sagittal plane (Fig. 1). HASTE is the half-Fourier variant of RARE allowing for faster acquisition of a heavily T2-weighted single slice within two seconds. HASTE can be applied as a single projection image or as a multislice sequence with thin sections.

Currently, 3-D TSE sequences or multislice HASTE sequences in the coronal or paracoronal plane are preferred for static-fluid MR urography (Fig. 2) (7–9,12,15). Combining those sequences with fat suppression has proved useful. Both types of pulse sequences generate multiple thin overlapping sections. Maximum intensity projection (MIP) images are postprocessed to obtain typical urographic views (Fig. 2). For acquisition of a multislice 2-D HASTE sequence, the breath-hold technique can be employed. The data acquisition time for a 3-D TSE sequence lasts between two and four minutes, which requires accurate compensation of respiratory motion of the kidneys. In 3-D TSE MR urography, respiratory triggering is preferred for motion artifact suppression. Note that the time necessary for respiratory compensation usually doubles the total sequence duration. With the use of modern multielement surface coils, parallel imaging techniques, such as SENSE, may be employed to reduce scan time significantly, which in turn can only be achieved at the expense of SNR. Typical sequence parameters for T2-weighted MR urography in adults and children are listed in Table 1.

Although T2-weighted 3-D TSE and multislice HASTE sequences are more time consuming than T2-weighted projection images, the analysis of multiple thin overlapping slices is regarded to be superior for the detection of pathologic details, which can be missed on an 80 mm thick projection MR urogram (6,8,9). On the other hand, MR projection images may be advantageous for use in babies and infants because of the very short acquisition time of approximately two seconds. In babies, the slice thickness of a projection MR image is reduced markedly (Table 1) and, thus, appears to be less problematic.

PRINCIPLES OF T1-WEIGHTED MR UROGRAPHY (GADOLINIUM EXCRETORY MR UROGRAPHY)

In the T1-weighted imaging approach in MR urography, the enhancement of the collecting system is based on the shortening of T1-relaxation time of the urine after renal excretion of an intravenously injected gadolinium agent (2,18). Unlike static-fluid MR urography, the feasibility of gadolinium-enhanced T1-weighted MR urography correlates with the renal function. Accordingly, the methodology of T1-weighted MR urography is similar to that of conventional urography and is therefore designated as excretory MR urography (2). T1-weighted MR urography provides both a morphologic depiction and a functional assessment of the urine excretion and flow through the urinary system. Several studies substantiate that

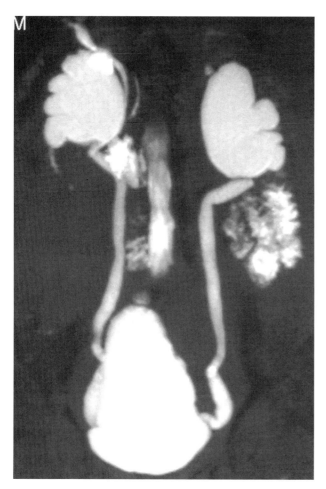

Figure 2 MIP reconstructed from the source images of a T2-weighted multislice HASTE sequence in a male patient with chronic infravesical obstruction and bilateral ureterohydrone-phrosis. *Abbreviations*: HASTE, half-Fourier acquisition single-shot turbo spin-echo; MIP, maximum intensity projection.

the gadolinium-enhanced technique achieves detailed MR urograms of nondilated and moderately obstructed urinary tracts, provided the renal excretory function is not severely impaired (2,4,19–31). Conversely, excretory MR urography is of no use in marked hydronephrosis associated with renal insufficiency.

An intravenous dose of 0.1 mmol/kg of bodyweight (kg-bw) of gadolinium is generally regarded the standard dose in clinical MR imaging and commonly recommended also for the use in excretory MR urography. Low–molecular weight gadolinium chelates eliminated by renal excretion are commercially available and have demonstrated a good safety profile, including a low nephrotoxicity at standard dose (32–35).

For the performance of gadolinium-enhanced renal MR imaging, it has to be taken into account that the kidneys physiologically are able to concentrate the excreted gadolinium load by a factor of 50 to 100 (33). For example, given an intra-venous dose of 0.1 mmol/kg-bw of gadolinium, gadolinium concentrations of more than 12.5 mmol/L of urine are possible (33). Such high endoluminal gadolinium

Table 1 Examples of Pulse Sequences Suited for T2-Weighted Static-Fluid MR Urography

Sequence[a]	Patient group	Respiratory compensation	TR/TE$_{eff}$ (msec)	TSE factor	FOV (mm); RFOV (%)	Matrix	No. of slices; slice thickness (mm)	Scan duration[b]; NSA
T2 HASTE[c] (projection image)	Adult	Breath-hold	−/200–500	128	350–390; 85	256 × 256	1; 60–80	2 sec; 1
T2 HASTE[d] (multislice)	Adult	Breath-hold or triggering	5000[e]/200	128	350–390; 85	256 × 256	30–40[f]; 3	2.5 min; 2
T2 2-D HASTE[d,g] (multislice)	Adult	Breath-hold	1500[e]/140	148	350–390; 100	236 × 256	15–20[f]; 3	23–30 sec; 1
T2 3-D TSE[d] (multislice)	Adult	Triggering	4000/400	85	350–390; 85	179 × 256	40–50[f]; 2	2.5–3.5 min; 1
T2 HASTE[c] (projection image)	Babies, infants	During expiration	−/200–500	128	170–300; 85	256 × 256	1; 30–40	2 sec; 1
T2 3-D TSE[d] (multislice)	Babies, infants	Triggering	4000/300	76	250–300; 85	179 × 256	30–40[f]; 1.5	2.0–2.5 min; 1

[a] All sequences with spectral fat-suppression.
[b] Without SENSE.
[c] Coronal or sagittal plane.
[d] Coronal or paracoronal plane.
[e] Time between two single-shots.
[f] Overlapping slices.
[g] Two consecutive stacks are necessary to cover the entire urinary tract.
Abbreviations: FOV, field of view; HASTE, half-Fourier acquisition single-shot turbo spin-echo; MR, magnetic resonance; NSA, number of signals averaged; RFOV, rectangular field of view; SENSE, sensitivity encoding; TE$_{eff}$, effective echo time; TR, repetition time; TSE, turbo spin-echo; 2-D, two-dimensional; 3-D, three-dimensional.

concentrations cause a paradoxical signal loss (contrast reversal) due to susceptibility effects (T2*-effects), which spoil the desired T1-enhancing urographic properties of gadolinium. The inherent renal ability to concentrate gadolinium up to one-hundred fold cannot be compensated simply by halving the intravenous gadolinium dose. Further reduction to a tenth of the standard gadolinium dose may help avoid T2*-effects, but the small amount of endoluminal contrast material leads to attenuated or even insufficient enhancement of the urinary tract. Moreover, if we intend to combine MR urography with conventional MRI of the kidneys or retroperitoneum in a single session, a standard gadolinium dose is usually necessary.

For achieving optimal T1-enhancement of the urine in excretory MR urography, it has proved very effective to inject the loop diuretic furosemide within one to five minutes prior to the administration of the standard gadolinium dose (2,4,18,21–25,29,30). The positive interaction between the diuretic and gadolinium fortunately occurs at very low doses of furosemide (0.1 mg/kg-bw) and is explained by the following three features (Fig. 3) (2,3):

1. The water retention inside the urinary system induced by low-dose furosemide increases the urine volume, which in turn leads to a mild distension of the pelvicalices and ureters.
2. The increase in endoluminal water load by furosemide causes the dilution of the subsequently excreted amount of gadolinium. Dilution of the urine prevents too high endoluminal gadolinium concentrations and, therefore, helps to avert the predominance of T2*-effects.
3. The increase in urine flow by furosemide leads to a rapid and uniform distribution of the excreted gadolinium agent throughout the entire urinary tract. This mechanism also prevents the possibility of excessively high gadolinium concentrations developing inside the urine.

These three "D-effects" of low-dose furosemide, "distension–dilution–distribution," act synergetically (36). Consequently, the contrast enhancement of the urinary tract may be less effective if we attenuate or omit one of these actions, for example, by using saline infusion instead of a diuretic or, alternatively,

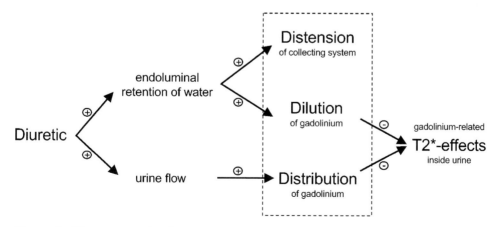

Figure 3 Three synergetic effects of low-dose furosemide in combination with gadolinium for use in excretory MR urography. The effects "dilution" and "distribution" are especially important for the suppression of undesired T2*-phenomena inside the gadolinium-enhanced urine. *Abbreviation*: MR, magnetic resonance.

a reduced dose of contrast agent without a diuretic (36,37). Especially the timing and the strength of hydration of the urinary system are better foreseeable with the use of low-dose furosemide than with infusion of saline solution. Because excretory MR urography is not a static examination and distribution of gadolinium-enhanced urine is a very important feature, the application of a compression device is not practical.

In general, the intravenous injection of a total amount of 10 mg of furosemide is at least as simple, harmless, and inexpensive as an infusion of 500 to 1000 mL of physiologic saline solution. Furosemide dosages not exceeding 0.1 mg/kg-bw usually provide a sufficient imaging window of around 30 minutes and do not impede significantly the patient's cooperation during the examination (2,22). In children, even a very low dose of 0.05 mg/kg-bw of furosemide injected via a 1 mL syringe has proved sufficient for combination with gadolinium (4,23).

Current experience with furosemide-enhanced excretory MR urography indicates that unless one ureter is completely obstructed, a sufficient gadolinium enhancement is normally attainable up to a serum creatinine level of 2 mg/dL (177 μmol/L) (2,4,21–23). This range, fortunately, already includes a large number of patients who are suited for undergoing excretory MR urography. Basically, the presence of ureterohydronephrosis is not a strict contraindication for the injection of low-dose furosemide. On the other hand, the use of furosemide is not indicated in patients presenting with an acute stone colic.

Anyway, with increasing degree of obstruction, the chances for achieving homogeneous gadolinium distribution with the help of furosemide diminish. The effectiveness of furosemide-enhanced excretory MR urography is limited in marked hydronephrosis. The impaired distribution of contrast material may cause undesired layers of gadolinium-enhanced and unenhanced urine inside the dilated calices and renal pelvis. Moreover, undistributed amounts of gadolinium allow susceptibility artifacts (T2*-effects) to develop inside the urine. In such a situation, additional mechanical mixing of gadolinium and urine is helpful and can be achieved by rotating the patient on the magnetic table from supine to prone and back.

PULSE SEQUENCES FOR T1-WEIGHTED MR UROGRAPHY

For the anatomic depiction of the gadolinium-enhanced urinary tract, fast T1-weighted, spoiled, 3-D gradient-echo (GRE) sequences performed in the coronal or paracoronal plane are well proven (Table 2) (2,4,20–26,29,30). Multiplanar MIP images are postprocessed from the source images of the 3-D data set (Fig. 4). In principle, sequence parameters used for excretory MR urography are quite similar to those applied in MR angiography. Repetition and echo times are set to minimal values (Table 2), which allows us to acquire the whole volumetric dataset within a breath-hold of less than 30 seconds. When used in combination with parallel imaging techniques (e.g., SENSE), the scan time can be minimized, to less than 20 seconds. Fast breath-hold imaging is the best method to avoid motion artifacts in the kidneys.

We usually start the 3-D GRE sequence within 10 minutes of injecting the contrast material (Table 3). A further advantage of fast scan times is that the 3-D GRE sequence may be repeated in short intervals so as to not miss the optimal moment of contrast enhancement of the urinary tract. In our examination protocol, we apply the 3-D GRE sequence with two modifications (Tables 2 and 3): On the one hand,

Table 2 Examples of T1-Weighted 3-D GRE Sequences Suited for Excretory MR Urography

Sequence[a]	Patient group	Respiratory compensation	TR/TE (msec); α	SENSE factor	FOV (mm); RFOV (%)	Matrix	No. of slices; Slice thickness[b] (mm)	Scan duration; NSA
T1 3-D GRE (survey MR urography)	Adult	Breath-hold	4–6/2–3; 30°	–	360–390; 85–100	179–196 × 256	50–60; 1.5	17–25 sec; 1
T1 3-D GRE (SENSE) (survey MR urography)	Adult	Breath-hold	5/2.5; 30°	2.0	400; 85–100	182 × 304	50–60; 1.5	13–18 sec; 1
T1 3-D GRE (detail MR urography)	Adult	Breath-hold	4–6/2–3; 30°	–	300–330; 85–95	196–212 × 256	35–45; 1.3	18–25 sec; 1
T1 3-D GRE (SENSE) (detail MR urography)	Adult	Breath-hold	6/3; 30°	2.0	400; 80	240 × 400	45; 1.3	16 sec; 1
T1 3-D GRE	Babies, infants	Gating	9/3; 30°	–	200–300; 70	192 × 256	40–50; 1.2	60–80 sec[c]; 2
T1 3-D GRE (SENSE)	Babies, infants	Gating	9/3; 30°	2.0	250–300; 100	192 × 256	40–50; 1.2	22–27 sec[c]; 1

[a]Coronal or paracoronal plane.

[b]Reconstructed slice thickness; original slice thickness is twice as high with 50% overlap.

[c]Minimum calculated acquisition time without considering duration of individual respiratory compensation.

Abbreviations: α, flip angle; FOV, field of view; GRE, gradient-echo; MR, magnetic resonance; NSA, number of signals averaged; RFOV, rectangular field of view; SENSE, sensitivity encoding; TE, echo time; TR, repetition time.

(A)

(B)

(C)

(D)

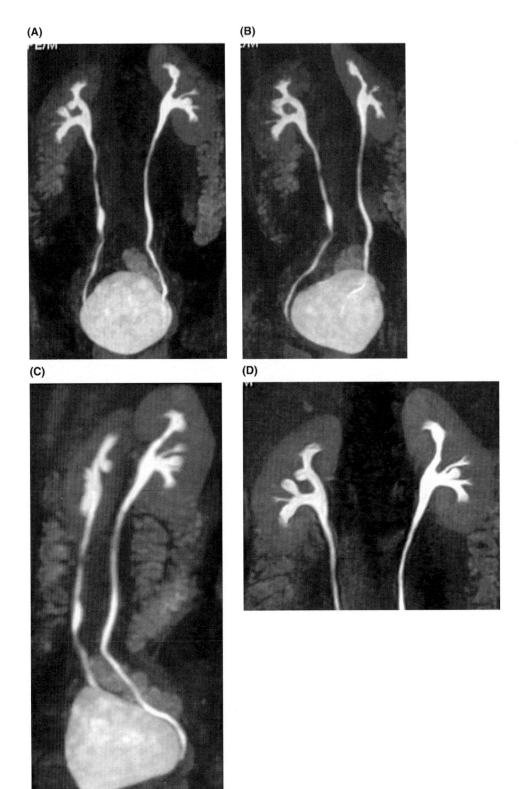

Figure 4   (*Caption on facing page*)

Table 3 General MR Urographic Examination Protocol Including Both T2- and T1-Weighted Sequences

Examination step	Pulse sequence	Comment
Precontrast	Optional: T2-weighted projection image	Initial assessment of fluid amount in bowel and urinary tract; scan time ~5 sec
Precontrast	3-D T2 TSE or multislice T2 HASTE	Scan time ~5 min
0.1 mg/kg furosemide IV		May alternatively be injected before step 2
0.1 mmol/kg gadolinium IV		Injection 1–5 min after furosemide
10 min postcontrast	T1 3-D GRE survey MR urogram	Scan time ~20 sec
15 min postcontrast	T1 3-D GRE survey MR urogram	
20 min postcontrast	T1 3-D GRE detail MR urogram	
After 25 min postcontrast	Optional: further T1 3-D GRE survey or detail urograms	

Abbreviations: GRE, gradient-echo; HASTE, half-Fourier acquisition single-shot turbo spin-echo; MR, magnetic resonance; TSE, turbo spin-echo.

survey MR urograms are acquired with a 256-matrix size and a large field of view (FOV) that display the entire urinary tract with moderate spatial resolution (Fig. 4A–C). On the other hand, a small FOV is used to obtain detail MR urograms with increased spatial resolution (Fig. 4D). The reduced FOV of a detail MR urogram may include either the kidneys and proximal ureters or the vesicoureteral junction and the distal ureters. Using a 512-matrix size is also feasible in MR urography to further improve spatial resolution, which, however, is obtained at the expense of SNR and scan time.

In critically ill patients or adolescents unable to suspend breathing during the acquisition of a 3-D GRE sequence, the navigator echo technique can be employed for avoiding respiratory motion artifacts. The resulting total sequence duration, however, is increased to several minutes. In babies and infants, breath-hold imaging is impossible, but sufficient compensation of motion artifacts may be achieved with conventional respiratory gating (4,23). Data acquisition without any motion artifact suppression may also be tried in small children but often results in inadequate urographic image quality.

Figure 4 (*Figure on facing page*) Normal gadolinium-enhanced excretory MR urogram. (**A–C**) Survey MR urography obtained using a 3-D GRE sequence with an FOV of 360 mm. MIPs display the urinary tract in different planes. (**A**) Coronal MIP. (**B,C**) Oblique MIP images visualize the vesicoureteral junction on either side separated from the bladder. (**D**) Detail MR urography of the pelvicalices obtained with an FOV of 300 mm permit better spatial resolution and delineation of caliceal fornices. *Abbreviations*: FOV, field of view; GRE, gradient-echo; MIP, maximum intensity projection; MR, magnetic resonance.

WHICH MR UROGRAPHY TECHNIQUE IN WHICH SITUATION?

The diverse facilities for imaging the urinary tract with MR provide a number of options of how to perform MR urography in the clinical routine. MR urography may be conducted using either exclusively T2-weighted pulse sequences or exclusively a gadolinium-enhanced T1-weighted technique. On the other hand, T2- and T1-weighted pulse sequences usually complement one another; thus, it is also possible that static-fluid and excretory MR urography be combined for obtaining a comprehensive examination of the urinary tract. For selecting the appropriate MR urographic examination procedure in each individual case, one may orientate oneself by the serum creatinine level and the degree of dilatation. The latter is often known from a preceding ultrasonography. If sonographic data are not available, a fast T2-weighted projection MR image (RARE or HASTE) may provide a quick scout view of the current state of dilatation at the very beginning of the MR urographic examination. In adult patients, we often encounter three typical clinical situations that favor a sophisticated MR urographic examination procedure (36,38):

Situation 1. *Sonographically, no hydronephrosis and no atrophy of the renal parenchyma are seen; the serum creatinine level is normal or slightly increased (below 2 mg/dL).*

Patients often present with uncharacteristic flank pain and/or microscopic hematuria. In this situation, T1-weighted gadolinium excretory MR urography in combination with only 5 to 10 mg of furosemide has proved excellent for achieving a complete and detailed depiction of the nondilated urinary tract with good SNR. A compression device is unnecessary.

Situation 2. *Slight or moderate hydronephrosis (grade 1 and 2) is known; there is no or minimal parenchymal atrophy and serum creatinine level is normal or slightly increased.*

Both MR urography techniques are well suited in this situation. We may start with T2-weighted MR urography, which readily identifies the level and degree of obstruction. If we are satisfied with the morphologic information seen on T2-weighted images, MR urography may be terminated at that point. Otherwise, gadolinium-enhanced T1-weighted MR urograms can be added easily, which often permit the best assessment of the configuration and length of a ureteral stenosis and provide functional information on the impaired urine flow through the obstructed ureter. Late MR urograms, beyond an acquisition delay of 30 minutes after injection of contrast material, are usually not necessary because the renal excretion is not reduced too severely. Actually, this situation favors the combination of static-fluid and excretory MR urography in one session (Table 3).

Situation 3. *A high-grade, often chronic hydronephrosis (grade 3 and 4) is known and associated with parenchymal atrophy and severe excretory malfunction.*

Because there is a large amount of static fluid present in this situation, T2-weighted MR urography is the imaging technique of choice for demonstrating the degree of hydronephrosis and the level of obstruction even in nonexcreting kidneys.

The only situation in which neither T2- nor T1-weighted MR urography really can help is in patients with shrunken kidneys and severely impaired excretory function not caused by obstruction. These patients often suffer from chronic renal insufficiency, for example caused by diabetes mellitus, glomerulonephritis, and analgetic nephropathy. Another exception to these three clinical categories is that of pregnant women, in whom solely T2-weighted static-fluid imaging is a useful MR urographic technique if ultrasonography is unconclusive.

APPLICATIONS FOR MR UROGRAPHY

Congenital and Acquired Anatomic Anomalies

There are a wide range of anatomic variants that can be imaged accurately with MR urography. The absence of ionizing radiation makes MR urography the method of choice for the detection of congenital anomalies in children. T2-weighted MR urography has proved excellent for imaging anomalies associated with an increased amount of fluid and/or kidney malfunction, such as ureteropelvic junction stenosis (Fig. 5), megaureter, and cystic kidney disease (4,23,39–42). T1-weighted excretory MR urography is preferred for the demonstration of anatomic variations in the nondilated collecting system, including malrotation of the collecting system (Fig. 6), caliceal diverticula, small ureteroceles, unobstructed bifid systems (Fig. 7), fusion anomalies, and medullary sponge kidneys (3,4). The diverse MR urographic techniques may even be applied for visualizing ectopic ureters (Fig. 8) (23). Furthermore, in children with urinary tract anomalies, it appears to be very promising to combine MR urography with MR nephrography for obtaining morphologic information plus quantitative functional data, including split renal function similar to scintigraphy (31,40–43).

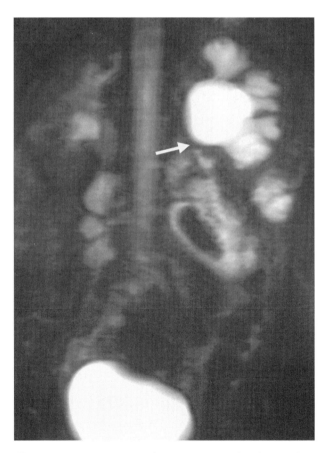

Figure 5 Four-year-old girl with a stenosis of the left UPJ. A T2-weighted MR urogram shows typical ballooning of the left pelvicaliceal system and missing dilatation of the ureter, indicating obstruction of the UPJ (*arrow*). *Abbreviations*: MR, magnetic resonance; UPJ, ureteropelvic junction.

(A)   **(B)**

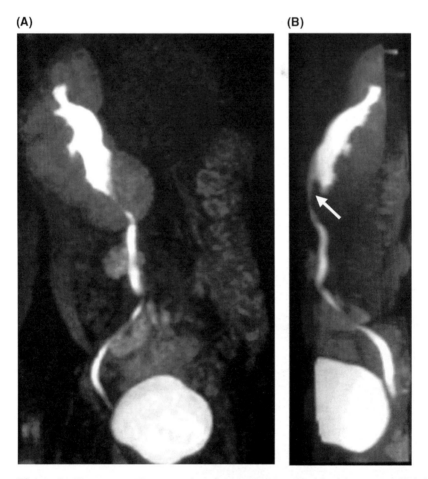

Figure 6 Excretory MR urography of a seven-year-old girl with a congenital single kidney.
(**A**) The coronal MIP from T1-weighted GRE sequence shows complete gadolinium-
enhancement of the nondilated urinary tract with abnormal configuration of the pelvicalices.
(**B**) The sagittal MIP demonstrates the malrotation of the pelvicalices with an anterior origin
of the UPJ (*arrow*). *Abbreviations*: GRE, gradient-echo; MIP, maximum intensity projection;
MR, magnetic resonance; UPJ, ureteropelvic junction.

This concept can be realized in a single session especially with the complementary use
of T2-weighted and gadolinium-enhanced T1-weighted imaging techniques.

In adult patients, variations of the urinary tract anatomy may not only be
congenital but also acquired. For example, MR urography is able to demonstrate
caliceal lesions associated with papillary necroses, caliceal diverticula, caliceal blunt-
ing in chronic pyelonephritis, and ureteric distortion caused by retroperitoneal
fibrosis (Fig. 9), radiotherapy, or surgery (2,3,22).

Imaging of the upper urinary tract anatomy may also be important in patients
who have undergone radical cystectomy and are referred for a postoperative follow-
up. MR urography is useful for achieving a complete overview of the postoperative
anatomy (Fig. 10). Assessment of the ureteral anastomoses is of special interest.
Intravenous supplementation of a spasmolytic agent, such as butylscopolammonium
bromide, has proved effective in suppressing motion artifacts resulting from peristalsis of a neobladder or an ileal conduit.

(A)   **(B)**

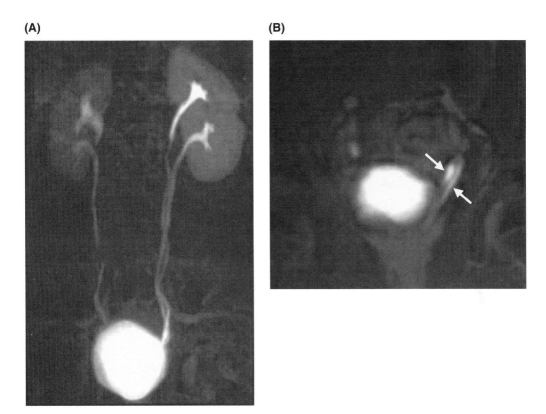

Figure 7 Seven-year-old girl with bifid pelvicalices on both sides. (**A**) The coronal MIP from excretory MR urography demonstrates a single ureter on the right and a duplex ureter on the left without dilatation. (**B**) The original source image of the T1-weighted 3-D dataset illustrates best that two separate ureteral orifices exist at the vesicoureteral junction on the left (*arrows*). *Abbreviations*: MIP, maximum intensity projection; MR, magnetic resonance.

Furthermore, T2-weighted static-fluid MR urography has proved useful in the visualization of the complicated urinary tract anatomy in patients with spinal dysraphism (44).

Another application for combining T2- and T1-weighted MR urography is the assessment of parapelvic cysts, which may distort the pelvicaliceal anatomy and occasionally simulate hydronephrosis in ultrasonography. Static-fluid MR urography depicts the configuration and dimensions of cysts that may completely fill the renal sinus (Fig. 11). Excretory MR urography discloses the true pelvicaliceal anatomy because T1-weighted imaging allows distinguishing between nonenhancing cysts and gadolinium-enhancing pelvicalices, which are typically displaced and compressed (Fig. 11) (38).

Apart from these general anatomic issues, MR urography also provides accurate depiction of the urinary tract morphology in chronic urolithiasis, tumor diseases, transplant kidneys, and live kidney donors, as outlined in the following sections.

Urolithiasis

In patients presenting with acute stone colic, plain abdominal radiography plus ultrasonography or, alternatively, unenhanced multislice CT are imaging modalities

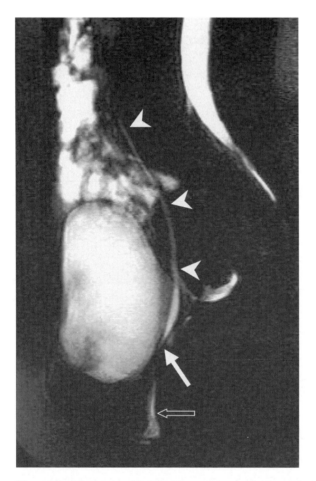

Figure 8 Nine-year-old girl with symptoms of urine dripping and enuresis. T2-weighted MR urography visualizes an ectopic ureter on the right side. The sagittal plane shows that the ureter (*arrowheads*) does not join the urinary bladder (*arrow*). After injection of furosemide, leakage of fluid into the vagina is detected (*open arrow*), indicating the presence of an ectopic ureteral orifice. The dysplastic right kidney is not seen on the MR urogram. *Abbreviation*: MR, magnetic resonance.

of choice, whereas MR urography plays only a minor role. One disadvantage of MRI in acute urolithiasis is the limited availability of in-bore times in emergency situations. Nevertheless, for those who already practice MR urography routinely, the detection of a pelvicaliceal calculus is not a rare finding (Fig. 11). Indeed, because urolithiasis is the major differential diagnosis in all urinary tract diseases, it is useful to know about the imaging features of stones in MRI.

Indirect signs of urolithiasis, such as uretrohydronephrosis and perinephric stranding, are readily seen on T2-weighted MR urograms. However, the main explanation for the limited value of MRI in urolithiasis is its poor capability for identifying small, calcified, soft-tissue structures, which is not a problem in CT. With MRI, we only have the chance to search for more or less typical filling defects. Most calculi present as round or branched signal voids (Figs. 11 and 12) inside the unenhanced or gadolinium-enhanced urine (2,5,7,20,24,29). However, such hypointense filling

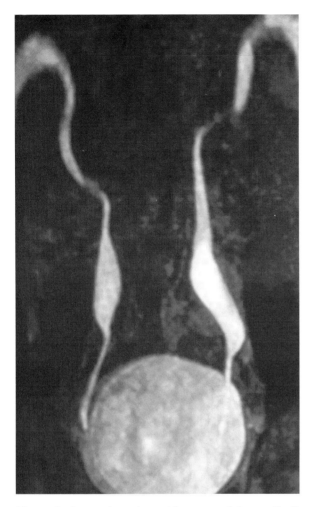

Figure 9 In a male patient with suspected Ormond's disease, excretory MR urography visualizes both ureters over their entire length with medial displacement and distinct variations in caliber. A stricture causing impaired gadolinium flow is not seen. *Abbreviation*: MR, magnetic resonance.

defects are unspecific, and distinguishing a small stone from a blood clot, a polyp, or a surgical clip may occasionally cause diagnostic pitfalls. Moreover, it has to be pointed out that especially nonobstructing filling defects, including stones, may be invisible on MIP images and must be diagnosed exclusively by reading the source sections of the MR urographic pulse sequence (3). On source images, the tip of a papilla protruding into a calix must not be misinterpreted as a caliceal stone (Fig. 12). Calculi typically show an excentric location inside a calix, whereas the tip of a papilla usually has a central position (45).

Literature references reporting the sensitivity of MR urography in ureteral stone disease are already available (20,24,29). Between 90% and 94% of ureteral calculi are detected as filling defects on MR urograms (20,29). In a comparative study investigating ureterolithiasis on MR urography and unenhanced CT (29), the sensitivity of MR urography (93.8%) was equal to that obtained with CT (90.6%).

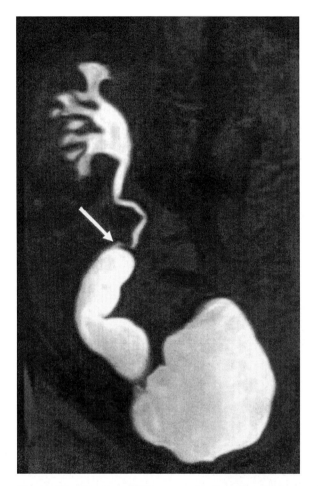

Figure 10 Excretory MR urography is performed in a male patient who underwent cystectomy and nephroureterectomy on the left with orthotopic neobladder reconstruction. The gadolinium-enhanced T1-weighted MIP accurately visualizes the postoperative urinary tract anatomy, including a nonstrictured uretero-ileal anastomosis (*arrow*). *Abbreviations*: MIP, maximum intensity projection; MR, magnetic resonance.

However, MR urography proved to be less exact than CT in determining the stone size (29). Corresponding data for nephrolithiasis are still unavailable, but it is very likely that MR urography will be inferior to unenhanced CT, especially in the detection of small caliceal calculi.

It would be justified if the question is raised as to whether there is any realistic application for MR urography in urolithiasis, apart from the limited value of MRI in acute stone disease. Especially in patients suffering from chronic or recurrent urolithiasis, MR urography is a potential alternative to CT for avoiding repeated radiation exposure (Figs. 11 and 13). In chronic nephrolithiasis resistant to treatment, MR urography provides detailed morphologic information about the complicated pelvicaliceal anatomy, which favors the formation of calculi and often leads to stone impaction (Fig. 13) (3,22). Unless there is an acute colic, the use of low-dose furosemide is actually not a problem in chronic stone disease. Prior to lithotripsy or endourologic stone removal, MR urography with multiplanar MIP images yields

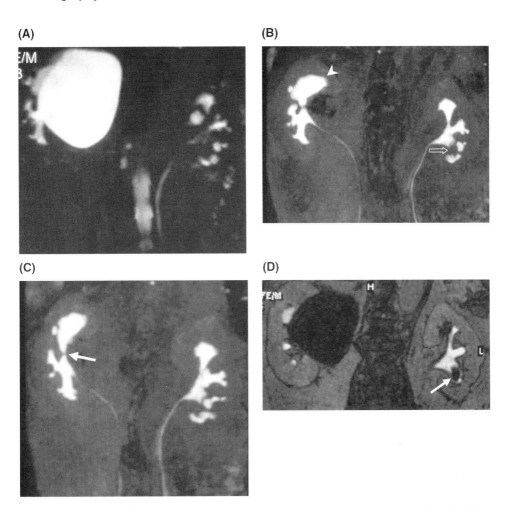

Figure 11 (**A**) T2-weighted MR urography shows a large parapelvic cyst on the right side with compression of the pelvicalices. (**B, C**) The coronal and oblique MIP images from T1-weighted excretory MR urography disclose the true anatomic situation of the displaced pelvicalices on the right. The upper caliceal group is markedly dilated (*arrowhead*) because of infundibular obstruction (*white arrow*). Note also the filling defect inside the lower caliceal group of the left kidney (*open arrow*). (**D**) The corresponding source image of the 3-D GRE sequence reveals a 2 cm sized calculus (*arrow*) obstructing the lower infundibulum. The cyst on the right displays a characteristic low signal on the T1-weighted source image and is not directly seen on MIP images. *Abbreviations*: GRE, gradient-echo; MIP, maximum intensity projection; MR, magnetic resonance.

a 3-D overview for determining the stone passage through a chronically affected collecting system (Fig. 13). Finally, T2-weighted MR urography can also be used for imaging of obstructive urolithiasis during pregnancy (13,46).

Transitional Cell Carcinoma

Many transitional cell carcinomas located in the pelvicalices or ureters can be detected noninvasively by standard contrast-enhanced CT or MRI without the need for a urographic phase. Nevertheless, the availability of thin urographic sections may

(A)

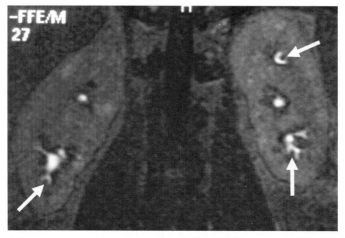

(B)

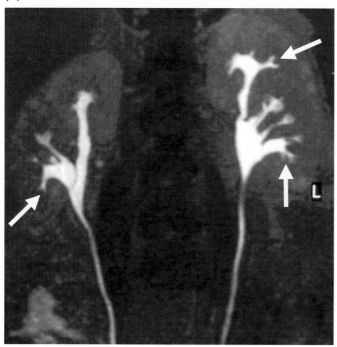

Figure 12 (**A**) On source images, hypointense "pseudo-filling-defects" extending into the center of calices (*arrows*) represent papillary tips and must not be confused with caliceal stones. (**B**) The corresponding MIP confirms the normal configuration of the calices with a typical papillary impression (*arrows*). *Abbreviation*: MIP, maximum intensity projection.

aid in finding small nonobstructing lesions and may also contribute information regarding local tumor staging. A urography is often mandatory for the planning of the appropriate operative therapy of a transitional cell carcinoma.

The propensity of transitional cell carcinomas for multicentric tumor growth favors the use of an imaging technique that enables a comprehensive bilateral

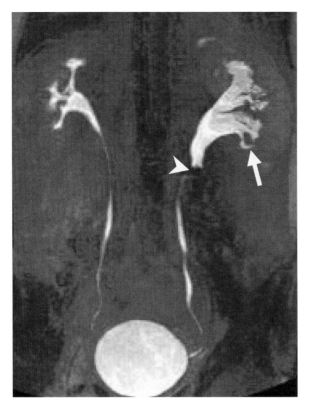

Figure 13 Excretory MR urography of a male patient with chronic left-sided nephrolithiasis and recurring flank pain. A calculus is obstructing the UPJ on the left (*arrowhead*), causing moderate dilatation of the pelvicalices. The lower calix on the left bears another calculus (*arrow*), which can potentially pass through the dilated infundibulum. MR urography accurately depicts the chronically distorted urinary system and provides a road map for lithotripsy or endourological stone removal. *Abbreviations*: MR, magnetic resonance; UPJ, ureteropelvic junction.

assessment of the upper urinary tract. Thus, MR urography performed in addition to conventional MR pulse sequences offers an alternative to CT or retrograde pyelography. Advanced-stage transitional cell carcinomas are often associated with severe renal malfunction, which especially suggests using T2-weighted static-fluid MR urography. On the other hand, the use of low-dose furosemide in T1-weighted excretory MR urography provides improved distension and a good SNR necessary in searching for small nonobstructing polyps.

In general, the imaging features of a transitional cell carcinoma in MR urography are similar to those seen in conventional urography or CT urography (3,36). A transitional cell carcinoma develops as a sessile plaque or exophyte with either irregular or smooth margins, urographically causing a more or less typical filling defect. Inside the renal pelvis, a transitional cell carcinoma can infiltrate the calices; thus, they appear to be ballooned, amputated, or completely filled out on MR urograms (Fig. 14). A ureteral transitional cell carcinoma typically causes the urographic "goblet sign," which denotes a cup-shaped dilatation of the prestenotic ureteral segment (Fig. 15) (2,3,20,47).

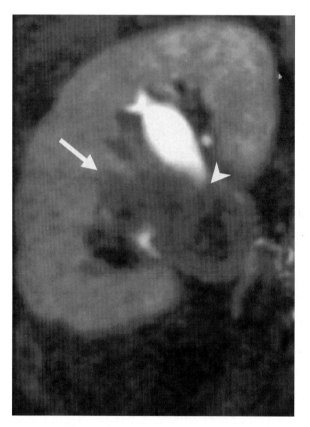

Figure 14 MR urography provides details about the endoluminal spread of an exophytic transitional cell carcinoma inside the renal pelvis. Secondary to infundibular tumor occlusion (*arrowhead*), a calix is dilated and appears amputated. Another calix is completely infiltrated with tumor invasion into the renal parenchyma (*arrow*), indicating a stage T3 carcinoma of the renal pelvis. *Abbreviation*: MR, magnetic resonance.

On both T1- and T2-weighted MR urographic source images, all kinds of filling defects usually display a hypointense signal. Therefore, it may occasionally be difficult with MR urography to distinguish a small transitional cell carcinoma from a blood clot, a calculus, or a surgical clip. Again, better differentiation is possible if MR urography is performed in conjunction with conventional axial pulse sequences, which helps avoid major pitfalls.

Although the exact value of MRI in the diagnosis of transitional cell carcinoma has not been defined in the literature, it seems realistic to predict that MR urography has the potential to reduce the total number of necessary retrograde pyelographies in the future.

MR Urography in Extrinsic Obstruction of the Urinary Tract

Numerous malignant and benign retroperitoneal disorders can affect the urinary tract extrinsically (Table 4). Ultrasonography usually shows a dilated urinary tract. Conventional CT or MRI is considered the standard imaging modality for making the diagnosis of a retroperitoneal tumor disease. Conventional MRI with axial

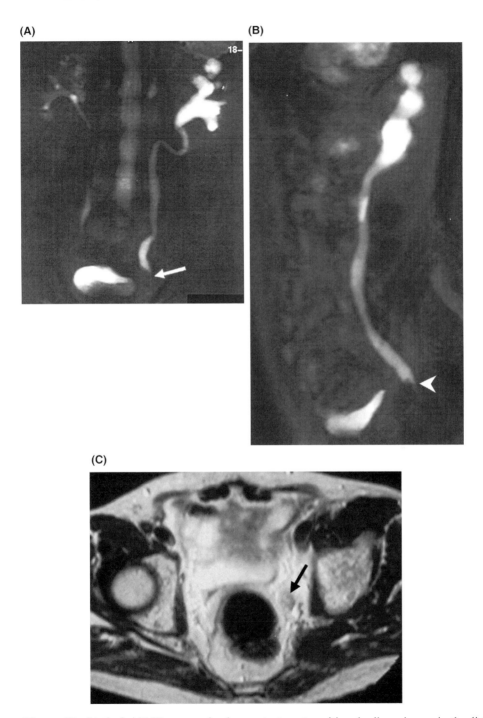

Figure 15 Static-fluid MR urography demonstrates a transitional cell carcinoma in the distal section of the left ureter. (**A**) Urographically, the tumor is characterized as a polypoid filling defect (*arrow*), causing moderate hydronephrosis. (**B**) On the sagittal MR urogram, the truncated ureter shows a concave widening (*arrowhead*), which is a quite typical urographic finding of endoureteral tumor growth. (**C**) The additional standard T2-weighted TSE sequence in the axial plane confirms that the filling defect is composed of a soft tissue mass (*black arrow*). The absence of any susceptibility-related signal void excludes the differential diagnosis of calculus disease. *Abbreviations*: MR, magnetic resonance; TSE, turbo spin-echo.

Table 4 Common Causes for Extrinsic Compression of the Urinary Tract

Benign causes	Malignant causes
Hematoma	Metastasis
Abscess	Sarcoma
Lymphocele	Lymphoma
Stricture (after surgery, radiation therapy, trauma)	Colorectal cancer
Retroperitoneal fibrosis	Uterine cancer
Aortic or iliac aneurysm	Ovarian cancer
Y-graft	Prostate cancer
Retrocaval ureter	

sections demonstrates location, size, and signal morphology of a retroperitoneal mass. As with imaging of transitional cell carcinoma, MR urography can be employed as an add-on to demonstrate the extent of urinary tract involvement, for example, in patients prior to gynecologic tumor surgery. Urographic signs for extrinsic compression are ureteral displacement and concentric stenosis either with gradual tapering or with abrupt truncation of the ureteral lumen (Fig. 16) (3,5,8,36). It is unclear whether MRI is able to differentiate ureteral tumor compression from extrinsic infiltration of the ureteral wall. A filling defect is missing, and a goblet sign is not seen.

Renal Transplantation

The combination of MR angiography and MR urography in a single session has the potential to replace IVU plus digital subtraction angiography in the preoperative assessment of live renal donors (27,48–50).

Moreover, imaging of the urinary tract of transplant kidneys may become a new domain of MR urography in the near future. Because the administration of nephrotoxic iodinated contrast agents is undesirable in transplant kidneys, conventional IVU or CT urography are often inapplicable imaging tools. Ultrasonography is of limited use for the assessment of transplant urinary tract disorders, which explains why urologists sometimes resort to antegrade pyelography. Thus, there exists a certain diagnostic gap with regard to conventional imaging of the urinary tract of the transplant kidneys. This gap may now be closed with the availability of modern MR urographic techniques (3,26,36,51). MIPs provide detailed urograms of the transplant urinary tract (Fig. 17).

Imaging of the transplant urinary tract is often related to complications affecting the ureter. Common causes of a ureteral stenosis may be a stricture, kinking, or extrinsic compression by a lymphocele. In the early postoperative phase, a urine leak may typically occur secondary to necrosis and perforation of the transplant ureter. Calculi and even intrinsic tumors are further urographically relevant pathologic findings encountered in transplant urinary systems.

MR urography offers sophisticated imaging features for the assessment of various disorders of the transplant urinary tract. The different T2- and T1-weighted MR urographic techniques can be performed either separately or complimentarily. T2-weighted MR urography usually permits exact localization of the site of obstruction in ureterohydronephrosis (51). Pathologic extraurinary fluid collections, such as

(A)

(B)

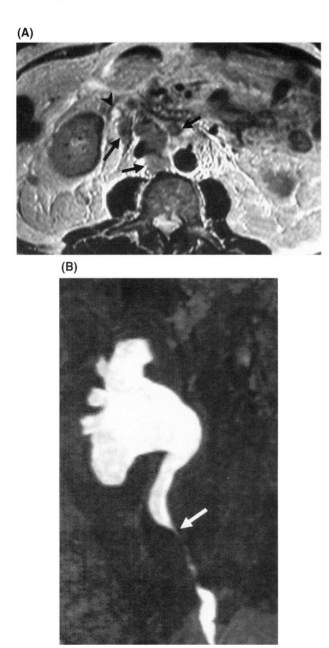

Figure 16 The combination of standard abdominal MRI plus MR urography is useful for the assessment of retroperitoneal tumor disease associated with extrinsic stenosis of the urinary tract. (**A**) In a male patient with abdominal lymphoma, the conventional axial T2-weighted TSE image reveals several enlarged para-aortic lymph nodes (*black arrows*), some of which are located next to the right ureter (*arrowhead*). (**B**) Excretory MR urography is performed as an add-on to conventional gadolinium-enhanced MRI. For this purpose, no extra injection of contrast material is necessary. The exact configuration, location, and length of the extrinsic stenosis is best seen on the MR urogram (*arrow*). Note that a fine stream of gadolinium-enhanced urine is still able to pass this stenosis, which also explains for the preserved excretory function of the right kidney. *Abbreviations*: MR, magnetic resonance; MRI, magnetic resonance imaging; TSE, turbo spin-echo.

(A)   (B)

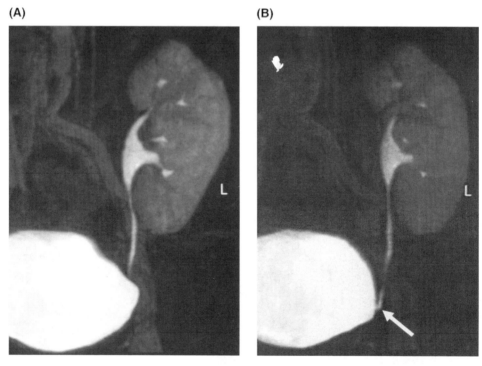

Figure 17 MR urography obtained as a follow-up examination after renal transplantation in a female patient. (**A**) Coronal and (**B**) oblique MIP images from excretory MR urography provide a good delineation of the nondilated pelvicalices and the entire course of the transplant ureter. The excretory function is not impaired. Abnormal ureteral kinking, obstruction, and leakage of urine are not detected. Even the vesicoureteral junction can be assessed without superposition of the bladder (*arrow*). *Abbreviations*: MIP, maximum intensity projection; MR, magnetic resonance.

lymphoceles, are easily identified with static-fluid MR urography (51). However, a compressed transplant ureter may not be demarcated from adjacent retroperitoneal fluid on T2-weighted images. Alternatively, good delineation of the transplant ureter can be achieved using gadolinium-enhanced T1-weighted MR urography, especially in conjunction with low-dose furosemide. Combining T2- and T1-weighted MR urography helps distinguish between a lymphocele and a urinoma. A urine leak is preferably diagnosed and localized with T1-weighted excretory MR urography by detecting extravasation of gadolinium-enhanced urine (3,22,26).

Anyway, disorders of the transplant urinary tract are usually associated with an increased serum creatinine level. Static-fluid MR urography is performed irrespective of the excretory function. Initial data tend to indicate that excretory MR urography seems to be feasible in transplant kidneys with serum creatinine levels greater than 2 mg/dL, provided the transplant kidney is still able to excrete a sufficient volume of urine per day (22).

For diagnostic follow-up after renal transplantation, MRI offers the interesting option of combining standard pulse sequences with MR angiography and MR urography, allowing the assessment of renal parenchyma, vasculature, and urinary tract during the same examination session with only a single injection of contrast material. Furthermore, it has been demonstrated that it is possible even in transplant kidneys to combine MR urography and MR nephrography for obtaining both morphologic information and the gadolinium excretion curve, similar to radionuclide studies (52).

REFERENCES

1. Friedburg HG, Hennig J, Frankenschmidt A. RARE-MR urography: a fast nontomographic imaging procedure for demonstrating the efferent urinary pathways using nuclear magnetic resonance. Radiologe 1987; 27:45–47.
2. Nolte-Ernsting CC, Bücker A, Adam GB, et al. Gadolinium-enhanced excretory MR urography after low-dose diuretic injection: comparison with conventional excretory urography. Radiology 1998; 209:147–157.
3. Nolte-Ernsting CC, Adam GB, Günther RW. MR urography: examination techniques and clinical applications. Eur Radiol 2001; 11:355–372.
4. Staatz G, Nolte-Ernsting CC, Adam GB, et al. Feasibility and utility of respiratory-gated, gadolinium-enhanced T1-weighted magnetic resonance urography in children. Invest Radiol 2000; 35:504–512.
5. Roy C, Saussine C, Jahn C, et al. Evaluation of RARE-MR urography in the assessment of ureterohydronephrosis. J Comput Assist Tomogr 1994; 18:601–608.
6. Rothpearl A, Frager D, Subramanian A, et al. MR urography: technique and application. Radiology 1995; 194:125–130.
7. Regan F, Bohlman ME, Khazan R, Rodriguez R, Schultze-Haakh H. MR urography using HASTE imaging in the assessment of ureteric obstruction. AJR 1996; 167:1115–1120.
8. Tang Y, Yamashita Y, Namimoto T, et al. The value of MR urography that uses HASTE sequences to reveal urinary tract disorders. AJR 1996; 167:1497–1502.
9. O'Malley ME, Soto JA, Yucel EK, Hussain S. MR urography: evaluation of a three-dimensional fast spin-echo technique in patients with hydronephrosis. AJR 1997; 168:387–392.
10. Reuther G, Kiefer B, Wandl E. Visualization of urinary tract dilatation: value of single-shot MR urography. Eur Radiol 1997; 7:1276–1281.
11. Hattery RR, King BF. Technique and application of MR urography. Radiology 1995; 194:25–27.
12. Balci NC, Mueller-Lisse UG, Holzknecht N, Gauger J, Waidelich R, Reiser M. Breath-hold MR urography: comparison between HASTE and RARE in healthy volunteers. Eur Radiol 1998; 8:925–932.
13. Grenier N, Pariente JL, Trillaud H, Soussotte C, Douws C. Dilatation of the collecting system during pregnancy: physiologic vs obstructive dilatation. Eur Radiol 2000; 10: 271–279.
14. Klein LT, Frager D, Subramanian A, Lowe FC. Use of magnetic resonance urography. Urology 1998; 52:602–608.
15. Rohrschneider WK, Hoffend J, Becker K, et al. Combined static-dynamic MR urography for the simultaneous evaluation of morphology and function in urinary tract obstruction. I. Evaluation of the normal status in an animal model. Pediatr Radiol 2000; 30:511–522.
16. Hennig J, Nauerth A, Friedburg H. RARE imaging: a fast imaging method for clinical MR. Magn Reson Med 1986; 3:823–833.
17. Aerts P, Van Hoe L, Bosmans H, Oyen R, Marchal G, Baert AL. Breath-hold MR urography using the HASTE technique. AJR 1996; 166:543–545.
18. Nolte-Ernsting C, Adam G, Bücker A, Berges S, Bjoernerud A, Günther RW. Contrast-enhanced magnetic resonance urography. First experimental results with a polymeric gadolinium bloodpool agent. Invest Radiol 1997; 32:418–423.

19. Farres MT, Gattegno B, Ronco P, Flahault A, Paula-Sauza A, Bigot JM. Nonnephrotoxic, dynamic, contrast enhanced magnetic resonance urography: use in nephrology and urology. J Urol 2000; 163:1191–1196.

20. Jung P, Brauers A, Nolte-Ernsting CA, Jakse G, Günther RW. Magnetic resonance urography enhanced by gadolinium and diuretics: a comparison with conventional urography in diagnosing the cause of ureteric obstruction. BJU Int 2000; 86:960–965.

21. Verswijvel GA, Oyen RH, Van Poppel HP, et al. Magnetic resonance imaging in the assessment of urologic disease: an all-in-one approach. Eur Radiol 2000; 10:1614–1619.

22. Nolte-Ernsting CC, Tacke J, Adam GB, et al. Diuretic-enhanced gadolinium excretory MR urography: comparison of conventional gradient-echo sequences and echo-planar imaging. Eur Radiol 2001; 11:18–27.

23. Staatz G, Rohrmann D, Nolte-Ernsting CC, et al. Magnetic resonance urography in children: evaluation of suspected ureteral ectopia in duplex systems. J Urol 2001; 166:2346–2350.

24. Sudah M, Vanninen R, Partanen K, Heino A, Voinio P, Ala-Opas M. MR urography in evaluation of acute flank pain: T2-weighted sequences and gadolinium-enhanced three-dimensional FLASH compared with urography. Fast low-angle shot. AJR 2001; 176:105–112.

25. Blandino A, Gaeta M, Minutoli F, et al. MR urography of the ureter. AJR 2002; 179:1307–1314.

26. Cohnen M, Brause M, May P, et al. Contrast-enhanced MR urography in the evaluation of renal transplants with urological complications. Clin Nephrol 2002; 58:111–117.

27. Israel GM, Lee VS, Edye M, et al. Comprehensive MR imaging in the preoperative evaluation of living donor candidates for laparoscopic nephrectomy: initial experience. Radiology 2002; 225:427–432.

28. Riccabona M, Simbrunner J, Ring E, Ruppert-Kohlmayr A, Ebner F, Fotter R. Feasibility of MR urography in neonates and infants with anomalies of the upper urinary tract. Eur Radiol 2002; 12:1442–1450.

29. Sudah M, Vanninen RL, Partanen K, et al. Patients with acute flank pain: comparison of MR urography with unenhanced helical CT. Radiology 2002; 223:98–105.

30. El-Diasty T, Mansour O, Farouk A. Diuretic contrast-enhanced magnetic resonance urography versus intravenous urography for depiction of nondilated urinary tracts. Abdom Imaging 2003; 28:135–145.

31. Grattan-Smith JD, Perez-Bayfield MR, Jones RA, et al. MR imaging of kidneys: functional evaluation using F-15 perfusion imaging. Pediatr Radiol 2003; 33:293–304.

32. Niendorf HP, Haustein J, Cornelius I, Alhassan A, Clauss W. Safety of gadolinium-DTPA: extended clinical experience. Magn Reson Med 1991; 22:222–228.

33. Krestin GP, Schuhmann-Giampieri G, Haustein J, et al. Functional dynamic MRI, pharmacokinetics and safety of Gd-DTPA in patients with impaired renal function. Eur Radiol 1992; 2:16–23.

34. Haustein J, Niendorf HP, Krestin G, et al. Renal tolerance of gadolinium-DTPA/dimeglumine in patients with chronic renal failure. Invest Radiol 1992; 27:153–156.

35. Arsenault TM, King BF, Marsh JW Jr, et al. Systemic gadolinium toxicity in patients with renal insufficiency and renal failure: retrospective analysis of an initial experience. Mayo Clin Proc 1996; 71:1150–1154.

36. Nolte-Ernsting CC, Staatz G, Tacke J, Günther RW. MR urography today. Abdom Imaging 2003; 28:191–209.

37. Nolte-Ernsting CC, Wildberger JE, Borchers H, Schmitz-Rode T, Günther RW. Multislice CT urography after diuretic injection: initial results. Fortschr Röntgenstr 2001; 173:176–180.

38. Nolte-Ernsting C, Staatz G, Wildberger J, Adam G. MR-urography and CT-urography: principles, examination techniques, applications. Fortschr Röntgenstr 2003; 175:211–222.

39. Sigmund G, Stoever B, Zimmerhackl LB, et al. RARE-MR-urography in the diagnosis of upper urinary tract abnormalities in children. Pediatr Radiol 1991; 21:416–420.

40. Borthne A, Nordshus T, Reiseter T, et al. MR urography: the future gold standard in paediatric urogenital imaging? Pediatr Radiol 1999; 29:694–701.

41. Borthne A, Pierre-Jerome C, Nordshus T, Reiseter T. MR urography in children: current status and future development. Eur Radiol 2000; 10:503–511.

42. Rohrschneider WK, Haufe S, Wiesel M, et al. Functional and morphologic evaluation of congenital urinary tract dilatation by using combined static-dynamic MR urography: findings in kidneys with a single collecting system. Radiology 2002; 224:683–694.

43. Rohrschneider WK, Haufe S, Clorius JH, Troger J. MR to assess renal function in children. Eur Radiol 2003; 13:1033–1045.

44. Maher MM, Prasad TA, Fitzpatrick JM, et al. Spinal dysraphism at MR urography: initial experience. Radiology 2000; 216:237–241.

45. Girish G, Chooi WK, Morcos SK. Filling defect artefacts in magnetic resonance urography. Eur Radiol 2004; 14:145–150.

46. Roy C, Saussine C, LeBras Y, et al. Assessment of painful ureterohydronephrosis during pregnancy by MR urography. Eur Radiol 1996; 6:334–338.

47. Daniels RE, 3rd. The goblet sign. Radiology 1999; 210:737–738.

48. Low RN, Martinez AG, Steinberg SM, et al. Potential renal transplant donors: evaluation with gadolinium-enhanced MR angiography and MR urography. Radiology 1998; 207:165–172.

49. Steinborn M, Wintersperger BJ, Heck A, et al. Contrast enhanced MR angiography in the preoperative evaluation of living kidney donors. Fortschr Röntgenstr 1999; 171:313–318.

50. Winterer JT, Strey C, Wolffram C, et al. Preoperative examination of potential kidney transplantation donors: value of gadolinium-enhanced 3-D MR angiography in comparison with DSA and urography. Fortschr Röntgenstr 2000; 172:449–457.

51. Schubert RA, Gockeritz S, Mentzel HJ, Rzanny R, Schubert J, Kaiser WA. Imaging in ureteral complications of renal transplantation: value of static fluid MR urography. Eur Radiol 2000; 10:1152–1157.

52. Knopp MV, Dorsam J, Oesingmann N, et al. Functional MR urography in patients with kidney transplantation. Radiologe 1997; 37:233–238.

9

MRI of Renal Anomalies and Pyelonephritis in Infants and Children

Deniz Altinok and J. Michael Zerin
Department of Pediatric Imaging, Children's Hospital of Michigan, Detroit, Michigan, U.S.A.

J. Damien Grattan-Smith
Department of Pediatric Radiology, Scottish Rite Children's Hospital, Atlanta, Georgia, U.S.A.

INTRODUCTION

The anatomic and functional imaging evaluation of congenital anomalies and infections of the upper urinary tract have traditionally been accomplished with some combination of renal–bladder ultrasonography, diuretic renal scintigraphy with Tc99m-MAG3 or Tc99m-diethylene-triaminepentaacetic (DTPA), renal cortical scintigraphy with Tc99m-dimercapto-succinic acid (DMSA), and voiding cystourethrography (VCUG). The roles of both computed tomography (CT) and magnetic resonance imaging (MRI) in pediatric renal imaging have historically been quite limited. Until recently, the only routine exceptions have been for the evaluation of patients with trauma and patients with tumors, and for the assessment of patients with complex multisystem anatomic abnormalities, in which these modalities can provide clinically useful information that cannot be obtained noninvasively by other means, such as in those with complicated duplication anomalies and ectopic ureters, anorectal malformations, extrophy, and cloacal anomalies (1–4).

Cross-sectional imaging has recently begun to play an increasingly important role in a widening spectrum of genitourinary disorders during childhood. MRI provides exquisite soft-tissue contrast resolution and direct multiplanar capabilities. MRI also does not require the administration of intravenous iodinated contrast material, and the patient is not exposed to ionizing radiation. The greater safety profile of gadolinium contrast agents, as compared with the iodinated media used for urography and CT, are additional important relative advantages of MRI over these other modalities (5–13). Both MRI and magnetic resonance (MR) urography can also be safely performed in patients with renal insufficiency (9,12,14). In contrast to CT, in which only direct axial imaging can be performed, direct coronal imaging with MRI permits rapid evaluation of large portions of the abdomen and pelvis at one time and provides images that simulate those obtained during conventional urographic examinations but with significantly more detailed anatomic and potentially functional information (2,4,9,15,16). Furthermore, MR urography (MRU) combines anatomic and functional evaluations of the urinary tract into a single test that does not use ionizing radiation. The MR urograms provide higher temporal, spatial, and contrast resolution when compared to traditional intravenous urograms. Nonetheless, interpretation of the MR images is still based on traditional urographic findings.

Even setting aside the increasing role of MRI and MRU in the primary imaging evaluation of infants and children suspected of having congenital urinary tract abnormalities, knowledge of the MRI appearances of these various renal malformations is also important because patients with these anomalies might have MR examinations for other reasons, whether directly related to their urinary tract disease or not.

Some potential technical difficulties are encountered when trying to obtain high-quality MR studies. The need for sedation remains an important limitation of MRI, particularly in infants and younger children, as well as in the developmentally challenged (8,12,13). All of these patients will likely not be able to lie still for the MR examination. Sedation is required because patient motion must be minimized to avoid degradation in image quality and presence of associated artifacts. Continuing improvements in MRI protocols resulting in decreasing acquisition times will hopefully eliminate this requirement or, at least, shorten the duration of sedation required in some children in the future.

NORMAL ANATOMY, ITS MR APPEARANCE, AND MRI TECHNIQUE

Normal Anatomy

The kidneys lie in the retroperitoneum, anterior to the psoas muscles within the perirenal space on each side. Anteriorly, the perirenal space is bounded by Gerota's fascia, posteriorly by the fascia of Zuckerkandl, and laterally by the lateral conal fascia. In the upper retroperitoneum, fusion of these fascial planes separates the anterior and posterior pararenal spaces. Inferiorly, the fascia remains open, resulting in potential communication between the anterior and posterior pararenal spaces.

In infants and younger children, the longitudinal axes of the kidneys are oriented roughly parallel to the spine, with the renal hila and the aortic origins of the renal arteries roughly at the level of the second lumbar vertebra. The right kidney lies directly posterior to the descending limb of the duodenum and pancreatic head and is usually slightly more caudally located than the left kidney. The right renal vein passes anteromedially from the renal hilum to enter the inferior vena cava (IVC), and the right renal artery courses rightward from its aortic origin behind the IVC to enter the renal hilum. The left kidney lies posterior to the tail of the pancreas. The left renal vein passes through the aorto-mesenteric angle to enter the IVC, whereas the left renal artery courses only for a short distance from its aortic origin to enter the left renal hilum. As the child grows, the psoas muscles enlarge and displace the lower renal poles anteriorly and laterally, causing the kidneys to lie somewhat more obliquely in relation to the spine in the adolescent and adult. In the coronal plane, the sizes of the kidneys can be assessed by comparison with the vertebral column, with each kidney normally spanning approximately three vertebral levels.

MRI

Although the presence of abundant perirenal fat surrounding the kidneys is usually seen as beneficial in MR renal imaging in older children and adults, MRI routinely provides excellent visualization of the kidneys, even in infants and younger children in whom there is relatively little perirenal fat. On spin-echo T1-weighted MR images, renal corticomedullary differentiation is well visualized, with the renal cortex typically having a higher signal intensity than the medullary pyramids (Fig. 1) (5,7,10, 13,17–19). The difference in signal intensity between the cortex and medulla is most pronounced in neonates and younger children. Corticomedullary differentiation is similarly accentuated on inversion recovery sequences (Fig. 1), but can vary depending on the state of hydration. Because infants and young children generally have less hilar fat than adults, the renal hilar regions are usually lower in signal intensity and, therefore, less conspicuous early in life. By early adolescence, their appearance is similar to that in adults.

On T1-weighted MR images, the renal collecting systems and ureters normally have a very low signal intensity on spin-echo sequences because of the long relaxation time of urine. The renal vessels also usually have a very low signal intensity related to rapid blood flow in and out of the kidney (20). When flow is slowed, intraluminal signal can be identified. Intraluminal signal can also appear artifactually secondary to flow-related enhancement in vessels that course within the plane of imaging.

On T2-weighted images in infants, the signal intensity of the renal medulla is increased when compared to that of the renal cortex (Fig. 1). In older children, the renal medulla and cortex both have increased signal intensities on T2-weighted sequences, although the cortex usually has a slightly higher signal intensity than the medulla (5,18,19). As a result, corticomedullary differentiation is less conspicuous on T2-weighted than on T1-weighted sequences. The perirenal fat also appears bright on T2-weighted sequences, and Gerota's fascia appears as a thin, lower-signal intensity line separating the perirenal fascia and pararenal spaces on either side. A chemical shift opposed-phase misregistration artifact at the interface between the kidney and the adjacent perirenal fat produces a characteristic low–signal intensity line along one side of the kidney with a symmetrically high–signal intensity line along the opposite side of the kidney. Recognition of this chemical shift artifact is critical to avoiding misattributing the appearance to calcification (21).

MRU and Evaluation of Renal Function

During MRU, visualization of the collecting system, ureter, and bladder can be obtained either by utilizing heavily T2-weighted sequences similar to MR cholangiopancreatography or on T1-weighted sequences after intravenous gadolinium administration (Fig. 2) (15,16,22–26). Gadolinium chelates, such as gadolinium diethylenetriamine pentaacetic acid (Gd-DTPA), are ideal for studying the morphology and function of the kidneys because they are filtered by the renal glomerulus and excreted by the renal tubules. The MRI evaluation of renal function is based on the assessment of the rate of excretion of gadolinium contrast media and the timing and relative intensity of enhancement of the renal cortex and medulla. The physiologic behavior of gadolinium is primarily governed by the biochemical properties of the ligand to which it is chelated. Like inulin, DTPA is freely filtered by the glomerulus and is neither reabsorbed nor secreted by the renal tubules, rendering it an ideal indicator

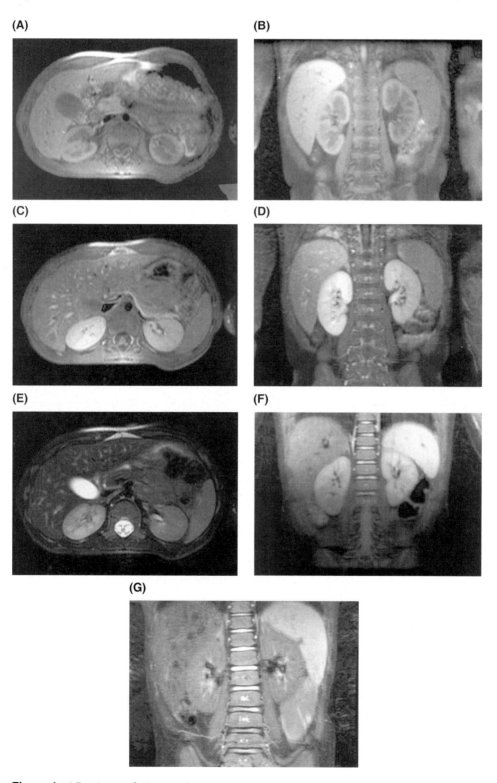

Figure 1   (*Caption on facing page*)

for glomerular filtration. When bound to gadolinium, the path of DTPA through the kidney can be followed easily on T1-weighted images. Renal cortical gadolinium enhancement primarily reflects renal perfusion and glomerular filtration, whereas enhancement of the medulla and opacification of the collecting system depends upon glomerular filtration as well as renal tubular secretion and absorption. The paramagnetic properties of gadolinium cause marked T1 and T2 shortening, which can be tracked on a time–activity curve, thereby generating a functional analysis analogous to that obtained during diuretic renal scintigraphy (8,18,25). However, the markedly superior spatial resolution of MRI (as compared with scintigraphy) enables one to differentiate cortical from medullary enhancement and, therefore, allows one to obtain more accurate measurements of renal perfusion and glomerular filtration. In addition, because of its ability to precisely separate cortical from medullary enhancement, MR renography has the unique potential to noninvasively distinguish glomerular from tubulointerstitial pathology (8,23). Differential renal function can be calculated by estimating the volumes of enhancing renal parenchyma for each kidney.

In its original application in pediatric imaging, contrast-enhanced MRU was designed to reproduce the conventional experience with diuretic renal scintigraphy (8,14–16,27). Although the protocol varied somewhat among investigators, the technique has been referred to as the "F+20" protocol because furosemide is administered 20 minutes after the contrast material is injected. The F+20 examination begins with spin-echo T1 and fat-suppressed fast spin-echo T2-weighted images of the kidneys, ureters, and bladder. A bolus of 0.1 mmol/kg of Gd-DTPA is then injected intravenously, immediately after which the entire urinary tract is continuously surveyed for three minutes using a dynamic volumetric gradient-echo technique with a time resolution of 15 seconds. The volumetric gradient-echo acquisition is then repeated at one minute intervals for 17 minutes, after which 1 mg/kg of furosemide is given and the imaging is continued for an additional 15 minutes again at one minute intervals.

The F+20 technique has two drawbacks (8,14,27). First, the imaging time is very long, such that some investigators have reported that sedated children frequently wake up before the examination is completed. Second, the very high concentrations of gadolinium in the renal collecting systems early during the excretion phase frequently produce severe magnetic susceptibility artifacts, which degrade image quality (8,18). In addition, although plots of signal intensity versus time graphically demonstrate delayed excretion in obstructed systems, they are of little value in quantifying wash-out of contrast material from the collecting system and ureters because signal intensity does not have a linear relationship with gadolinium concentration. As a result, gadolinium signal intensity remains constantly high throughout the examination (8).

These limitations of the F+20 MRU technique led to the development of the "F-15" protocol in which furosemide is given 15 minutes before the contrast material rather than afterward. With the F-15 technique, noncontrast-enhanced T1-weighted

---

Figure 1 (*Figure on facing page*) Normal MRI of the kidneys with different pulse sequences. (**A**) Axial and (**B**) coronal noncontrast T1-weighted, fat-saturated images of the kidneys. (**C**) Axial and (**D**) coronal postcontrast T1-weighted, fat-saturated images of the kidneys. (**E**) Axial noncontrast T2-weighted, fat-saturated image of the kidneys. (**F**) Coronal noncontrast fast spin-echo inversion recovery image of the kidneys. (**G**) Coronal postcontrast fast spin-echo inversion recovery image of the kidney. *Abbreviation*: MRI, magnetic resonance imaging.

(A)

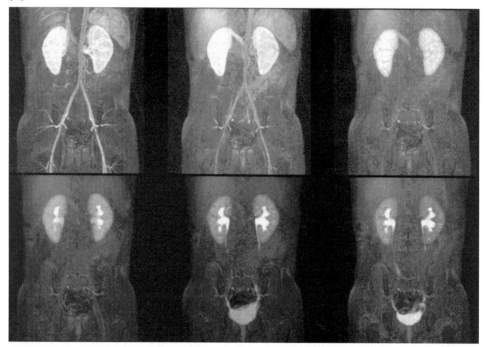

(B)

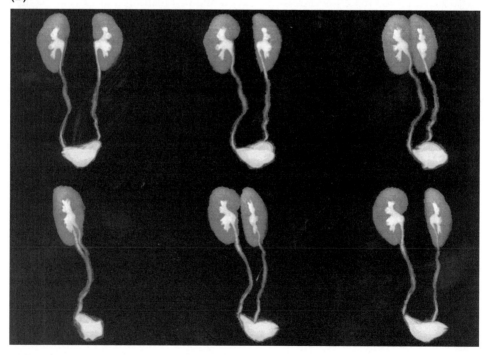

Figure 2 Normal postcontrast T1-weighted MR urogram. (**A**) A series of six coronal post-contrast T1-weighted images during the cortical, excretory, and delayed phases show normal cortical enhancement and excretion bilaterally. Urinary bladder appears normal. (**B**) A series of six coronal MIP images rotated through 360° show the normal appearance of both kidneys and the bladder. *Abbreviations*: MIP, maximum intensity projection; MR, magnetic resonance.

and T2-weighted images are acquired just after furosemide administration (8,27). Gadolinium is then injected 15 minutes after the furosemide, and dynamic imaging commences immediately. A high-resolution volumetric sequence is then obtained with the patient prone, to promote mixing of the excreted contrast material with urine as well as drainage of contrast material into dilated collecting systems (if dilatation is present). The F-15 technique dramatically shortens the imaging time. It also eliminates the appearance of any gadolinium-related magnetic susceptibility artifacts. In addition, the F-15 protocol makes it possible to quantitatively trace the passage of contrast material from its appearance in the calyces to the renal pelvis and into the ureter. In this fashion, the diagnosis of obstruction can be based on functional asymmetry in excretion rather than solely on such morphologic abnormalities as pelvocaliectasis, ureterectasis, or persistent ureteral narrowing (8,27). Also, differential renal function can be estimated based on the volume of enhancing renal parenchymal volume during the corticomedullary phase prior to appearance of contrast material in the collecting systems. In the future, using assessments of differential function that are based on time–activity analysis of corticomedullary gadolinium transit will likely be more precise than those that rely on morphologic assessments of functioning renal parenchymal volume alone (8,27).

MRU performed without gadolinium enhancement using heavily T2-weighted sequences generates images in which static fluid in the renal collecting systems has a very high signal intensity (4,8,9,14–16,22–29). On these images, signal intensity in the renal parenchyma is relatively suppressed because it normally has a shorter T2 relaxation time. One of the most widely used T2-weighted urographic techniques is performing a series of single-shot, fast spin-echo sequences with half-Fourier acquisitions, with reconstruction of multiple thin slice images or a single thick section image. Steady-state free precession sequences are also becoming more popular in adults.

T2-weighted MRU provides excellent visualization of the urinary tract in patients with dilated collecting systems and ureters (22–24,28) and is, therefore, usually able to identify the precise site of any obstruction when such dilatation is present. T2-weighted MRU is also useful for evaluating patients with impaired renal function because imaging is not dependent upon excretion of gadolinium by the kidney. When used in conjunction with contrast-enhanced imaging, ureteric anatomy can be delineated in almost every case, even when there are nonfunctioning systems. The most significant limitations of this technique are its inability to consistently demonstrate nondilated systems and its inability to provide any direct functional data. Superimposition of fluid-filled extra-urinary structures, such as bowel loops and the gallbladder, can also be a problem. Some investigators have suggested that visualization of nondilated collecting systems and ureters can be improved with the administration of furosemide (15,16). It must be remembered that visualization of urinary calculi is also limited on MRI, because these appear as filling defects or signal voids on both conventional MRI and on MRU techniques (14,23,24,26,28).

MR Angiography

The intrinsic sensitivity of MRI to motion allows for the depiction of vessels and for the assessment of flow both quantitatively and qualitatively when several specific sequences are employed (6,20,25,30). Ironically, vascular flow phenomena were initially considered to represent undesirable artifacts, and considerable effort was aimed at eliminating them. Subsequently, the diagnostic importance of these flow-related signal changes was realized and rapidly led to the development of MR angiographic imaging protocols that permitted direct imaging of vascular morphology and quantification of flow (even in the absence of contrast material administration). Flow-sensitive techniques, such as phased contrast MR angiography (MRA) and time-of-flight MRA, were developed, although both techniques do have some limitations, including artifactual signal dropout caused by turbulent blood flow, degradation of image quality secondary to respiratory motion, and saturation of in-plane blood flow. These effects limit the visualization of small vascular structures, which can particularly be a problem in infants and smaller children. 3-D gadolinium (3D-Gd) MRA overcomes the limitations by acquiring a 3-D dataset within a single breath hold. Continuing improvements in 3D-Gd MRA will likely reduce the necessity of utilizing imaging modalities that require intravascular administration of potentially nephrotoxic iodinated contrast material, such as CT angiography or conventional catheter angiography (25,30).

CONGENITAL ANOMALIES OF THE KIDNEYS AND URETERS

Variations in Renal Shape

Nonpathological variations in renal shape can be developmental or can result from the compression or displacement of the kidney by adjacent normal or abnormal structures (13,31). The spleen can flatten the upper pole of the left kidney and produce a prominent lateral renal bulge, commonly referred to as a dromedary hump. In patients with splenomegaly, the displacement and compression of the left kidney can be quite pronounced, but the resulting renal deformity should not be mistaken for a renal mass.

Persistent fetal lobation is a common developmental variant in renal shape that should be readily recognized and should not be confused either with a renal mass or with cortical scarring. The indentations in the renal contour due to fetal lobation lie between the medullary rays and occur throughout the kidney, in contrast to cortical scars due to chronic atrophic pyelonephritis, where the areas of parenchymal loss directly overlie the pyramids and also have a strong polar predilection (32).

The junctional cortical defect is a common sonographic finding on the lateral surface of the upper third of the kidney, usually extending inferomedially for a variable distance into the renal sinus (33–35). It is also occasionally visible on other modalities and should not be mistaken for a cortical scar or infarct. This common normal defect represents the anterior site of fusion of the superior and inferior reniculi, the two primitive nephrogenic masses that combine to form the kidney.

Anomalies of Renal Position, Rotation, and Fusion

During nephrogenesis, the developing kidneys normally ascend from the pelvis to the retroperitoneum until they reach their normal positions in the flanks. As each kidney ascends, it rotates along its sagittal axis such that the renal hilum is redirected anteromedially where the advancing ureteral bud invaginates into the developing renal sinus. Renal ascent is normally completed by the ninth gestational week. When a kidney fails to ascend normally, in addition to being abnormal in location, it is also frequently malrotated and the renal sinus is poorly developed (36,37).

The sagittal renal axis in the supine patient is normally at an approximately 30° angle relative to the long axis of the body, with the lower poles located anterior to the upper poles. On either a frontal radiograph from an intravenous urogram or on a coronal image from an MRU, lines representing the longitudinal axes of the kidneys should intersect superiorly at approximately the level of the 10th to 11th thoracic vertebra.

There are a wide range of anomalies of renal rotation, from nonrotation (in which the renal pelvis is located anteriorly) to incomplete rotation (in which the renal pelvis is located between 30° and 90° from horizontal), to reverse rotation (in which the renal pelvis is located laterally), to transverse rotation (in which the renal pelvis is located superiorly or inferiorly) (36–39). Whereas ectopic kidneys are frequently malrotated, otherwise normally positioned kidneys can also occasionally be malrotated. Whereas the position and orientation of the kidney are usually readily apparent on MRI, differentiation between anterior and posterior malrotation and between superior and inferior transverse malrotation depends on the identification of the courses of the main renal vessels as they emerge from the renal hilum and continue along the external surface of the kidney to reach the aorta and IVC.

Renal ectopia occurs in 1 in 500 to 1200 individuals (13,36,37). Most ectopic kidneys lie caudal to the normal renal fossa. Although all caudally ectopic kidneys are often referred to generically as pelvic kidneys, the actual degree of ectopia is quite variable. It is generally accepted that ptotic kidneys are located only slightly caudal to the normal renal position, lumbar kidneys located somewhat more caudally, but still intra-abdominal, and sacral kidneys located completely caudal to the lumbosacral junction. In patients who have anterior abdominal wall defects, such as gastroschisis or omphalocele, the kidneys can be located cephalad to the normal renal fossa, just beneath the diaphragm. In patients with congenital diaphragmatic hernia, the ipsilateral kidney rarely is intrathoracic (13,37,40,41). Ectopic kidneys typically have an anomalous arterial supply related to their final position at the point of arrest of normal renal ascent (13,36,37,42,43). Horseshoe, crossed ectopic, and pelvic kidneys typically receive their blood supply from renal arteries originating from the midabdominal aorta and also from the distal abdominal aorta, iliac vessels, or even branches of the inferior mesenteric artery. Multiple renal arteries are frequently present in these patients.

Horseshoe kidney is the most common renal fusion anomaly, with an incidence of 1 in 400 to 1800 individuals (Fig. 3) (44,45). In nearly all cases, the kidneys lie on either side of the midline, and their lower poles are joined by an isthmus composed of renal parenchyma and fibrous tissue in variable proportions. Upper pole fusion is exceedingly rare. The horseshoe kidney is typically located somewhat more caudally than normal, with the isthmus passing between the inferior mesenteric artery and the aortic bifurcation. The renal axes are reversed, with the lower poles being located more medially than the upper poles. Also, the kidneys are anteriorly malrotated (13,31). As a result, the pelves and ureteropelvic junctions (UPJs) are located anteriorly, and the ureters are displaced laterally by the isthmus. UPJ obstruction occurs in 30% of patients with horseshoe kidney and can be caused by intrinsic stenosis, by a high ureteral insertion, or by extrinsic compression by the isthmus or an anomalous vessel (46).

Crossed renal ectopia represents a spectrum of anomalies of renal ascent in which the ectopic kidney is located both caudal and medial to its normal location, either overlying the midline or completely on the opposite side of the abdomen (13,36,37,43,47,48). Usually the ectopic kidney is fused to its contralateral mate, a condition referred to as "crossed-fused renal ectopia." Crossed ectopia without fusion accounts for less than 10% of cases. Solitary crossed renal ectopia, i.e., crossed

(A)

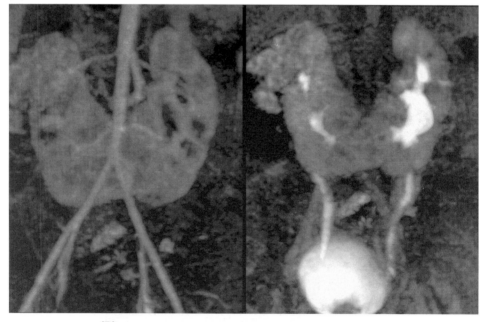

(B)

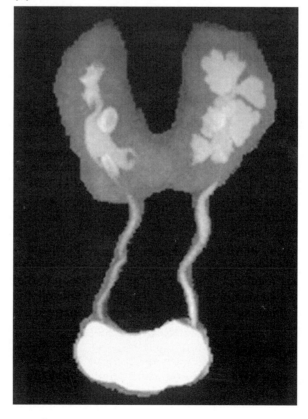

Figure 3 (*Caption on facing page*)

ectopia with contralateral renal agenesis and bilateral crossed renal ectopia, are very rare. In all cases of crossed renal ectopia, whether fused or unfused, the ureter draining the ectopic kidney crosses the midline to insert on its proper side on the trigone of the bladder.

Variations in the extent of renal fusion, as well as in the timing of the fusion in relation to renal ascent and rotation, result in a wide spectrum of potential anatomic configurations in crossed renal ectopia (13,36,37,47). The most common form is the unilateral fused type, in which the upper pole of the ectopic kidney is fused to the lower pole of its normally or nearly normally positioned contralateral mate. In another common configuration, the ectopic kidney assumes a transverse, inferior position, spanning the midline, with its upper pole fused to the medial aspect of the lower pole of the more vertically oriented contralateral kidney resulting in an "L-shaped kidney." Occasionally, the extensive fusion of the kidneys in the midline results in a single, amorphous renal structure, usually located in the lower abdomen or pelvis, referred to variably in the literature as a "lump," "cake," or "disk" kidney (Fig. 4). Although crossed renal ectopia is reported to be less common than horseshoe kidney, crossed ectopia and horseshoe kidney very likely represent a continuum of anomalies in renal ascent, position, and fusion rather than being truly distinct entities.

In children with myelomeningocele and severe thoracolumbar kyphoscoliosis, the lower poles of the kidneys can be oriented more medially, thereby falsely simulating a horseshoe kidney. A mistaken diagnosis of horseshoe kidney is thus most likely in children with caudal regression syndrome, in which the two kidneys lie directly apposed to one another, mimicking the appearance of a single, fused, midline kidney. This problem was originally described on intravenous urography (49); however, the appearance can also be confusing when other imaging modalities are used, including renal scintigraphy, CT, or even potentially MRI (13,31,50).

Patients with ectopic, malrotated, or fused kidneys are usually asymptomatic. However, renal ectopia is frequently associated with other congenital urinary tract malformations, including duplication anomalies, vesicoureteral reflux, multicystic dysplastic kidney, and UPJ obstruction (36,37). Symptoms, when present, are usually related to collecting-system dilatation, infection, or urolithiasis. Renal ectopia, renal agenesis, and multicystic dysplastic kidney are present in half of patients with cloacal malformation and are also the most common renal malformations that are associated with the VACTERL [vertebral anomalies, anal atresia, cardiac defects, tracheoesophageal fistulae, renal abnormalities, limb abnormalities (usually radial dysplasia)] anomalad (13,37,51). Anomalies of renal position and fusion, including horseshoe kidney, crossed renal ectopia, and pelvic kidney, are also the most common renal anomalies in Turner syndrome (52).

Figure 3 (*Figure on facing page*) A two-year-old with horseshoe kidney. (**A**) Coronal postcontrast T1-weighted images during the cortical phase (*left*) and excretion phase (*right*) show the typical morphology of a horseshoe kidney with abnormally vertical renal axes and a well-defined isthmus extending between the two lower poles. Note that the isthmus overlies the aortic bifurcation and proximal common iliac vessels. (**B**) Coronal 3-D postcontrast T1-weighted MIP image showing the typical morphology of a horseshoe kidney with abnormally vertical renal axes and a well-defined isthmus extending between the two lower poles. Note that the collecting systems are rotated laterally and the proximal ureters overlie the lower poles of the kidneys. *Abbreviation*: MIP, maximum intensity projection.

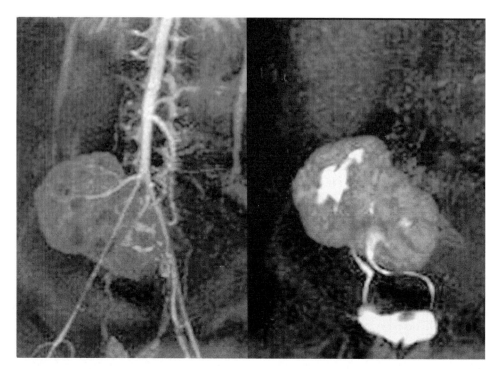

Figure 4 Infant with crossed fused renal ectopia in the pelvis (lump kidney). Coronal postcontrast T1-weighted images during the cortical phase (*left*) and excretion phase (*right*) show both kidneys fused, with a single renal structure lying in the right pelvis and separate right and left ureters, each inserting normally into the trigone on their respective sides. Note the vascular supply to the right kidney arises from the origin of the right common iliac artery and the vascular supply to the left kidney from the left common iliac artery.

Renal Agenesis

Bilateral renal agenesis is a rare, lethal condition that is typically associated with oligohydramnios, pulmonary hypoplasia, and musculoskeletal and facial deformation anomalies secondary to severe intrauterine fetal compression—i.e., Potter syndrome (36,37,53,54). The patient is characteristically anuric and rapidly develops clinical and biochemical characteristics consistent with severe renal insufficiency. Diagnosis is usually readily established based upon portable ultrasonographic evaluation and confirmed with renal scintigraphy (13,31,54). Renal scintigraphy can confirm the absence of functioning renal parenchyma, although this is usually unnecessary when the diagnosis is straightforward based on clinical and sonographic features. Affected newborns usually die of respiratory failure within a few hours or days following birth, due to associated pulmonary hypoplasia. Given the invariably lethal nature of this disorder and the availability of bedside ultrasound (US) examinations, MRI plays no role in the diagnosis of this condition in the newborn (13,31).

Unilateral renal agenesis, on the other hand, is by comparison relatively common (1 in 1000 live births) (Fig. 5) (13,31,37,54,55). In this disorder, only a solitary functioning kidney is identifiable on all imaging studies. Unilateral renal agenesis is likely not a single disorder, because it has become clear that a number of embryological abnormalities can result in unilateral absence of a kidney. Unilateral renal

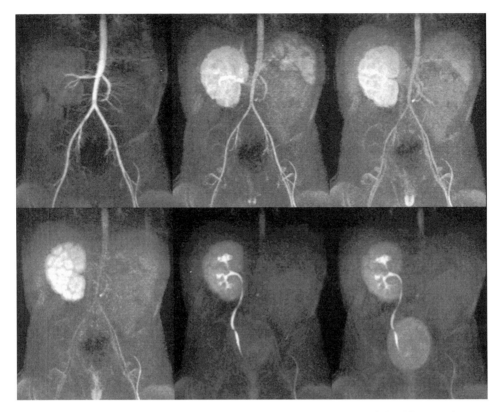

Figure 5 Infant with left renal agenesis. A series of six coronal T2-weighted images show no evidence of a left kidney anywhere in the abdomen or pelvis. The left renal artery is also not identified. The right kidney appears normal.

agenesis can result from a spectrum of embryological defects during nephrogenesis as well as from vascular insults to the developing fetal kidney (37). Although multi-cystic dysplastic kidney (MCDK) is discussed in greater detail in section "Renal Dysplasia and MCDK," it is important to mention in the current context that involution of MCDK can be indistinguishable from unilateral renal agenesis in the absence of earlier documentation of a cystic dysplastic kidney (13,31,54,55).

Because there is no function on the affected side in patients with unilateral renal agenesis and MCDK, scintigraphy is not helpful in distinguishing between these entities, and there is probably considerable overlap in diagnosis as a result. Occasionally, MRI can be used to detect a small, poorly functioning or nonfunctioning kidney in a child who appears to have unilateral agenesis on US and renal scintigraphy (13,31). In such cases, however, the reason for the atrophic appearance and poor function of the kidney frequently cannot be established through imaging in the absence of associated known lower genitourinary anomalies, such as an ectopic ureter (that might suggest MCDK) or a history of a previous severe vascular renal insult. Additionally, severe congenital or infantile renal artery stenosis can have a similar imaging appearance.

MRI in patients with an absent kidney may not be justifiable in the absence of any symptoms. On the other hand, in a child who presents with a history of an "absent kidney" and incontinence or hypertension, MRI can be invaluable in

(A)

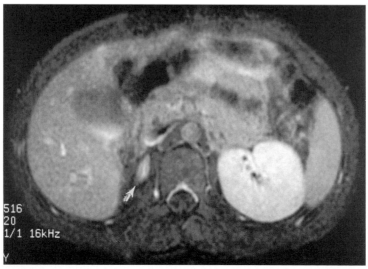

(B)

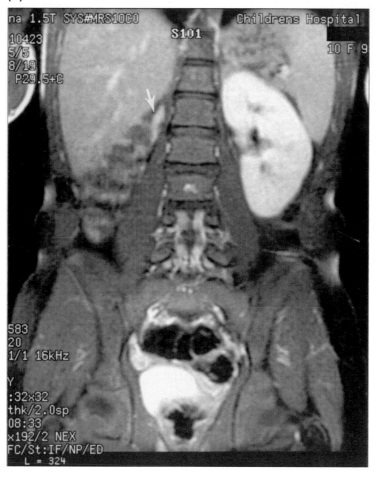

Figure 6 (*Caption on facing page*)

identifying a tiny renal remnant. Nephrectomy in these symptomatic patients can, in some instances, lead to resolution of incontinence or improvement or even complete resolution of hypertension (Fig. 6) (13,31).

Compensatory renal hypertrophy is a well-established, albeit poorly understood, trophic response of the solitary kidney in a child to the lack of a contralateral functioning organ (31,56,57). In 1971, Griscom et al. (56) showed that in neonates and young infants born with a solitary functioning kidney, this kidney will usually be larger than normal, as a consequence of an acceleration in the rate of renal growth that begins early in life. This period of accelerated growth is time limited and is followed by a restoration of the normal rate of renal growth that parallels the growth curve for normally paired kidneys. Subsequent prenatal and postnatal studies with US have confirmed the generally larger size of solitary kidneys in children in a variety of congenital and acquired disorders that result in the absence of a contralateral functioning kidney.

Failure to visualize a kidney in its normal location can also be suspected to be the result of a congenital abnormality when the ipsilateral adrenal gland has an abnormal configuration. The normal "arrowhead" configuration of the adrenal gland results from its elevation and deformation by the subjacent kidney. When a kidney is absent or ectopic, the ipsilateral adrenal gland assumes an elongated, linear configuration. In some cases, its appearance can superficially mimic that of a small, hypoplastic, atrophic, or dysplastic kidney (58,59). This is particularly true in the fetus and neonate, who have relatively larger-sized adrenal glands (compared with the other abdominal visceral organs) than do adults. There is a useful trick to avoid this mistake: The adrenal gland will always be present even when the kidney is absent. Therefore, if the adrenal gland cannot be identified separately from a retroperitoneal structure that is initially misidentified as a small kidney, the structure in question can be assumed to represent the adrenal gland instead, with the ipsilateral kidney either being absent or being located somewhere else in the abdomen or pelvis.

Renal Dysplasia and MCDK

MCDK is a nonhereditary, developmental disorder of the kidney in which atresia of the ureteral bud at or below the UPJ results in a severely dysplastic, nonfunctioning, cystic kidney (Fig. 7) (23,36,37,54,60). This entity was first described in 1836 by the French pathologist Cruveilhier based on an autopsy of a three-year-old boy. Before the development of US and renal scintigraphy, reliable noninvasive diagnosis of MCDK was not possible. Because most patients presented with a palpable flank mass that could not be distinguished from a renal tumor based on the then available imaging techniques, nearly all MCDK patients underwent nephrectomy, as much for diagnosis as for treatment (31,61). Today, the presence of the abnormal multicystic

---

Figure 6 (*Figure on facing page*) A nine-year-old girl with malignant hypertension and secondary cardiomyopathy secondary to severe right congenital renal artery stenosis (renal angiodysplasia). Previous US and MAG-3 renal scans showed no right kidney and were interpreted as being consistent with right renal agenesis. (**A**) Axial and (**B**) coronal noncontrast-enhanced T1-weighted fast spin-echo images show a normal left kidney and a very tiny right kidney (*arrows*) in the right renal fossa. Following laparascopic right nephrectomy, her blood pressure normalized. *Abbreviation*: US, ultrasound.

(A)   **(B)**

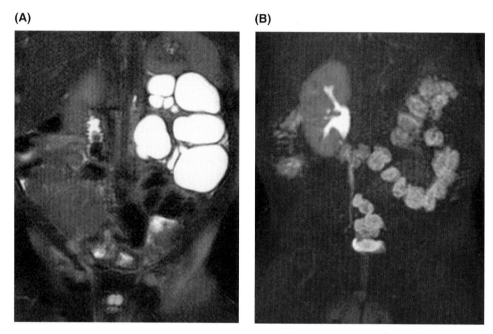

Figure 7 A six-month-old girl with left MCDK. (**A**) Coronal T2-weighted image showing a large multicystic structure in the left renal fossa with no visible normal parenchyma. A normal right kidney is present. (**B**) Coronal postcontrast, excretory phase MIP image showing a normally functioning right kidney with no functioning renal parenchyma on the left. *Abbreviations*: MCDK, multicystic dysplastic kidney; MIP, maximum intensity projection.

kidney is usually first detected at antenatal sonography (in more than 80% of patients). A specific diagnosis of MCDK is now most commonly made noninvasively in the newborn period based on the characteristic imaging findings on US combined with renal diuretic or cortical scintigraphy. Together, these two imaging tests demonstrate that the kidney is nonfunctioning and has been replaced by multiple noncommunicating cysts (31,57,62,63). On US, the cysts in MCDK are usually noted to be of different sizes, with the largest cyst rarely located centrally. This feature distinguishes MCDK from severe pelvocaliectasis. When the cystic areas are produced by renal collecting system dilatation, the largest centrally located "cyst" actually represents the dilated renal pelvis. The pelvis can be seen to be surrounded by smaller, radially arranged dilated calyces. The lack of a visible mantle of parenchyma around the MCDK cysts can also be used to differentiate this entity from pelvocaliectasis, where at least a thin rim of renal parenchyma is usually identified.

Patients with MCDK who are not diagnosed in the neonatal period present either later in childhood or as an adult with a palpable abdominal mass or have the diagnosis made as an incidental finding during imaging that is performed for an unrelated reason. On CT or MRI, the appearance is similar to that previously described for US. The affected kidney is readily visible, again being replaced by multiple cysts of different sizes that are separated by a small amount of abnormal-appearing soft tissue.

Several less common variants of MCDK are worth mentioning. In the hydronephrotic variant of MCDK (60), also referred to as pelvo-infundibular atresia (56), the kidney is nonfunctioning and contains one or more smaller peripheral cysts with a large central cyst. This appearance is due to the fact that in the hydronephrotic variant, the large central cyst does, in fact, represent the central portion of a dysmorphic and dilated collecting system. In the segmental MCDK, only one moiety of a partially or completely duplicated collecting system is affected (64,65). When the multicystic dysplastic segment of the kidney involutes, recognition that there is a duplex collecting system is difficult in the absence of a tell-tale ureterocele or ectopic ureter (65). Bilateral multicystic renal dysplasia is incompatible with life and is accompanied by severe oligohydramnios, pulmonary hypoplasia, and other characteristics of Potter syndrome (36,37,53).

The tendency for prenatally diagnosed MCDK to involute, both before and after birth, has been well documented. Fluid in the cysts is frequently absorbed, and the cysts collapse (62,63,66). Eventually, there is only a tiny, solid remnant. Because the kidney is not functioning, it will not be visible on either urography or renal scintigraphy, and the small amount of residual dysplastic parenchyma is often undetectable on US. In this situation, confusion with unilateral renal agenesis is likely if the patient's first imaging examination is performed only after the cystic kidney has involuted (55). In circumstances in which differentiation between these disorders is clinically valuable, MRI is the most reliable imaging modality for demonstrating the small dysplastic remnant of an otherwise occult involuted MCDK (13,31,67).

Associated Anomalies in Renal Agenesis and MCDK

MRI and MRU can be of particular value in the evaluation of children of both genders who have renal agenesis or MCDK, because these studies can also detect the various lower genitourinary anomalies that are occasionally associated with these entities (4,67,68).

In girls, both unilateral renal agenesis and MCDK are occasionally associated with uterovaginal anomalies. Although a wide spectrum of anatomic variations have been reported in this situation, the classical description is of uterovaginal duplication, with unilateral vaginal obstruction and hemihydrocolpos on the same side as the absent or involuted kidney (68). An ectopic ureter to the obstructed uterovaginal unit is occasionally present, in which case there is also usually a small renal remnant, either in the renal fossa or elsewhere in the abdomen or pelvis (4,67,68).

In boys, both unilateral renal agenesis and MCDK can be associated with an ipsilateral seminal vesicle cyst, often with an atretic, ectopic ureter (Fig. 8) (69). Occasionally, the ipsilateral vas deferens and testes are absent.

Duplications and Other Anomalies of the Renal Collecting System and Ureter

Duplication anomalies of the renal collecting system and ureter are quite common (1 in 160 live births), with a strong familial association (36,37,54,70,71). Partial duplications, including bifid collecting systems in which the two ureters join before inserting into the bladder at a single orifice, are more common than are complete duplications in which the duplicated ureters have separate distal orifices. In complete duplications, the upper pole ureter inserts medial and distal to the lower pole ureter.

Most duplications of the renal collecting system and ureters, either partial or complete, are not complicated by collecting system or ureteral dilatation, reflux,

(A)   **(B)**

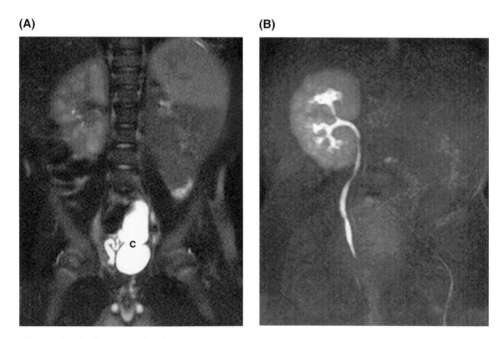

Figure 8   A three-month-old boy with left renal agenesis and a right seminal vesicle cyst. (**A**) A coronal T2-weighted image demonstrates a normal right kidney with bowel in the left renal fossa. Note the large retrovesical cystic structure representing a giant left seminal vesicle cyst (c). (**B**) A coronal postcontrast T1-weighted, excretory phase MIP image shows a single functioning kidney on the right with no visible left kidney. *Abbreviation*: MIP, maximum intensity projection.

or obstruction, and the presence of the duplication is, therefore, clinically unimportant. Occasionally, however, there are associated abnormalities of the upper pole or the lower pole renal collecting systems and ureters, or both. Abnormalities associated with the upper pole renal collecting system and ureter include ureterocele and ectopic intra-vesical or extravesical ureteral insertion.

Ureteroceles occur mostly in girls and are usually associated with upper pole pelvocaliectasis and ureterectasis (Fig. 9) (36,37,54,72,73). Most ureteroceles are located at an ectopic site of insertion of the upper pole ureter into the bladder, often at the bladder neck. The ectopic insertion site can also be in the urethra (Fig. 10).

Ureteroceles in boys are usually associated with nonduplicated collecting systems. Single-system ureteroceles can have a normal ureteral insertion site or can insert ectopically. Irrespective of their location, they are almost always associated with ureterovesical junction (UVJ) obstruction and pelvocaliectasis and ureterectasis or MCDK (72,74). The nonobstructing adult type "simple" ureterocele is very rare in childhood.

When the upper pole ureter of a duplex collecting system inserts outside the bladder in a girl—at the bladder neck, into the urethra or vagina, or onto the peri-neum—she will be continually wet despite being normally toilet-trained (75,76). This anomaly is usually unilateral but can be bilateral. The same syndrome can also occur with a single, extravesical, ectopic ureter that drains a nonduplicated collecting system, although this is less common (77,78). Unfortunately, diagnosis of this anomaly is frequently delayed, by months or even years, either because this entity is not

(A)   (B)

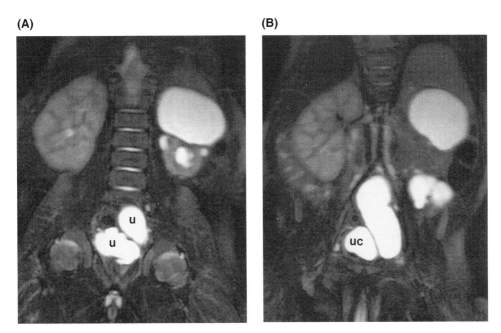

Figure 9 A nine-month-old girl with a left duplex kidney with upper pole ureterocele. (**A**) A coronal T2-weighted image shows a duplicated left collecting system with severe upper pole pelvocaliectasis and mildly dilated lower pole calyces. Portions of the left upper pole megaureter are visible in the pelvis (u). (**B**) A more anterior coronal T2-weighted image shows the markedly dilated left upper pole, multiple segments of the left upper pole megaureter, and a large left ureterocele in the bladder (uc).

suspected or because the requested imaging studies are not those that are usually capable of making the correct diagnosis (76).

In the past, diagnosis of extravesical upper pole ureteral ectopia has traditionally been made on intravenous pyelography, although the findings can be very subtle (75,76,79). Renal US will occasionally reveal a dilated upper pole collecting system and ureter; however, very often, US findings are not diagnostic. In many cases, the US examination will be normal. With VCUG, the only two potentially contributory findings are lower pole reflux, which might suggest the presence of a duplication or, much more rarely, reflux directly into an ectopic ureter that inserts into the urethra. Contrast-enhanced CT performed with thin (5 mm) sections through the kidneys is more reliable than either excretory urography or US but requires administration of intravenous contrast material as well as the use of ionizing radiation (75,76). The diagnosis of extravesical upper pole ureteral ectopia is readily made on MRU (4,67,80). In addition to demonstrating the presence of the duplication anomaly and dysplastic upper pole moiety, MRU frequently also allows for identification of the precise site of insertion of the distal upper pole orifice (4,14,24,67,80). Although extravesical ectopic ureters also rarely occur in boys, incontinence does not result because in boys, the ectopic ureter always inserts proximal to the external urethral sphincter (36,37,81).

Complications in the lower poles of duplex collecting systems are generally the same as the more commonly observed childhood abnormalities seen in nonduplicated collecting systems and ureters: vesicoureteral reflux, UPJ obstruction, and primary megaureter (82). Lower pole ureteroceles are extremely rare (83).

(A)

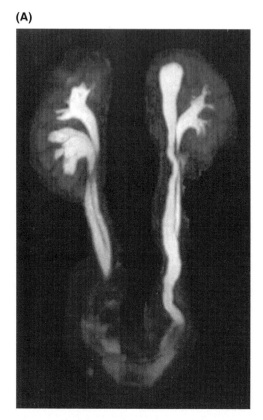

(B)

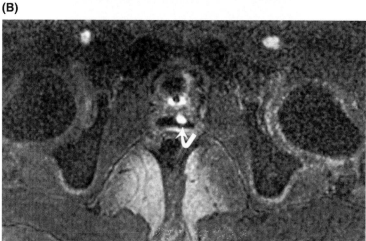

Figure 10 A 10-year-old girl with persistent incontinence. (**A**) A coronal postcontrast T1-weighted, excretory phase MIP image shows a complete left duplex kidney with a dilated upper calyx with minimal overlying cortex. Proximally, the upper pole megaureter lies medial to the nondilated lower pole ureter. Distally, the upper pole megaureter extends caudally below the bladder. On the right there is a partial duplication anomaly with the right upper and lower pole ureters joining near the pelvic brim to form a single nondilated distal right ureter. (**B**) An axial T2-weighted image of the pelvis confirms the ectopic insertion of the left upper pole ureter posterior to the bladder base into the vagina (*arrow*). *Abbreviation*: MIP, maximum intensity projection.

Calyceal Diverticulum ("Congenital Calyceal Cyst")

A calyceal diverticulum is a congenital saccular outpouching of the collecting system (36,37,84–86). The neck of the diverticulum usually communicates with the calyceal fornix but can arise from any site within the calyces, infundibula, renal pelves, or even ureters. On US, calyceal diverticula appear as solitary or multiple cystic lesions within the renal parenchyma and are usually relatively centrally located within the kidney, adjacent to the renal pyramids and collecting system. Although many calyceal diverticula are less than 1 cm in diameter, they can occasionally be quite large. Calyceal diverticula can also vary in size when measured from one imaging study to the next, depending upon the degree of distention of the diverticulum.

Most calyceal diverticula communicate freely with the renal collecting systems and will become opacified during antegrade or retrograde urography, as well as during excretory urography and contrast-enhanced CT (on images obtained after renal excretion has occurred). Occasionally, however, the neck of the diverticulum is stenotic, in which case the diverticulum will become only faintly opacified or, in some cases, will remain completely unopacified. Detection of faint opacification in a calyceal diverticulum on CT can be assisted by comparing the attenuation of the fluid in the "cyst" on delayed imaging sequences when the patient lies supine and prone.

The ability of MRI to specifically identify calyceal diverticula is similar to that of CT. Typically, the diverticulum is indistinguishable from a simple renal cyst on unenhanced MR images or on enhanced MR images obtained prior to excretion of gadolinium into the renal collecting systems (Fig. 11). The signal characteristics of the fluid within the diverticulum are usually the same as those of the urine in the adjacent collecting system, although these can vary depending on the content of the diverticulum, such as when it contains debris, milk of calcium, or pus (87). Following gadolinium administration, enhancement of the fluid in the diverticulum provides proof of communication between the diverticulum and the collecting system and establishes the diagnosis. Calculi within a calyceal diverticulum are often more easily visualized on US (where they appear echogenic and demonstrate posterior shadowing) or nonenhanced CT (where they are of high attenuation) than on MRI (where they appear as signal-void filling defects).

UPJ Obstruction

Unilateral or bilateral pelvocaliectasis without ureteral dilatation is the most common sonographic appearance in the fetus and neonate with a dilated urinary tract. In some cases, the diagnosis of UPJ obstruction is straightforward and can be made with the combination of US and nuclear scintigraphy (the latter demonstrating asymmetric washout). However, in the neonate, imaging differentiation between obstruction and transient hydronephrosis of the neonate is often difficult (31,88–93). Numerous sonographic grading systems have been proposed to aid in more rapidly identifying those patients who would benefit from surgical intervention, although none is foolproof. Consensus on criteria for obstruction is still elusive (91,92,94,95). Progression of renal collecting system and ureteral dilatation and deterioration in renal function are uncommon in neonates and infants with milder dilatation. When the anteroposterior renal pelvic diameter exceeds 10 mm, the risk of developing classical scintigraphic findings of obstruction or deterioration in renal function increases with the severity and extent of the infundibular and calyceal dilatation. However, even moderately severe dilatation will sometimes regress spontaneously (91,95).

(A)

(B)

(C)

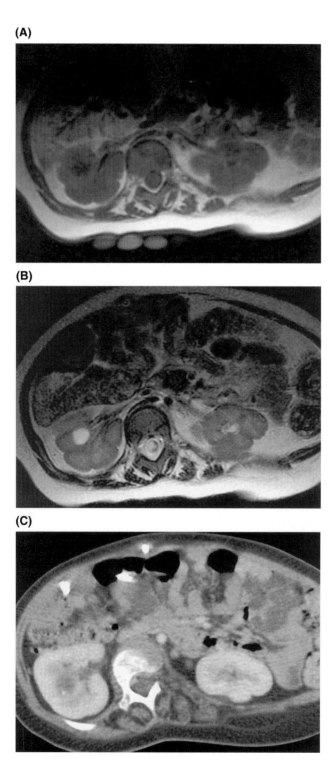

Figure 11 (*Caption on facing page*)

In older children with UPJ obstruction who present with flank pain, vomiting, or hematuria, the diagnosis is generally straightforward (13,36,37,54,96). Pelvocaliectasis is often severe, and cortical atrophy is frequently present. As a result, functional evaluation with excretory urography or diuretic renal scintigraphy is typically diagnostic of obstruction. The diagnosis can be more difficult in those patients who have intermittent UPJ obstruction secondary to extrinsic compression by a crossing vessel or band because the kidney can appear nearly or entirely normal when the patient is asymptomatic (96–98). In these patients, timing the examination to coincide with the patient's symptoms is more important in arriving at the correct diagnosis than is the choice of imaging modality.

T2-weighted MRU is particularly suited for imaging congenital anomalies that cause urinary tract obstruction and dilatation, such as UPJ or UVJ obstruction, because the urine in the dilated collecting system and ureter produces a very high signal with excellent signal-to-noise ratio (4,8,9,14–16,22–29). Although it is also possible to get excellent quality images with T1-weighted spin-echo-imaging sequences following administration of gadolinium-based contrast material (Figs. 12 and 13) (15,16,22–26), T2-weighted MRU has the advantage of not requiring the use of MR contrast agents. With T2-weighted MRU, the urographic effect is based solely on the presence of water (i.e., urine) in the renal collecting systems and ureters and is independent of renal excretory function. For this reason, T2-weighted MRU can be used to visualize a dilated obstructed collecting system of a poorly or even nonfunctioning kidney. T2-weighted MRU has also been used to visualize congenital obstructive uropathy affecting the fetal urinary tract. The major limitations of T2-weighted MRU are that it provides little information regarding renal function and that it is less useful in patients with obstructed, but nondilated, urinary tracts because these nondilated tracts are not well seen. Gadolinium-enhanced T1-weighted spin-echo MRU images are generally of much better quality in all patients with nondilated renal collecting systems and ureters.

Thus, T2-weighted (noncontrast) and T1-weighted (gadolinium-enhanced) MRU examinations have different advantages and disadvantages. The choice of which type of study to perform should be tailored to each individual patient. MRU can also be utilized to follow patients with UPJ obstructions after they have been treated (Fig. 14).

Ureteral and UVJ Obstruction

As is the case in patients with UPJ obstructions, T2-weighted MRU is particularly helpful in patients with ureterectasis, because the urine in the dilated ureter will be

---

Figure 11 (*Figure on facing page*) An eight-year-old boy with right calyceal diverticulum containing several small calculi that could be identified on CT but not MRI. (**A**) An axial T1-weighted image shows a rounded, low–signal intensity, centrally located lesion in the lateral aspect of the mid-right kidney, consistent with either a cyst or a calyceal diverticulum. (**B**) An axial T2-weighted image shows a rounded, high–signal intensity, centrally located lesion in the lateral aspect of the mid-right kidney, consistent with either a cyst or a calyceal diverticulum. (**C**) An axial noncontrast-enhanced CT image shows a rounded, low attenuation, centrally located lesion in the lateral aspect of the mid-right kidney. The location of the lesion between two calyces and the presence of two small calculi within the lesion suggest it is a calyceal diverticulum, rather than a renal cyst. *Abbreviations*: CT, computed tomography; MRI, magnetic resonance imaging.

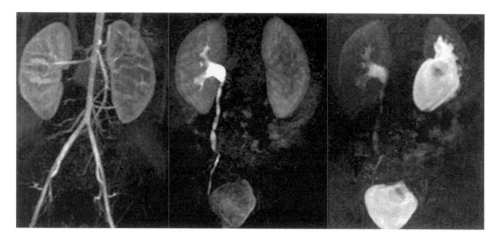

Figure 12 A 15-month-old boy with left UPJ obstruction. Coronal postcontrast T1-weighted images during the cortical (*left*), excretory (*middle*), and delayed (*right*) phases show normal left cortical perfusion with delayed medullary enhancement and prolongation of the left nephrogram. In the delayed phase, there is marked left pelvocaliectasis with no visualization of the left ureter. The pattern matches the classic obstructive urogram appearance on excretory urography. *Abbreviation*: UPJ, ureteropelvic junction.

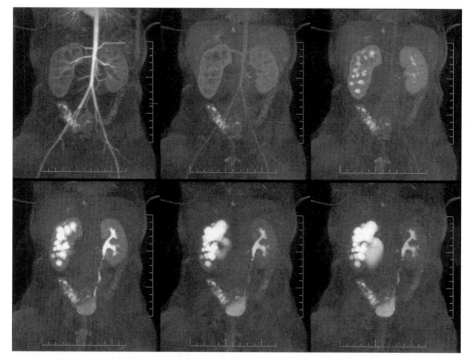

Figure 13 A six-month-old boy with right UPJ obstruction. A series of six coronal postcontrast T1-weighted images show normal cortical perfusion bilaterally, with the dilated right calyces appearing as low–signal intensity filling defects on the early images. During the excretion phase, the calyces have a high signal intensity bilaterally, with severe right pelvocaliectasis and diffuse right cortical thinning. Visualization of the right renal pelvis is delayed and the right ureter is never seen. The left kidney appears normal. *Abbreviation*: UPJ, ureteropelvic junction.

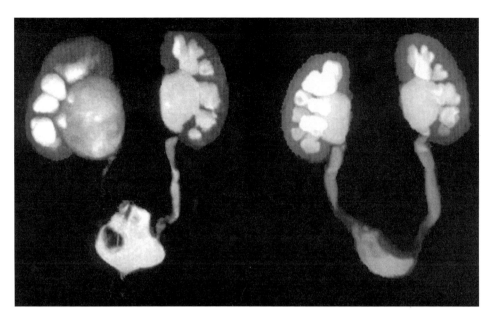

Figure 14   A 15-month-old boy with congenital right UPJ obstruction, before and after right dismembered pyeloplasty. (*Right*) Coronal 3-D postcontrast T1-weighted excretory phase MIP images show severe right pelvocaliectasis with diffuse cortical thinning and no visualization of the right ureter, consistent with right UPJ obstruction. Renal transit time on the right side was greater than 15 minutes. The left kidney appears normal. (*Left*) A coronal 3-D postcontrast T1-weighted excretory phase MIP image following right dismembered pyeloplasty shows a markedly improved right pelvocaliectasis with some residual calyceal clubbing. Cortical thickness is also somewhat improved on the right. Transit time on the right is also normal (less than five minutes). *Abbreviations*: MIP, maximum intensity projection; UPJ, ureteropelvic junction.

readily visualized and the precise site of the obstruction can almost always be demonstrated (8,27).

Primary megaureter is a nonprogressive disorder characterized by functional obstruction at the UVJ, with ureterectasis secondary to an adynamic distal ureteral segment (99). The ureter typically dilates from "the bottom up," with the distal ureter often being most severely affected. Pelvocaliectasis is frequently absent. The abnormal distal adynamic segment of the ureter is characteristically narrowed and has a "beaklike" appearance. Hyperperistalsis of the mid- and upper-ureter are usually present and can be seen with US and on MRU studies.

Nonobstructive megaureter and megacystis can also occur in children, including in severe vesicoureteral reflux with aberrant micturition (100,101) and in prune belly syndrome.

Congenital mid-ureteral obstructions, the so-called "ureteral valves," occur rarely and are believed to result from either the failure of the normal complete ureteral canalization or vascular insufficiency, resulting in stricture formation (36,37,102). Congenital fetal ureteral folds have been implicated by some authors (8,27) as the cause of midureteral obstruction, although this remains controversial because nonobstructing focal redundancies are occasionally seen on urography and VCUG in the upper- and midureter in normal neonates and in infants without proximal dilatation.

Retrocaval ureter (103) is an uncommon developmental anomaly of the IVC, not the ureter, which results from persistence of the fetal subcardinal or posterior cardinal venous system. The right ureter passes medially and behind the IVC, cephalad to the confluence of the iliac veins, emerges between the IVC and the aorta, and then passes over the anterior surface of the IVC before descending to the bladder. On excretory urography, the retrocaval right ureter characteristically deviates over the superior margin and medial to the fourth lumbar pedicle, where it is compressed behind the IVC with a variable degree of obstruction and proximal dilatation. Acquired ureteral strictures can also occur secondary to adjacent inflammatory disease, neoplasm, or following trauma to the ureter. Ureterocele is the most common cause of congenital UVJ obstruction.

RENAL INFECTIONS

Acute Pyelonephritis and Renal Scarring

Most upper urinary tract infections in children originate from bacterial contamination of the perineum and lower urinary tract by uropathogenic fecal flora. Although vesicoureteral reflux is the most widely described mechanism for upward transport of bacteria from the bladder to the renal collecting systems and kidneys, it is not invariably present in patients who develop ascending pyelonephritis. Other, as yet uncharacterized, mechanisms for upward conveyance of bacteria clearly exist. Pyelonephritis secondary to hematogenous seeding of the kidney is, by comparison, quite rare in childhood and generally occurs only in the context of serious extra-urinary disease of the cardiovascular, gastrointestinal, or musculoskeletal system that predisposes to recurrent bacteremia.

Ascending pyelonephritis in children is typically segmental in distribution and occurs most frequently at the renal poles. Although pyelonephritis can be unifocal, multifocal involvement is much more common. Bilateral disease is often present. The polar predilection in ascending pyelonephritis is thought to be due to the greater tendency of the papillary orifices at the renal poles to be incompetent, thereby allowing for "intrarenal" reflux of infected urine from the collecting system back into the collecting tubules. This phenomenon of intrarenal reflux is also commonly referred to as pyelotubular backflow.

Frequently, it can be difficult to reliably differentiate between upper and lower urinary tract infections in children based upon clinical and laboratory parameters alone.

Imaging modalities that have been used for diagnosing acute pyelonephritis in children who have fever and bacteriuria include DMSA renal cortical scintigraphy, power Doppler ultrasonography, CT, and MRI (29,93) (104–112). With each of these modalities, the diagnosis of acute pyelonephritis depends on the demonstration of both anatomic and physiologic changes in the appearance of the kidneys. Anatomic changes include parenchymal edema resulting in local or generalized renal enlargement, often with focal alterations in the renal contours, as well as alterations in renal parenchymal imaging characteristics, such as changes in tissue echogenicity, attenuation, or signal intensity. Alterations in the appearance of the renal collecting systems, such as urothelial thickening secondary to edema, pelvocaliectasis from bacterial endotoxins, vesicoureteral reflux, and the presence of debris in the collecting systems, ureters, or bladder are also common. Physiologic changes include segmental or lobar reduction in renal parenchymal perfusion and excretory function in the affected areas.

The vast majority of upper urinary tract infections in children are bacterial, with more than 90% being due to *Escherichia coli*. Nevertheless, the imaging appearance of acute pyelonephritis is not microbiologically specific and is frequently the same in fungal disease, as in bacterial disease. The abnormal pattern of enhancement of the infected areas can persist for several months after completion of antibiotic therapy, before resolving or progressing to visible scar formation. In the event of scar formation, evolution in the appearance and size of the scar can continue for years following the inciting infection, with the scar becoming increasingly conspicuous as the surrounding unaffected tissue continues to grow. The sensitivity of CT in acute pyelonephritis is comparable with that of DMSA nuclear scintigraphy and superior to that of combined power Doppler and conventional gray-scale US (93,104). The ability of CT or MRI to differentiate between scars and areas of acute infection in the absence of a previous examination is a significant advantage over conventional DMSA nuclear scintigraphy (12,113).

US is the most widely used imaging modality for evaluating children who have acute urinary tract infection. Inflammatory renal edema secondary to acute pyelonephritis can produce local or generalized renal enlargement, as well as focal alterations in the renal contours and cortical echogenicity (13,31,87,105,106). Focal polar enlargement can be dramatic and can occasionally be misinterpreted as being due to the presence of a renal mass. Areas of pyelonephritis typically appear abnormally hyperechoic with reduced or absent corticomedullary differentiation. However, areas that are severely hypovascular and those that are undergoing necrosis can appear hypoechoic and can be difficult to distinguish from early abscess development (13,31,114).

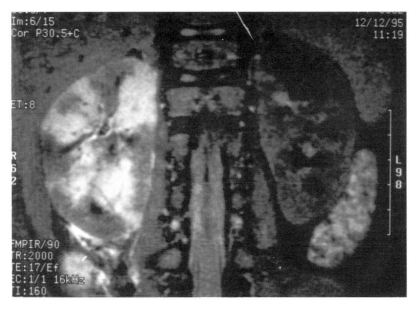

Figure 15   An infant girl with acute multifocal pyelonephritis. A coronal postcontrast inversion recovery image shows multiple wedge-shaped, high-intensity and, therefore, nonenhancing lesions throughout the right kidney, consistent with acute multifocal pyelonephritis. A very small amount of perinephric fluid is present around the lower pole with adjacent edema of the perinephric fat.

(A)

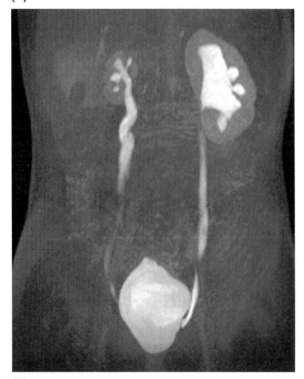

(B)

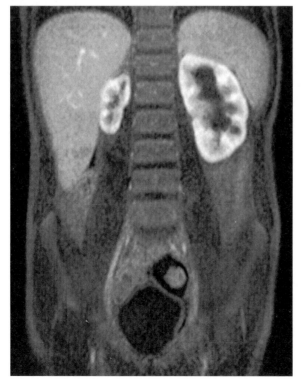

Figure 16 (*Caption on facing page*)

On nonenhanced CT, the diagnosis of acute pyelonephritis is often more diffi-cult because infected segments are generally isodense or only slightly hypodense in relation to adjacent normal parenchyma. Increased attenuation in a focus of acute pyelonephritis on nonenhanced CT is consistent with localized hemorrhage secondary to segmental venous thrombosis and parenchymal infarction, an appearance frequently associated with scarring and severe parenchymal atrophy (13,31,114). On contrast-enhanced CT, acute pyelonephritis usually produces one or more wedge-shaped or triangular areas of decreased parenchymal enhancement (13,31,87,93,104,106,112). The infected areas in the kidney appear edematous, typi-cally having convex margins and causing the renal contour to bulge, occasionally even mimicking an intrarenal mass. With more extensive involvement, the affected portion of the kidney appears enlarged, although it usually still maintains its reniform shape, with patchy enhancement of the less involved areas. The need for intravenous contrast enhancement as well as for exposure to ionizing radiation are both drawbacks to using CT. In addition, some authors have suggested that multiple contrast-enhanced imaging series are necessary to assure maximum sensitivity in detecting acute pyelone-phritis. They have observed that in some patients, the diagnosis is not apparent on early contrast-enhanced "cortical" phase CT images (12,108). In comparison, in these patients the findings are frequently more apparent on delayed enhanced images.

The use of MRI for the diagnosis of acute pyelonephritis and renal cortical scar-ring has been studied in both piglets and humans (12,107–110,113). On gadolinium-enhanced fast spin-echo T2 and inversion recovery sequences, normally enhancing renal parenchyma have a much reduced signal intensity due to the shortening of the T1 and T2 relaxation times by gadolinium. In contrast, areas of pyelonephritis remain bright because of the lower gadolinium concentration in these areas (Fig. 15). The infected areas in the kidney are also typically edematous and can produce a localized bulge in the renal contour. As with CT, edema of the perinephric fat is common. In addition, small amounts of perinephric fluid are occasionally visible on MRI. Their presence does not necessarily indicate the presence of a perinephric abscess that requires drainage (13,31).

In a comprehensive study of acute pyelonephritis in a piglet model, Majd et al. (108) compared the accuracy of DMSA–single photon emission CT (SPECT), MRI, CT, and power Doppler ultrasonography, using histology as the reference standard. In this study, there were no statistically significant differences between DMSA–SPECT, MRI, and CT either in the diagnosis of pyelonephritis or in the localization of lesions within the kidneys. The sensitivity for the diagnosis of pyelonephritis exceeded 90% for all three modalities. Power Doppler ultrasonography, on the other hand, was significantly less sensitive than any of these other modalities.

Post-pyelonephritis renal cortical scarring and atrophy are also usually readily visualized on MRI as areas of parenchymal loss without change in signal intensity between pre– and postgadolinium inversion recovery sequences (12,13,31,108,113).

Figure 16 (*Figure on facing page*) A 10-year-old girl with a history of recurrent urinary tract infections and bilateral vesicoureteral reflux resulting in bilateral reflux nephropathy with marked right renal atrophy and malignant hypertension. (**A**) A coronal postcontrast T1-weighted MIP image shows a markedly atrophic right kidney with clubbed calyces bilaterally. (**B**) A coronal 2 mm thick slice through the kidneys postcontrast demonstrates the marked par-enchymal loss on the right. Both kidneys are excreting the contrast material, but the right kidney contributes only 14% of total renal function. *Abbreviation*: MIP, maximum intensity projection.

Retraction of the renal contour is often evident in affected areas and can progress as the scar matures, with loss of renal parenchymal volume (Fig. 16) (113). The sensitivity of MRI using fat-saturated, T1-weighted, and an enhanced inversion recovery sequence is comparable with that of DMSA renal cortical scintigraphy in detecting renal scarring (108,113). Whether perfusion imaging of the renal cortex in the early contrast-enhanced phase is more sensitive in detecting renal scarring than is either DMSA or conventional MRI has not yet been studied objectively.

Complicated Renal Infections

Renal abscess and other serious acute complications of pyelonephritis are, fortunately, very rare in healthy children with ascending pyelonephritis. Renal abscesses are more commonly seen in children with hematogenous pyelonephritis, in those who are immunocompromised (115), and where infection occurs in an obstructed collecting system. Distinguishing between uncomplicated acute pyelonephritis and abscess is important because uncomplicated infection is typically treated with antibiotics alone, whereas an abscess usually requires surgical drainage (116).

Renal abscesses can be perirenal or intraparenchymal. Intraparenchymal abscesses appear as round or irregular cystic intrarenal structures, which may be unilocular or multilocular. On sonography, abscesses typically contain echogenic purulent debris. Although CT remains the most widely used modality for the evaluation of complicated renal infections in children, as in adults (116,117), MRI is equally efficacious and would be the preferred modality in patients with a significantly impaired renal function or with a history of contrast allergy, in whom the use of iodinated contrast media may be contraindicated. CT and MRI can detect even small amounts of perinephric fluid. Careful monitoring of the clinical course of patients with such fluid is warranted to ensure that this fluid does not develop into a discrete abscess. If patients remain septic or febrile, close imaging follow-up is also critical. Sometimes, CT and MRI can suggest that perinephric fluid is infected. Debris within infected fluid may alter its attenuation or signal characteristics. Also, when contrast material is administered, an enhancing wall can often be seen around the fluid.

Both bacterial endotoxin and vesicoureteral reflux can produce transient dilatation of the renal collecting systems and ureters, mimicking obstructive renal collecting system and ureteral dilatation, or even pyonephrosis (when collecting system debris is also present). US, CT, and conventional MRI are not definitive in differentiating between an uninfected dilated collecting system and true pyonephrosis. Echogenic (as seen on US), high-attenuation (as seen on CT), or high-signal (as seen on MRI) debris in the renal collecting systems and ureters of children with pyelonephritis does not necessarily indicate either obstruction or pyonephrosis, even when the collecting system is dilated. Similarly, desquamated cells and crystalline material in chronically obstructed, but uninfected systems cannot necessarily be differentiated from purulent urine on standard imaging studies.

Diffusion-weighted MRI has been applied extensively in neuroimaging for evaluating patients with acute cerebral strokes and intracranial neoplasms and in demyelinating disorders, as well as in differentiating between cerebral abscess and cystic or necrotic neoplasms (118). Until recently, applications of diffusion-weighted imaging (DWI) have been quite limited outside of the central nervous system because of significant image degradation related to respiratory and cardiac motion. Ultrafast, single-shot echo planar imaging techniques now permit the application of DWI elsewhere in the body, including the urinary tract. By revealing the micromolecular motion of water within tissues, DWI provides information on the velocity and direction of movement of the water molecules in tissue under the influence of a diffusion gradient (119). Marked hyperintensity on diffusion-weighted sequences consistent with restricted diffusion has been reported in pyelonephritis and renal abscesses in animals and adult humans. Restricted diffusion in pyelonephritis is thought to be primarily a result of cytotoxic edema, as is the case in the central nervous system (119,120). However, intratubular inspissation of inflammatory cells might also be important. DWI also might be useful in differentiating between noninfected dilatation and pyonephrosis (119). Differences in the relative mobility or viscosity of water molecules in tissues create the contrast in DWI. Because pus is a thick, high-viscosity fluid consisting of water, inflammatory cells, necrotic tissue, and proteinaceous exudates causing a marked restriction of water proton mobility, the fluid in a renal abscess or pyonephrotic collecting system has a very low apparent diffusion coefficient (ADC). As a result, the fluid in the pyonephrotic collecting system has a very high signal intensity on diffusion-weighted images and relative signal hypointensity of ADC maps. Either acute or subacute hemorrhage into the collecting system or within a renal cyst can also produce a very high signal intensity because the very long T2 relaxation time of blood can mimic the appearance of purulent material. However, the ADC maps, which are free of this T2 effect, will differentiate between hemorrhage and pus. Nevertheless, at the current time, percutaneous puncture of the collecting system remains the only definitive procedure for the diagnosis or exclusion of pyonephrosis. In pyonephrosis and renal abscess, drainage is necessary and is usually accomplished percutaneously with US guidance. Although DWI is being utilized increasingly in pediatric neuroimaging, applications for this imaging approach in pediatric uroradiology are still limited.

REFERENCES

1. Appignani BA, Jaramillo D, Barnes PD, Poussaint TY. Dysraphic myelodysplasias associated with urogenital and anorectal anomalies: prevalence and types seen with MR imaging. Am J Roentgenol 1994; 163:1199–1203.
2. Avni FE, Nicaise N, Hall M, et al. The role of MR imaging for the assessment of complicated duplex kidneys in children: preliminary report. Pediatr Radiol 2001; 31: 215–223.
3. McHugh K. The role of radiology in children with anorectal anomalies; with particular emphasis on MRI. Eur J Radiol 1998; 26:194–199.
4. Riccabona M, Riccabona M, Koen M, et al. Magnetic resonance urography: a new gold standard for the evaluation of solitary kidneys and renal buds? J Urol 2004; 171:1642–1646.
5. Dietrich RB, Kangarloo H. Kidneys in infants and children: evaluation with MR. Radiology 1986; 158:313–317.
6. Dietrich RB. Genitourinary system. In: Cohen MD, Edwards MK, eds. Magnetic Resonance Imaging of Children. Philadelphia, PA: BC Decker Inc., 1990:679–723 (chapter 21).
7. Hricak H, Crooks L, Sheldon P, Kaufman L. Nuclear magnetic resonance imaging of the kidney. Radiology 1983; 146:425–432.
8. Grattan-Smith JD, Perez-Bayfield MR, Jones RA, et al. MR imaging of kidneys: functional evaluation using F-15 perfusion imaging. Pediatr Radiol 2003; 33:293–304.
9. Leppert A, Nadalin S, Schirg E, et al. Impact of magnetic resonance urography on preoperative diagnostic workup in children affected by hydronephrosis: should IVU be replaced? J Pediatr Surg 2002; 37:1441–1445.

10. Leung AW, Bydder GM, Steiner RE, Bryant DJ, Young IR. Magnetic resonance imaging of the kidneys. Am J Roentgenol 1984; 143:1215–1227.
11. Siegel MJ. MR imaging of the pediatric abdomen. MRI Clin North Am 1995; 3:161–182.
12. Weiser AC, Amukele SA, Leonidas JC, Palmer LS. The role of gadolinium enhanced magnetic resonance imaging for children with suspected acute pyelonephritis. J Urol 2003; 169:2308–2311.
13. Zerin JM. CT and MRI of the kidneys in children. In: Haaga JR, Lanzieri CF, Gilkeson RC, eds. Computed Tomography and Magnetic Resonance Imaging of the Whole Body. 4th ed. Mosby, 2003.
14. Avni EF, Bali MA, Regnault M, et al. MR urography in children. Eur J Radiol 2002; 43:154–166.
15. Rohrschneider WK, Haufe S, Clorius JH, Troger J. MR to assess renal function in children. Eur Radiol 2003; 13:1033–1045.
16. Rohrschneider WK, Haufe S, Wiesel M, et al. Functional and morphologic evaluation of congenital urinary tract dilatation by using combined static-dynamic MR urography: findings in kidneys with a single collecting system. Radiology 2002; 224:683–694.
17. Boechat MI. Magnetic resonance imaging of abdominal and pelvic masses in children. Top Magn Reson Imaging 1990; 3:25–41.
18. Semelka RC. Kidneys. In: Abdominal-Pelvic MRI. New York, NY: Wiley-Liss, 2002:741–865.
19. Glazer GM. MR imaging of the liver, kidneys, and adrenal glands. Radiology 1988; 166:303–312.
20. Bradley, Waluch V. Blood flow: magnetic resonance imaging. Radiology 1985; 154: 443–450.
21. Soila KP, Viamonte M Jr, Starewicz PM. Chemical shift misregistration effect in magnetic resonance imaging. Radiology 1984; 153:819–820.
22. Borthne AS, Pierre-Jerome C, Gjesdal KI, et al. Pediatric excretory MR urography: comparative study of enhanced and non-enhanced techniques. Eur Radiol 2003; 13:1423–1427.
23. Kawashima A, Glockner JF, King BF Jr. CT urography and MR urography. Radiol Clin North Am 2003; 41:945–961.
24. Nolte-Ernsting CC, Staatz G, Tacke J, Gunther RW. MR urography today. Abdom Imaging 2003; 28:191–209.
25. Zhang J, Pedrosa I, Rofsky NM. MR techniques for renal imaging. Radiol Clin North Am 2003; 41:877–907.
26. Zielonko J, Studniarek M, Markuszewski M. MR urography of obstructive uropathy: diagnostic value of the method in selected clinical groups. Eur Radiol 2003; 13: 802–809.
27. Perez-Brayfield MR, Kirsch AJ, Jones RA, Grattan-Smith JD. A prospective study comparing ultrasound, nuclear scintigraphy and dynamic contrast enhanced magnetic resonance imaging in the evaluation of hydronephrosis. J Urol 2003; 170:1330–1334.
28. Hughes J, Jan W, Goodie J, Lund R, Rankin S. MR urography: evaluation of different techniques in non-dilated tracts. Clin Radiol 2002; 57:989–994.
29. Rodriguez LV, Spielman D, Herfkens RJ, Shortliffe LD. Magnetic resonance imaging for the evaluation of hydronephrosis, reflux and renal scarring in children. J Urol 2001; 166:1023–1027.
30. Edelman RR, Mattle HP, Atkinson DJ, Hoogewoud HM. MR angiography. Am J Roentgenol 1990; 154:937–946.
31. Zerin JM. Postnatal renal sonographic screening. In: Gearhart JP, Rink RC, Mouriquand PDE, eds. Pediatric Urology. Philadelphia, PA: WB Saunders Co, 2001.
32. Zerin JM. Reflux nephropathy. In: Pollack HM, McClennan BL, eds. Clinical Urology. Philadelphia, PA: WB Saunders Co, 2000.
33. Hoffer FA, Hanaberg AM, Teele RL. The interrenicular junction: a mimic of renal scarring on normal pediatric sonograms. Am J Roentgenol 1985; 145:1075–1078.

34. Currarino G, Lowichik A. The Oddono's sulcus and its relation to the renal "junctional parenchymal defect" and the "interrenicular septum." Pediatr Radiol 1997; 27:6–10.

35. Carter AR, Horgan JG, Jennings TA, Rosenfield AT. The junctional parenchymal defect: a sonographic variant of renal anatomy. Radiology 1985; 154:499–502.

36. Gray SW, Skandalakis JS. The kidney and ureter. In: Gray SW, Skandalakis JS, eds. Embryology for Surgeons. Philadelphia, PA: WB Saunders Co, 1972:43–518.

37. Nino-Murcia M, DeVries P, Friedland G. Congenital anomalies of the kidney. In: Pollack HM, McClennan BL, eds. Clinical Urography. 2nd.Philadelphia,PA: WB Saunders Co, 2000:690–763.

38. Brasch WF. Anomalous renal rotation and associated anomalies. J Urol 1971; 25:9–21.

39. Weyrauch HM Jr. Anomalies of renal rotation. Surg Gynecol Obstet 1939; 69:183.

40. Serena A, Duque JJ, Cotero A, Llorens V, Fombellida JC. Radionuclide visualization of a thoracic renal ectopia. Clin Nucl Med 1994; 19:1021–1022.

41. N'Guessen G, Stephens FD, Pick J. Congenital superior ectopic (thoracic) kidney. Urology 1984; 24:219–228.

42. Gulsun M, Balkanci F, Cekirge S, Deger A. Pelvic kidney with an unusual blood supply: angiographic findings. Surg Radiol Anat 2000; 22:59–61.

43. Rubinstein ZJ, Hertz M, Shahin N, Deutsch V. Crossed renal ectopia: angiographic findings in six cases. Am J Roentgenol 1976; 126:1035–1038.

44. Grainger R, Murphy DM, Lane V. Horseshoe kidney: a review of presentation, associated congenital anomalies and complications in 73 patients. Ir Med J 1983; 76:315–317.

45. Mostafavi MR, Prasad PV, Saltzman B. Magnetic resonance urography and angiography in the evaluation of a horseshoe kidney with ureteropelvic junction obstruction. Urology 1998; 51:484–486.

46. Schuster T, Dietz HG, Schutz S. Anderson-Hynes pyeloplasty in horseshoe kidney in children: is it effective without symphysiotomy? Pediatr Surg Int 1999; 15:230–233.

47. Abeshouse BS, Bhisitkul I. Crossed renal ectopia with and without fusion. Urol Int 1959; 9:63–91.

48. Kakei H, Kondo A, Ogisu BI, Mitsuya H. Crossed ectopia of solitary kidney: a report of two cases and a review of the literature. Urol Int 1976; 31:470–475.

49. Fernbach SK, Davis TM. The abnormal renal axis in children with spina bifida and gibbus deformity—the pseudohorseshoe kidney. J Urol 1986; 136:1258–1260.

50. Wong JC, Clarke SE, Bingham JB. Fusion or apposition? A case of a broken horseshoe kidney. Clin Nucl Med 1997; 22:63–64.

51. Weaver DD, Mapstone CL, Yu PL. The VATER association analysis of 46 patients. Am J Dis Child 1986; 140:225–229.

52. Lippe B, Geffner ME, Dietrich RB, Boechat MI, Kangarloo H. Renal malformations in patients with turner syndrome: imaging in 141 patients. Pediatrics 1988; 82:852–856.

53. Curry CJ, Jensen K, Holland J, Miller L, Hall BD. The Potter sequence: a clinical analysis of 80 cases. Am J Med Genet 1984; 19:679–702.

54. Barnewolt CE, Paltiel HJ, Lebowitz RK, Kirks DR, eds. Genitourinary Tract in Kirks. Practical Pediatric Imaging. 3rd ed. Philadelphia, PA: Lippincott-Raven Publishers, 1998:1042–1106.

55. Hitchcock R, Burge DM. Renal agenesis: an acquired condition? J Pediatr Surg 1994; 29:454–455.

56. Griscom NT, Vawter FG, Fellers FX. Pelvoinfundibular atresia: the usual form of multicystic kidney; 44 unilateral and two bilateral cases. Semin Roentgenol 1975; 10:125–131.

57. Zerin JM, Leiser J. The impact of vesicoureteral reflux on contralateral renal length in infants with multicystic dysplastic kidney. Pediatr Radiol 1998; 28:683–686.

58. Hadar H, Gadoth N, Gillon G. Computed tomography of renal agenesis and ectopy. J Comput Tomogr 1984; 8:137–143.

59. Bronshtein M, Amit A, Achiron R, Noy I, Blumenfeld Z. The early prenatal sonographic diagnosis of renal agenesis: techniques and possible pitfalls. Prenat Diagn 1994; 14:291–297.

60. Felson B, Cussen LJ. The hydronephrotic type of congenital multicystic disease of the kidney. Semin Roentgenol 1975; 10:113–123.

61. Bloom DA, Brosman S. The multicystic kidney. J Urol 1978; 120:211–215.

62. Avni EF, Thoua Y, Lalmand B, et al. Multicystic dysplastic kidney: natural history from in utero diagnosis and postnatal follow-up. J Urol 1987; 138:1420–1424.

63. Strife JL, Souza AS, Kirks DR, et al. Multicystic dysplastic kidney in children: US follow-up. Radiology 1993; 186:785–788.

64. Jeon A, Cramer BC, Walsh E, Pushpanathan C. A spectrum of segmental multicystic renal dysplasia. Pediatr Radiol 1999; 29:309–315.

65. Share JC, Lebowitz RL. Ectopic ureterocele without ureteral and calyceal dilatation (ureterocele disproportion): findings on urography and sonography. Am J Roentgenol 1989; 152:567–571.

66. Rottenberg GT, Gordon I, De Bruyn R. The natural history of the multicystic dysplastic kidney in children. Br J Radiol 1997; 70:347–350.

67. Gylys-Morin VM, Minevich E, Tackett LD, et al. Magnetic resonance imaging of the dysplastic renal moiety and ectopic ureter. J Urol 2000; 164:2034–2039.

68. Tanaka YO, Kurosaki Y, Kobayashi T, et al. Uterus didelphys associated with obstructed hemivagina and ipsilateral renal agenesis: MR findings in seven cases. Abdom Imaging 1998; 23:437–441.

69. King BF, Hattery RR, Lieber MM, et al. Congenital cystic disease of the seminal vesicle. Radiology 1999; 178:207–211.

70. Caldamone AA. Duplication anomalies of the upper tract in infants and children. Urol Clin North Am 1985; 12:75–91.

71. Whitaker J, Danks DM. A study of the inheritance of duplication of the kidneys and ureters. J Urol 1966; 95:176–178.

72. Zerin JM, Baker DR, Casale AJ. Single system ureteroceles in children: imaging aspects. Pediatr Radiol 2000; 30:139–146.

73. Glassberg KI, Braren V, Duckett JW, et al. Suggested terminology for duplex systems, ectopic ureters and ureteroceles. Report of the Committee on Terminology, Nomenclature and Classification, American Academy of Pediatrics. J Urol 1984; 132:1153–1154.

74. Blane CE, Ritchey ML, DiPietro MA, Sumida R, Bloom DA. Single system ectopic ureters and ureteroceles associated with dysplastic kidney. Pediatr Radiol 1992; 22:217–220.

75. Braverman RM, Lebowitsz RL. Occult ectopic ureter in girls with urinary incontinence: diagnosis by using CT. AJR 1991; 156:365–366.

76. Carrico C, Lebowitz RL. Incontinence due to an infrasphincteric ectopic ureter: why the delay in diagnosis and what can the radiologist do about it? Pediatr Radiol 1998; 28:942–949.

77. Gharagozloo AM, Lebowitz RL. Detection of a poorly functioning malpositioned kidney with single ectopic ureter in girls with urinary dribbling: imaging evaluation in five patients. AJR 1995; 164:957–961.

78. Prewitt LH Jr, Lebowitz RL. The single ectopic ureter. Am J Roentgenol 1976; 127:941–948.

79. Stannard MW, Lebowitz RL. Urography in the child who wets. Am J Roentgenol 1978; 130:959–962.

80. Staatz G, Rohrmann D, Nolte-Ernsting CC, et al. Magnetic resonance urography in children: evaluation of suspected ureteral ectopia in duplex systems. J Urol 2001; 166:2346–2350.

81. Williams DI, Royle M. Ectopic ureter in the male child. Br J Urol 1969; 41:421–427.

82. Fernbach SK, Zawin JK, Lebowitz RL. Complete duplication of the ureter with ureteropelvic junction obstruction of the lower pole of the kidney: imaging findings. Am J Roentgenol 1995; 164:701–704.

83. Harb JF, Tiguert R, Hurley PM, Gheiler EL, Smith C. Ureterocele arising from a lower-pole moiety. Urol Int 1999; 63:245–246.

84. Krzeski T, Witeska A, Borowka A, Pypno W. Diverticula of renal calyces. Int Urol Nephrol 1981; 13:231–235.

85. Feeks EF, Maino TJ, Proctor JG, Bower EA. An abscess that wasn't: renal calyceal diverticulum in a student naval aviator. Aviat Space Environ Med 1998; 69:785–787.

86. Kavukcu S, Cakmakci H, Babayigit A. Diagnosis of caliceal diverticulum in two pediatric patients: a comparison of sonography, CT, and urography. J Clin Ultrasound 2003; 31:218–221.

87. Marotti M, Hricak H, Fritzsche P, et al. Complex and simple renal cysts: comparative evaluation with MR imaging. Radiology 1987; 162:679–684.

88. Garcia-Peña BM, Keller MS, Schwartz DS, Korsvik HE, Weiss RM. The ultrasonographic differentiation of obstructive versus nonobstructive hydronephrosis in children: a multivariate scoring system. J Urol 1997; 158:560–565.

89. King LR. Hydronephrosis: when is obstruction not obstruction? Urol Clin North Am 1995; 22:31–42.

90. Maizels M, Reisman ME, Flom LS, et al. Grading nephroureteral dilatation detected in the first year of life: correlation with obstruction. J Urol 1992; 148:609–614.

91. Onen A, Jayanthi VR, Koff SA. Long-term followup of prenatally detected severe bilateral newborn hydronephrosis initially managed nonoperatively. J Urol 2002; 168:1118–1120.

92. Maizels M, Mitchell B, Kass E, Fernbach SK, Conway JJ. Outcome of nonspecific hydronephrosis in the infant: a report from the registry of the society for fetal urology. J Urol 1994; 152:2324–2327.

93. Dacher JN, Boillot B, Eurin D, et al. Rational use of CT in acute pyelonephritis: findings and relationship with reflux. Pediatr Radiol 1993; 23:281–285.

94. Homsy YL, Saad F, Laberge I, Williot P, Pison C. Transitional hydronephrosis of the newborn and infant. J Urol 1990; 144:579–583.

95. Palmer LS, Maizels M, Cartwright PC, Fernbach SK, Conway JJ. Surgery versus observation for managing obstructive grade 3 to 4 unilateral hydronephrosis: a report from the society for fetal urology. J Urol 1998; 159:222–228.

96. Zerin JM. Uroradiologic emergencies in infants and children. Radiol Clin North Am 1997; 35:897–919.

97. Rooks VJ, Lebowitz RL. Extrinsic ureteropelvic junction obstruction from a crossing renal vessel: demography and imaging. Pediatr Radiol 2001; 31:120–124.

98. Hoffer FA, Lebowitz RL. Ureteropelvic junction obstruction caused by a crossing renal vessel. Radiology 1985; 156:655–658.

99. Meyer JS, Lebowitz RL. Primary megaureter in infants and children: a review. Urol Radiol 1992; 14:296–305.

100. Willi UV, Lebowitz RL. The so-called megaureter-megacystis syndrome. Am J Roentgenol 1979; 133:409–416.

101. Burbige KA, Lebowitz RL, Colodny AH, Bauer SB, Retik AB. The megacystis-megaureter syndrome. J Urol 1984; 131:1133–1136.

102. Docimo SG, Lebowitz RL, Retik AB, et al. Congenital midureteral obstruction. Urol Radiol 1989; 11:156–160.

103. Uthappa MC, Anthony D, Allen C. Case report: retrocaval ureter: MR appearances. Br J Radiol 2002; 75:177–179.

104. Dacher JN, Pfister C, Monroc M, Eurin D, LeDosseur P. Power Doppler sonographic pattern of acute pyelonephritis in children: comparison with CT. Am J Roentgenol 1996; 166:1451–1455.

105. Klar A, Hurvitz H, Berkun Y, et al. Focal bacterial nephritis (lobar nephronia) in children. J Pediatr 1996; 128:850–853.

106. Lee JK, McClennan BL, Melson GL, Stanley RJ. Acute focal bacterial nephritis: emphasis on gray scale sonography and computed tomography. Am J Roentgenol 1980; 135:87–92.

107. Lonergan GJ, Pennington DJ, Morrison JC, et al. Childhood pyelonephritis: comparison of gadolinium-enhanced MR imaging and renal cortical scintigraphy for diagnosis. Radiology 1998; 207:377–384.
108. Majd M, Nussbaum Blask AR, Markle BM, et al. Diagnosis of experimental pyelonephritis in piglets: comparison of 99m Tc DMSA SPECT, spiral CT, MRI and power Doppler sonography. Radiology 2001; 218:101–108.
109. Pennington DJ, Lonergan GJ, Flack CE, Waguespack RL, Jackson CB. Experimental pyelonephritis in piglets: diagnosis with MR imaging. Radiology 1996; 201:199–205.
110. Pennington DJ, Zerin JM. Imaging of the urinary tract in children. Ann Pediatr 1999; 28:678–686.
111. Rushton HG. The evaluation of acute pyelonephritis and renal scarring with technetium 99m-dimercaptosuccinic acid renal scintigraphy: evolving concepts and future directions. Pediatr Nephrol 1997; 11:108–120.
112. Soulen MC, Fishman EK, Goldman SM, Gatewood OMB. Bacterial renal infection: role of CT. Radiology 1989; 171:703–707.
113. Chan YL, Chan KW, Yeung CK, et al. Potential utility of MRI in the evaluation of children at risk of renal scarring. Pediatr Radiol 1999; 29:856–862.
114. Rigsby CM, Rosenfield AT, Glickman MG, Hodson J. Hemorrhagic focal bacterial nephritis: findings on gray-scale sonography and CT. Am J Roentgenol 1986; 146: 1173–1177.
115. Zinn HL, Haller JO. Renal manifestations of AIDS in children. Pediatr Radiol 1999; 29:558–561.
116. Mendez G Jr, Ishikoff MB, Morillo G. The role of computed tomography in the diagnosis of renal and perirenal abscesses. J Urol 1979; 122:582–586.
117. Soulen MC, Fishman EK, Goldman SM. Sequelae of acute renal infections: CT evaluation. Radiology 1989; 173:423–426.
118. Warach S, Chien D, Li W, Ronthal M, Edelman RR. Fast magnetic resonance diffusion-weighted imaging of acute human stroke. Neurology 1992; 42:1717–1723.
119. Chan JH, Tsui EY, Luk SH, et al. MR diffusion-weighted imaging of kidney: differentiation between hydronephrosis and pyonephrosis. Clin Imaging 2001; 25:110–113.
120. Verswijvel G, Vandecaveye V, Gelin G, et al. Diffusion-weighted MR imaging in the evaluation of renal infection: preliminary results. JBR-BTR 2002; 85:100–103.

10

New Developments in MRI in Assessment of Parenchymal Renal Diseases

Nicolas Grenier and Olivier Hauger
*Service d'Imagerie Diagnostique et Thérapeutique de l'Adulte,
Groupe Hospitalier Pellegrin, and ERT CNRS Imagerie Moléculaire et Fonctionnelle,
University Victor Segalen-Bordeaux 2, Bordeaux, France*

Yahsou Delmas and Christian Combe
*Department of Nephrology, Groupe Hospitalier Pellegrin, and INSERM,
University Victor Segalen-Bordeaux 2, Bordeaux, France*

INTRODUCTION

Acute and chronic nephropathies are responsible for morphological and functional changes of the kidney. Imaging techniques today play a minor role in assessing these diseases because the main changes are microscopic and functional. Currently, standard imaging techniques offer mainly macroscopic morphological information, such as kidney size and corticomedullary differentiation (CMD), but functional information is obtained by scintigraphic techniques.

Recent developments in the magnetic resonance imaging (MRI) systems, providing higher signal-to-noise ratio and higher spatial and/or temporal resolution, and the specific MR contrast agents have the potential to offer morphological and functional information that are relevant for establishing the diagnosis, determining the prognosis, and monitoring response to treatment of various renal diseases.

PARENCHYMAL SIGNAL INTENSITY CHANGES

$T1$-weighted ($T1$w) spin-echo and gradient-echo sequences show a CMD in normal kidneys, with lower signal intensity (SI) within the medulla, which is enhanced by fat suppression. On $T2$-weighted ($T2$w) sequences, CMD is reversed with a higher SI within the medulla. These effects are presumably due to higher water content per unit of tissue mass within pyramids. CMD is decreased on $T1$w images, nonspecifically, when serum creatinine is increased (Fig. 1) (1). Proposed mechanisms are either owing to a decreased cortical SI caused by edema or to an increased medullary SI caused by a decreased tubular flow or deposition of proteinaceous or bloody materials. The intensity of CMD decrease was initially shown to be correlated with

(A)   (B)

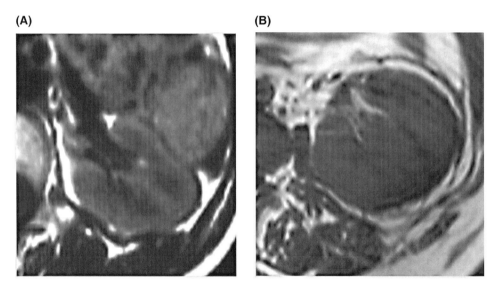

Figure 1 CMD on T1w MR images: examples of (**A**) normal and (**B**) absent CMD. These changes are not specific and independent of renal function. *Abbreviations*: MR, magnetic resonance; CMD, corticomedullary differentiation; T1w, T1-weighted.

the degree of renal failure and was supposedly absent when serum creatinine reached 3.0 mg/dL (1). However, in acute renal failure (ARF), CMD may remain preserved at least within two weeks of developing ARF, and its degree independent of serum creatinine level (2).

Other types of parenchymal SI changes have been described in some specific diseases. These changes essentially concern cases of decrease of cortical or medullary SI on T2w images (3). Ischemia and hemosiderin deposition are the most frequent causes of such changes. Where hemosiderin is concerned, hemolysis is the first mechanism to be proposed. It may occur either within the cortex or within the medulla (Fig. 2). The three main causes of cortical decrease of SI on T2w images related to hemosiderin deposition are: paroxysmal nocturnal hemoglobinuria (Fig. 2A), sickle-cell disease, and causes of mechanical hemolysis (e.g., patients with certain types of artificial heart valves). Within the medulla, hemosiderin deposition may occur after episodes of hemorrhagic congestion, mainly within the outer medulla, which is more sensitive to hypoxic injury. The main causes of these MR features are hemorrhagic fever with renal syndrome, ischemic ARF (Fig. 2B), and renal vein thrombosis. Besides hemosiderin, a decrease of SI on T2w images may also be due to ischemia, as shown in infarction and in cortical necrosis. In this case, no enhancement is noted on post–gadolinium (Gd) contrast administration using T1w sequences.

MORPHOLOGICAL BIOMARKERS OF KIDNEY FUNCTION

Actually, there is a growing interest in validating accurate and reproducible methods for calculation of renal volume, which may be an index of functional renal parenchyma (4). Follow-up of chronic nephropathies would be simplified for patients by such measurements. Today, the most widely used marker is the renal length, which is measured with sonography. However, its correlation with renal size is far from perfect (5,6). Measurement of parenchymal thickness has received little attention (7,8),

(A)

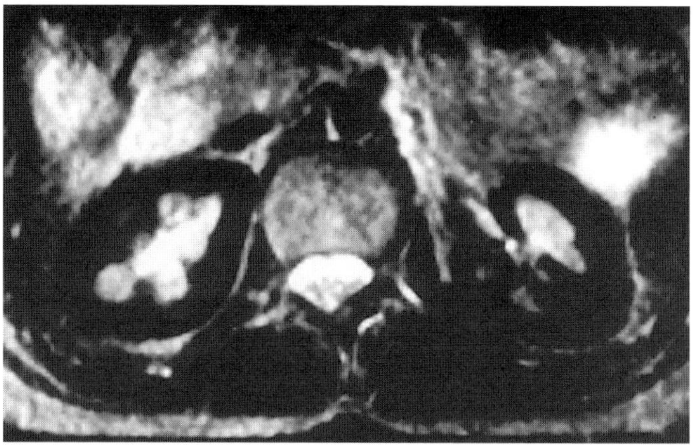

(B)

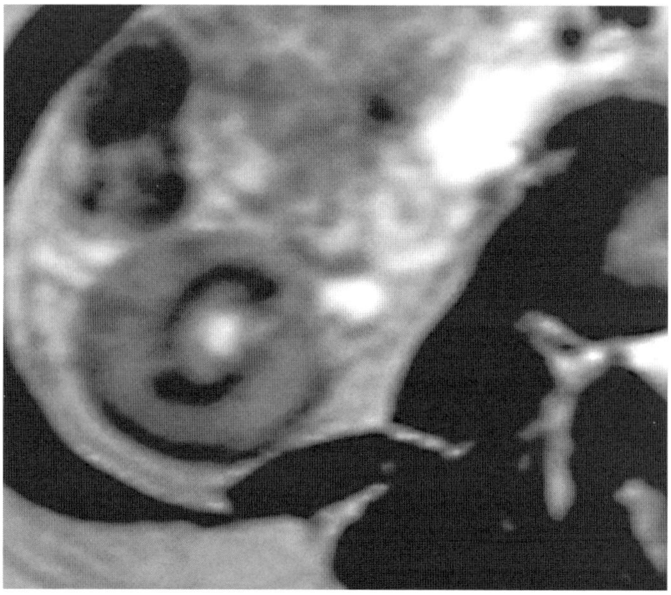

Figure 2 Parenchymal hypointensity on $T2$w images: (**A**) Paroxysmal nocturnal hemoglobinuria. Axial $T2$w image obtained at 2 T shows that the SI of the renal cortex is decreased, whereas it remains normal in the medulla. (**B**) Acute ischemic nephropathy. Decrease of SI on a $T2$w image within the outer medulla on axial view. Pathologic examination of the outer medulla showed iron in the interstitium compatible with hemosiderin deposition. *Abbreviations*: $T2$w, $T2$-weighted; SI, signal intensity. *Source*: Part (**A**) from Ref. 3.

and its reproducibility is hampered by its heterogeneity throughout each kidney. The best method would be a volumetric technique applied to the entire parenchyma, excluding the sinus, or to the cortex. Coulam et al. (9) reported an excellent correlation between MRI measurement of total renal parenchymal volume and autopsy volume and weight, using coronal multiphasic contrast-enhanced three-dimensional (3-D) sequences in pigs. However, the segmentation was manual, done slice-by-slice. The cortical volume seems to be the most useful parameter because it is directly related to the filtration capabilities of the kidney. In our institution, we developed an automatic segmentation technique of the renal cortex applied to a contrast-enhanced 3-D dataset obtained at the vascular phase. This technique demonstrated its feasibility (unpublished data) but still requires validation.

New medical therapies for inherited polycystic diseases are emerging, with encouraging results in animal models (10). These treatments are able to slow established diseases, indicating that clinical trials should be considered. Increased renal volume predicts and is associated with loss of renal function in autosomal-dominant polycystic kidney disease (11), and renal cystic volume predicts renal outcome more reliably than the total renal volume (12). Therefore, measurement of renal cystic volume would be worthwhile to follow the effect of treatment. Computer-assisted detection software will be necessary for that purpose, with automatic detection of cyst walls and automatic volume calculations based on 3-D datasets, and used as an accurate surrogate marker, mostly when renal function is still preserved (11).

FUNCTIONAL IMPACT OF RENAL DISEASES

Renal perfusion and glomerular filtration (GFR) are major functional parameters, which are involved in many renal parenchymal diseases. Noninvasive and accurate measurement of renal perfusion could have a major impact in understanding physiopathology of renovascular diseases and in their follow-up. GFR is used as an index of functioning renal mass, representing the sum of filtration rates in each functioning nephron. A decrease in GFR may be the earliest and only clinical sign of renal disease, and its serial monitoring allows estimating the severity and following the course of kidney diseases.

These functional measurements with MRI are nowadays limited to semiquantitative evaluation due to several reasons. First, it is difficult to obtain accurate and reproducible information in a mobile organ that is submitted to respiratory movements and magnetic susceptibility artifacts arising from the surrounding bowel. In addition, the complexity of the relationship between the observed signal changes and the concentration of the contrast agent makes quantitative analysis difficult. Use of relative SI only precludes quantification of these parameters but allows instead calculation of parameters that, to some extent, reflect blood flow or filtration without being in absolute units. These parameters can only be used intraindividually to compare different renal areas or one kidney from the other. Therefore, nuclear medicine remains at present the reference method for quantification of most renal functional parameters, but MRI could compete soon in many fields. These parameters are calculated from MRI measurements using either such exogenous contrast agents as Gd-chelates or iron oxide particles, or endogenous contrast agents, such as water protons.

Technical Issues for Contrast-Enhanced Studies

Extensive reviews of all technical problems related to quantitative GFR measurement have been published recently (13,14). Most of these approaches are based on dynamic contrast-enhanced acquisitions, either with $T1$ weighting ($R1$ relaxation-enhanced), using paramagnetic Gd-chelates, or with $T2^*$-weighting ($R2^*$ susceptibility-enhanced), using superparamagnetic iron oxide particles (SPIO). Because both types of agents have a concomitant effect on all components of relaxivity, Gd-chelates may produce $T2$ and $T2^*$ effects at a high concentration, and, conversely, iron oxide particles may produce $T1$ effects at a low concentration. Therefore, according to the type of agent used, specific optimization of the injected dose and of the imaging sequence is necessary.

T1w Dynamic Contrast-Enhanced MRI (with Gd-Chelates)

When Gd-chelates are used, a reasonable $T1$ weighting can be achieved using spoiled gradient-echo (type FLASH—Fast Low Angle Shot). Nonselective magnetization preparation, combined with very short repetition time (TR) and echo time (TE) values, make it possible to obtain a heavy $T1$ weighting with very short acquisition times. Absolute measurement of renal perfusion and filtration requires accurate sampling of the vascular phase of the kidney in order to measure the arterial input function (AIF). The AIF is the signal-time-curve observed in the suprarenal abdominal aorta, used for different kinetic models in order to compensate for the noninstantaneous bolus injected into the blood. Recent advents in MR instrumentation and hardware facilitate coverage of the entire kidneys with several slices using 3-D sequences while maintaining a temporal resolution around 1.5s (15).

The concentration of Gd within the kidney has to be decreased to reduce the $T2^*$ contribution occurring at high concentration within the aorta and renal medulla. This can be achieved by decreasing the injected dose (0.025 and 0.05 mmol/kg) and by hydrating the patient.

To convert changes in SI into changes in $R1$, different approaches can be used. A commonly used method is based on a phantom of tubes filled with Gd solutions at various concentrations, which is then imaged with the sequence used for the dynamic study. The acquired SI values are plotted against measured $R1$ values, and a polynomial fit is made to obtain a calibration curve. However, this approach has some drawbacks, including the assumption that the relaxivity k is equivalent in solution and in tissues. Another method of conversion is to use the relationship between SI and $R1$ given by the equation driven by the sequence used (16), which unfortunately is not straightforward. In addition, some sequences may not even have an analytical formula that can be used for this method (17). The tissue concentration of contrast agent (C) can then be calculated by following the linear relationship to the $T1$ relaxation rate ($R1 = 1/T1$) and the specific relaxivity of the agent within the tissue (k, proportionality constant that depends on the properties of tissue, the type of microvasculature and the contrast agent, and the sequence used), $C = (R1 - R1_0)/k$, where $R1_0$ is the bulk $R1$ relaxation rate of the tissue without contrast agent.

This mathematically complex conversion from SI to $R1$ can be avoided using direct dynamic measurement of $R1$ (instead of SI). Very fast dynamic measurements of $R1$ based on the Look-Locker sequence (18) providing dynamic $T1$ mapping of kidneys and aorta is one possibility to eliminate this problem (19,20). Preliminary renal studies appear extremely encouraging (21), but their accuracy in dynamic quantification are yet to be investigated.

T2*w Dynamic Contrast-Enhanced MRI (with Iron Oxide Particles)

The passage of magnetopharmaceuticals leads to differences in the local magnetic susceptibility between vessels and the surrounding tissue. Thus, both intra- and extravascular spins undergo a reduction in $T2^*$, which leads to a significant transient signal loss. When iron oxide particles are used, the increased magnetic susceptibility caused by the ferromagnetic atom causes a relative large spin dephasing, and thus, $T2^*$w sequences can conveniently be used to detect the passage of the agent through a tissue of interest. Because these compounds are currently restricted to experimental studies in animals, $T2^*$w perfusion with these agents has received little attention in clinical practice.

These studies have predominantly been performed using snapshot FLASH-type sequences, with small TR and TE values together with a relative small flip angle in order to facilitate $T2^*$ weighting.

Dynamic susceptibility contrast imaging ($T2^*$w) does not make quantification of SI into concentration units possible. However, a relative measure of the concentration for iron oxide particles can be estimated using the linear proportionality between the concentration of the contrast agent and $R2^*$ changes given by the equation:

$$\Delta R2^*(t) = C(t)/k$$

where k is the relaxivity (proportionality constant that depends on the properties of tissue, the type of microvasculature and the contrast agent, and the sequence used). Measured SI is then converted into changes in $R2^*$ by the following relationship:

$$\Delta R2^*(t) = -\ln[S(t)/S_0]/\mathrm{TE}$$

where TE is the echo time of the sequence and S_0 the baseline signal before arrival of the tracer.

Impact of Diseases on Renal Flow Rate and Renal Perfusion

Renal blood flow (RBF), or flow rate, refers to the global amount of blood reaching the kidney per unit of time, normally expressed in mL/min. Renal perfusion refers to the blood flow that passes through a unit mass of renal tissue (mL/min/g) in order to vascularize it and exchange with the extravascular space. In clinical practice, measurement of RBF or perfusion may become important for the evaluation of renal artery stenosis (RAS) or nephropathies with microvascular involvement (22) and help in monitoring intravascular interventions.

Renal Flow Rate

Similar to Doppler sonography, the cine-phase-contrast MR method is useful to evaluate the intra-arterial velocity profile and to quantify the RBF in each renal vessel without the injection of a contrast agent. This parameter is usually measured alternatively either on a renal artery or a renal vein and in the abdominal aorta as the difference of flow above and below the renal arteries. The technique is well described in the literature (23) and is based on the measurement of phase shifts of flowing spins along one direction (usually perpendicular to the vessel of interest). For accurate flow measurements in the human arteries, the imaging plane is usually positioned 10 to 15 mm downstream from the ostium where respiratory movements are minimal, and perpendicularly to the renal artery.

With a time resolution of 32 msec per time frame, Schoenberg et al. (24–26) showed that either a normal velocity curve or a partial loss of the early systolic peak (ESP) was consistent with low-grade stenosis; complete loss of the ESP and decrease of the midsystolic peak indicated moderate stenosis (50%); flattened flow profile with no systolic velocity components was representative of high-grade stenosis

(Fig. 3). Using this classification, the combined approach of 3-D Gd-enhanced MR angiography (MRA) and phase-contrast flow sequence revealed the best interobserver and intermodality agreement. Sensitivity and specificity of detection of significant RAS ($>50\%$) were 100% and 93%, respectively. Therefore, this technique has been considered to be a useful complement to MRA of renal arteries (Fig. 4). This method is also capable to measure the RBF in the renal artery below a stenosis, as the product of the mean velocity within the artery and the cross-sectional area of the renal artery.

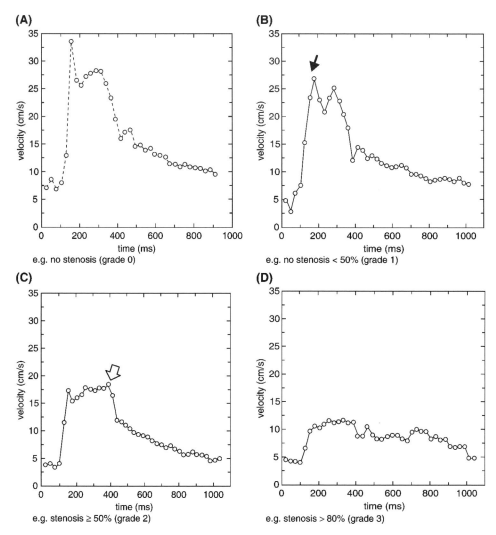

Figure 3 Cine-phase-contrast flow curves for different degrees of RAS. A semiquantitative grading scheme is applied on the basis of distinct changes in the waveform pattern. This scheme was shown to the readers as a guideline for the grading of hemodynamic changes. Note that the absolute scaling is the same for all four flow curves. (**A**) Normal flow profiles reveal a characteristic ESP and a midsystolic maximum. (**B**) Low-grade stenoses typically reveal only a partial loss of the ESP (*solid arrow*). (**C**) Moderate stenoses demonstrate an almost complete loss of the ESP and a decrease of the midsystolic maximum (*open arrow*). (**D**) High-grade stenoses have a featureless flattened flow profile. *Abbreviations*: RAS, renal artery stenosis; ESP, early systolic peak. *Source*: From Ref. 26.

(A)

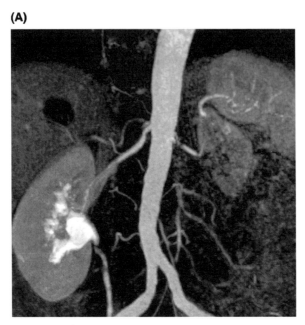

(B)

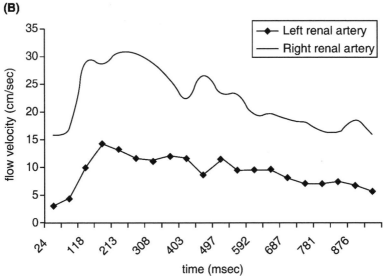

Figure 4 (**A**) A 75-year-old female patient with high-grade left renal artery stenosis and scarring of the kidney demonstrated on MR angiogram. (**B**) In the phase-contrast MR-flow measurement, a substantially altered flow profile of the affected side with loss of the systolic velocity components becomes visible. *Abbreviation*: MR, magnetic resonance. *Source*: Courtesy of Dr. Stefan O. Schoenberg and Dr. Henrik Michaely, Department of Clinical Radiology, Ludwig-Maximilians-University, Munich, Germany.

Renal Perfusion with Contrast-Enhanced Dynamic Studies

The degree of perfusion depends on both the arterial flow rate and such local factors as regional blood volume and vasoreactivity. Theory of perfusion calculation as well as imaging methods depends on the type of contrast agent used. Diffusible Gd-chelates as well as two categories of agents without interstitial diffusion or GFR (iron oxide particles and blood-pool Gd-chelates: macromolecular or albumin bound) have been proposed for renal perfusion (27,28).

First-Pass Dynamic Studies Using Intravascular Agents with a T2* Effect. Because absolute quantification of regional perfusion is not straightforward with iron oxide particles and requires several signal processing steps together with several assumptions, most studies have been conducted using either qualitative or semiquantitative indices; maximal signal decrease (MSD), time to MSD (T_{MSD}), or wash-in and wash-out slopes can be measured for comparison from right to left kidney, from cortex to medulla, or from one territory to another.

Because these agents are considered having a unicompartmental distribution within the kidney, absolute regional RBF can be calculated (in mL/min/g) according to Stewart and Hamilton's central volume theorem:

$$rRBF = rRBV \times MTT,$$

where rRBF is the regional RBF, rRBV is the regional renal blood volume, and MTT is the mean transit time. Calculation of rRBV (in mL/g of renal tissue) corresponds to the area under the fitted first-pass concentration–time curve, denoted as $C(t)$, normalized to AIF denoted as $C_a(t)$, and to the mean renal density ($\rho = 1.04$ g/mL), and taking into account the difference (k_h) in arterial and capillary hematocrits (29):

$$rRBV = k_h/\rho \int C(t)dt \Big/ \int Ca(t)dt$$

The real MTT is difficult to measure because it would require a better understanding of the range of microvasculature structure within the tissues. However, it has been shown that the first moment of the renal-fitted concentration–time curve is a reasonable estimation of the relative MTT (30).

Application of this quantitative technique to a series of patients with RAS have been reported recently (31). A decreased rRBF was noted only for severe stenosis (Fig. 5) or in kidneys suffering from chronic damage related to other renal diseases, illustrating the complementary role of morphological information provided by MRA and hemodynamic data.

First-Pass Dynamic Studies Using Diffusible Gd-chelates. Renal perfusion can also be evaluated with standard Gd-chelates that are freely diffusible within the interstitial space and excreted exclusively by GFR. First-pass studies with these agents allow measurement of both the renal perfusion and the GFR during the same acquisition protocol. Renal perfusion is calculated from the first-pass renal curve following an instantaneous bolus of the contrast agent, which requires a high temporal resolution.

The most widely used perfusion model is derived from Peters's model, developed for nuclear medicine with ^{99m}Tc-diethylene-triamine-pentacetate (DTPA) as radiopharmaceutical (32). Because ^{99m}Tc and these Gd-chelates have similar pharmacokinetical properties, the obtained dynamic uptake curves by MRI is comparable with that obtained with a gamma camera. The simple kinetic description of microspheres can be applied to the initial wash-in of the renal MR signal–time curve (33). Introducing the arterial changes of $R1$ allows [$\Delta(R1)_{art}$] calculation of renal perfusion per unit of volume and can be extracted from the mathematical expression:

$$RBF/vol = \max slope_{renal}/\max \Delta(R1)_{art}$$

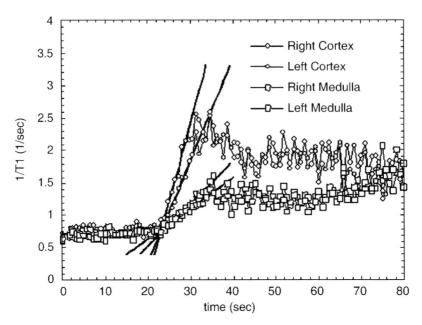

Figure 5 Measurement of renal perfusion with $T1w$ dynamic Gd-enhanced sequence in a patient with right renal artery stenosis. Renal transit curves after injection of Gd-DTPA show a decreased ascending slope on the right cortex. Blood flow measured from the slope of renal perfusion curve and the peak enhancement in the aorta were 1.29 and 1.89 mL/min/g in the right and left cortex, respectively. *Abbreviations*: $T1w$, $T1$-weighted; Gd, gadolinium; DTPA, diethylene-triamine-pentacetate. *Source*: From Ref. 32.

Using this method, with a small bolus of contrast (0.025 mmol/kg) and a $T1w$ gradient-echo sequence, Vallée et al. (32) were able to measure cortical blood flow (BF) in 16 patients with normal kidneys (254 ± 116 mL/min/100 g), decreasing to 109 ± 75 mL/min/100 g in case of RAS (Fig. 10) and to 51 ± 34 mL/min/100 g in case of renal failure. Unfortunately, no reference measurements with radiopharmaceutical techniques were used.

Renal Perfusion Without Contrast Agents

Renal perfusion can alternatively be measured using pulsed arterial spin labeling (or spin tagging) using endogenous water as a diffusible tracer (Fig. 6) (34). With this technique, a perfusion-weighted image can be generated by the subtraction of an image in which inflowing spins have been labeled from an image in which spin labeling has not been performed. Quantitative perfusion maps can then be calculated (in mL/min/100 g of tissue) when T1 of the tissue and efficiency of labeling are known. Several pulse-sequence strategies have been described to tag arterial flowing spins, which can be divided into two groups (continuous or pulsed labeling) with different advantages and drawbacks as described in detail by Calamante et al. (35).

An experimental study, with the echo planar imaging with signal targeting with alternating radio frequency (EPISTAR) sequence, on a model of RAS in pigs, showed that a decrease of blood flow was 100% sensitive and specific for detection of 70% renal artery stenoses (36). The flow-sensitive alternating inversion recovery (FAIR) preparation sequence applied to a 24 volunteers and 46 patients with a

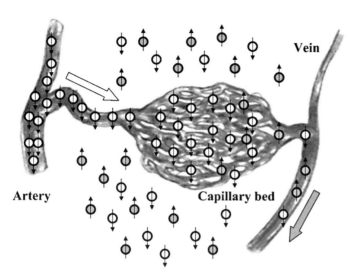

Figure 6 Schematic description of the principles of freely diffusible tracer theory. Inverted magnetization (white) comes from the arterial tree (*white arrow*) and diffuses at the capillary level. There, spins are exchanged with the tissue magnetization (gray) and reduce its local intensity. The degree of attenuation is a direct measure of perfusion. Remaining tagged magnetization as well as exchanged water molecules flow out of the voxel of interest through the venous system (*gray arrow*). *Source*: From Ref. 34.

RAS or a renal disease, allowed to significantly separate normal and diseased kidneys by measuring cortical signal-to-noise ratio (Fig. 7) (37). Recently, a technique associating a FAIR preparation and true–fast imaging with free precession data acquisition provided very encouraging quantitative results because of shorter echo time and fewer saturation effects (38). However, these methods are complex to implement in clinical systems and have never been poorly correlated to established methods. Hence, its impact in clinical practice remains uncertain.

Impact of Diseases on GFR

Impact of nephropathies on GFR can be assessed semiquantitatively or quantitatively. Measurement of GFR is difficult to obtain accurately as a routine. Semiquantitative evaluation of renal function, as split (or differential) renal function, is usually not useful in daily assessment and follow-up of renal diseases. Split renal function assessment is sufficient in urological management of most patients with obstructive uropathies (39). In addition, information about split renal function can be helpful when renal function is reduced and associated with renal asymmetry or renovascular disease, and before renal surgery or renal biopsy in patients with renal impairment.

If the time resolution of the sequence is sufficiently high, normal SI–time curve following Gd-injection can be characterized by three phases: a first abrupt, ascending segment followed by a first peak, corresponding to the *vascular-to-glomerular first-pass* or *cortical vascular phase*; a second slowly ascending segment, ended by a second peak, corresponding to the *glomerulotubular phase*; and a slowly descending segment, corresponding to the predominant excretory function, the so-called *excretory phase* (Fig. 8).

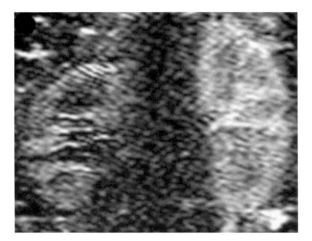

Figure 7 Example of perfusion measurement with the arterial spin-labeling (ASL) technique in a 52-year-old female patient with right-sided renal artery stenosis of 60%. The ASL perfusion-weighted image shows reduced SI of the right kidney. The signal-to-noise ratio of the affected kidney is 4.8 vs. 8.6 in the healthy kidney. *Abbreviations*: ASL, arterial spin-labeling; SI, signal intensity. *Source*: From Ref. 37.

Semiquantitative Measurement of Split Renal Function

It has been shown that the functional parameters calculated from the SI–time curves obtained with a $T1w$ sequence were in terms of simple parameters, such as the maximum peak value, time-to-peak, and the area under the curve (40,41). In these approaches, conversion from SI to concentration of contrast agent is not necessary.

Rohrschneider et al. (42) obtained calculations of the percentage of the single-kidney "activity" comparable to those derived with gamma camera scintigraphy (43,44). These studies were based on a dynamic radio frequency (RF)-spoiled gradient-echo sequence and half of a standard clinical accepted dose of Gd-DTPA. A region of interest (ROI) was positioned around the renal parenchyma (omitting pelvis), and calculation of the relative renal function was then based on the equation:

$$RF = AUC(mm)^2 \times S(mm^2)$$

where AUC corresponds to the area under the glomerulotubular segment of the time–intensity curve and S is the ROI area (Fig. 8). The split renal function (in percentage) corresponds, for each kidney, to the product:

$$RF(\%) = RF/RF_{total} \times 100$$

where RF_{total} is the sum of RFs of both kidneys.

Lee et al. (45) proposed a GFR index (μmol) measured, after conversion of SI into concentration, by multiplying the average concentration of Gd (μmol/mL) between two and three minutes by the volume of interest (volume of the cortex, medulla, or both, in mL). The correlation with ^{99m}Tc-DTPA plasma clearance was not perfect ($r = 0.72$).

Quantitative Methods

The indications of true GFR measurements in nephrology may include follow-up of renal transplants, evaluation of living donors when measurement of creatinine

(A)

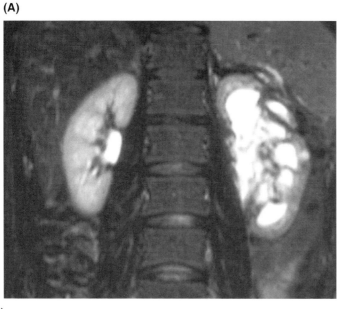

(B)

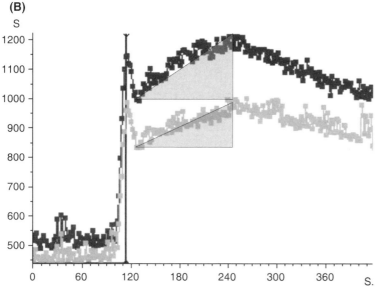

Figure 8 SI–time curves obtained in a patient with left urinary obstruction. (**A**) Anatomic image showing dilatation of the left pyelocaliceal system. (**B**) SI–time curves obtained from regions-of-interest drawn on the entire renal parenchyma (excluding pyelocaliceal system) on each side, showing three phases: a first abrupt ascending segment followed by a first peak, corresponding to the "vascular-to-glomerular first-pass" or cortical vascular phase; a second slowly ascending segment, ended by a second peak, corresponding to the glomerulotubular phase; and a slowly descending segment, corresponding to the predominant excretory function and the so-called "excretory phase." Areas under the curve have been drawn to calculate split renal function. *Abbreviation*: SI, signal intensity.

clearance is not reliable (low muscle mass, obese, etc.) (46), and clinical protocols requiring a reliable and reproducible renal function estimation.

GFR measurement can be obtained by two types of techniques.

1. Creatinine clearance estimated from formulae that avoid urinary collection, such as the Cockcroft and Gault and the Modification of Diet in Renal Disease study. However, these formulae have several limitations related to variations of plasma creatinine level, which are around 10%; tubular secretion of creatinine in advanced renal failure may lead to overestimation of GFR and reduction of creatinine excretion that occurs with age due to a decrease in skeletal muscle mass. Furthermore, in acute or rapidly progressing renal failure, these formulae provide inaccurate information when GFR is rapidly changing (47).
2. Tracer clearance, using either nonradioactive (such as inulin or iothalamate) or radioactive tracers (^{51}Cr–ethylenediamine tetraacetic acid or ^{99m}Tc-DTPA). These procedures are not widely used because they are time consuming and require several blood samplings, with or without urine collection.

SKGFR Based on Intrarenal Kinetics.   The requirements to quantify GFR are identical to those previously listed for perfusion measurements using $T1$ agents. By introducing advanced models that take into account both the first passage of blood and the filtration part, it is possible to simultaneously calculate both RBF and single-kidney GFR (SKGFR).

To calculate GFR, several compartmental models have been proposed: the Rutland-Patlak model (16,48), the cortical compartment model (49), and an extensive multicompartmental model (45) including several cortical and medullary compartment models. According to Annet et al. (50), the cortical compartment model seems to provide more accurate results than the Patlak plot applied to the cortex alone or to the entire parenchyma. However, results from these studies are precluded by some limitations, which include nonuniform SI either from section to section (48) or between time-points (45), inaccurate or absence of movement correction, and inadequate conversion of SI into concentration (49). Developments are progressing for using sequences providing uniform SI in space and time, for applying automatic movement correction to improve the quality of SI time curves, and to display 3-D maps of GFR on a voxel-by-voxel basis (Fig. 9). However, these methods still require validation with reference methods in large human populations with normal and decreased renal function.

Single-Kidney Extraction Fraction.   A quantitative method of in vivo measurement of the single-kidney extraction fraction (EF) and SKGFR was proposed by Dumoulin et al. (51) and applied to experimental studies by Niendorf et al. (52–54). This method is based on the measurement of $T1$ within flowing arterial and venous blood (Look-Locker method) during continuous Gd infusion where the steady-state equation can be used:

$$SKGFR = EF \times RBF \times (1 - Hct)$$

where RBF is the renal blood flow and Hct is the hematocrit value of the blood. The EF is calculated from the equation:

$$EF = (1/T1a - 1/T1v)/(1/T1a - 1/T1_0)$$

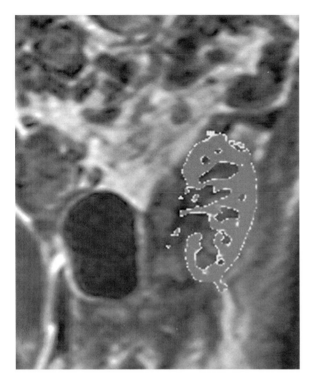

Figure 9 GFR map of a kidney transplant obtained after dynamic $T1w$ Gd-enhanced sequence and application of the Rutland-Patlak plot on a voxel-by voxel basis. *Abbreviations*: $T1w$, $T1$-weighted; GFR, glomerular filtration; Gd, gadolinium.

where $T1a$ is $T1$ in the renal artery, $T1v$ is $T1$ in the vein, and $T1_0$ is the $T1$ in the blood without Gd. Once EF is calculated for each kidney, values of SKGFR can be calculated if RBF is known. Preliminary animal studies have shown concordant results compared to those calculated from inulin clearance.

PROGNOSTIC FACTORS OF RENAL IMPAIRMENT

Several pathophysiological factors that are of significance for the prognosis of renal diseases can be assessed in the near future with specific MR techniques and contrast agents. These factors in acute renal diseases include cell viability, degree of glomerular or interstitial inflammation, and tubular dysfunction. In chronic renal diseases they include medullary hypoxia and development of glomerular or interstitial fibrosis.

Prognostic Factors in Acute Renal Diseases

Criteria of Cell Viability

In ARF, direct toxicity to the cells or ischemic damage may lead to apoptosis or necrosis of tubular cells. Therefore, identification of these cellular events could help in assessing the severity and the reversibility of diseases. Several methods could be promoted, such as diffusion-sensitized sequences or MR-targeting of apoptotic cells.

MR Diffusion of Acute Renal Diseases. SI observed on diffusion-weighted sequences depends on molecular movements within intra- and extracellular spaces, which depend essentially on local temperature and biological barriers present in the tissue (cellular membranes, fibers, organelles, macromolecules, etc.). In addition, "external" factors, such as perfusion, magnetic susceptibility of tissues, cardiac pulsations, and respiratory movements, influence this technique (55). The "external" factors are relatively well controlled within the brain but difficult to nullify in abdominal applications, particularly artifacts due to bowel peristalsis and respiratory movements. Technical details of MR diffusion imaging are beyond the scope of this chapter and have been discussed elsewhere (56).

Using appropriate acquisition methods, cortical values of apparent diffusion coefficient (ADC) appear higher in the cortex than in the medulla (Fig. 10) (57). In acute renal disease, diffusion-weighted imaging could be useful to separate cellular edema from cellular necrosis, i.e., reversible versus irreversible renal damage. Reversible cellular edema is characterized by decreased ADC values, due to a reduction of the size of extracellular diffusion spaces and of the exchanges between intra- and extracellular spaces (so-called restricted diffusion). Irreversible cellular necrosis is characterized by increased ADC values because of destruction of cell membranes enlarging extracellular diffusion spaces. In an experimental model of diabetic nephropathy, we showed that the regional ADC values were decreased within the outer medulla when tubular cell edema occurred (58). However, the exact role of this method in evaluating prognosis of acute renal diseases has still to be defined.

MRI of Apoptosis. Apoptosis and its regulatory mechanisms contribute to cell number regulation in ARF (59). Tubular cells apoptosis is promoted by both exogenous factors such as nephrotoxic drugs and bacterial products, and endogenous factors, such as lethal cytokines. Conversely to necrosis, which is a nonreversible process, apoptotic pathways are potentially accessible to therapeutic modulation (60).

There is growing interest in using MRI for detection of apoptosis, mainly in the field of oncology and in ischemic diseases. This approach needs to label apoptotic cells using ultrasmall particles iron oxides (USPIOs) as markers and phosphatidylserine as a target. This requires to link the superparamagnetic nanoparticle with annexin V or synaptotagmin I, which both bind to the phosphatidylserine that appears on the outer leaflet of the plasma membrane of apoptotic cells (61). To our knowledge, this approach has never been applied to an ischemic kidney model.

Degree of Tubule Dysfunction

In ARF models, the primary site of renal injury whether in the proximal or distal part of the nephron remains uncertain (62). Using Gd-dendrimer chelates, which are cleared by GFR, some authors were able to demonstrate proximal tubule dysfunction in acute tubular damage induced by cisplatin in mice (63). This contrast agent accumulates within the outer medulla, where the proximal straight tubules are located (Fig. 11A). In diseased kidneys, the bright SI of the outer medulla does not show, and the gradation of tubular damage assessed by dynamic MRI correlates with renal function (Fig. 11B and C).

Intrarenal Inflammation

Macrophages are virtually absent in normal kidneys but may infiltrate renal tissues in certain nephropathies, such as acute proliferative types of human and experimental

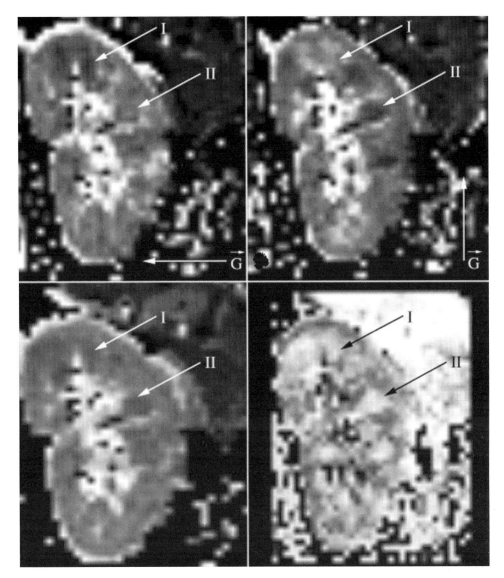

Figure 10 Calculated ADC maps with a diffusion weighting in two orthogonal directions demonstrate the radial-shaped anisotropy of the medulla. The pyramid cell in the upper part of the kidney (I) shows a lower ADC with an applied diffusion weighting in the left–right direction (*top left*), while the ADC obtained in the superior–inferior direction is elevated (*top right*). The pyramid cell in the center part of the kidney (II) has a lower ADC in the superior–inferior direction, while the ADC in the left–right direction is elevated. On the ADC$_{trace}$ maps (*bottom left*) both pyramids are clearly depicted as regions with a lower ADC than the cortical tissue, and on the FA map (*bottom right*) both regions can be identified by the elevated FA. *Abbreviations*: ADC, apparent diffusion coefficient; FA, fractional anisotropy. *Source*: From Ref. 57.

glomerulonephritides (64), renal graft dysfunctions (rejection and acute tubular necrosis) (65), in acute ischemic disease (66), and such nonspecific kidney diseases as hydronephrosis (67). This macrophagic attraction is a dynamic process under the control of chemotactic molecules and expression level of leucocytes adhesion

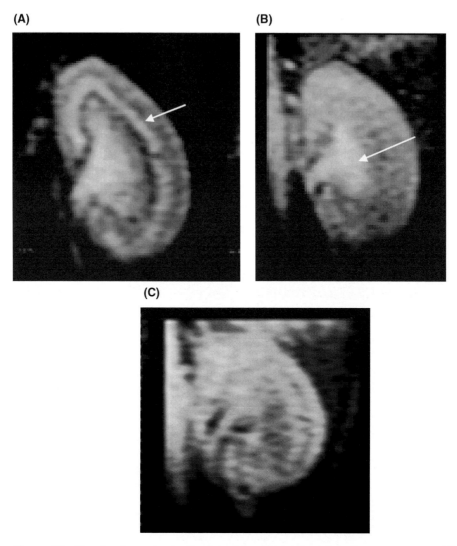

Figure 11 Renal enhancement after injection of dendrimer-based contrast agent. (**A**) In a normally functioning kidney, we note a bright band within the outer stripe of outer medulla (*arrow*) where proximal straight tubules are located. (**B**) In mildly damaged kidney, this bright band disappears and late enhancement of inner medulla predominates. (**C**) Severely damaged kidneys showed no appearance of medullary enhancement. *Source*: From Ref. 63.

molecules. In animals, the degree of macrophagic infiltration and proliferation is correlated with the severity of renal disease, whereas it remains unclear if macrophages produce direct renal insults or if they are a consequence of the disease in order to regulate the inflammatory response. Their role is complex, contributing to glomerular and tubulointerstitial injury through the secretion of various cytokines and proteases, which induce changes in extracellular matrix and progressive fibrotic changes (glomerulosclerosis, tubulointerstitial fibrosis, etc.) (68).

Today, in clinical practice, the degree of inflammatory response in the kidney can be only approached by renal biopsy. Therefore, noninvasive and reproducible identification and quantification of intrarenal inflammation has great potential because it could participate in characterization of the kidney disease and assessment of prognosis and monitor response to treatment.

Depending on the type of kidney disease and its severity, macrophagic activity may predominate within the glomeruli (i.e., within the cortex), or within the interstitium (i.e., diffuse, within all kidney compartments), or in the medullary ascending vasa recta (i.e., within the medulla). USPIO are small-sized nanoparticles that have a long half-life in the blood stream (two hours in rats and 36 hours in humans) and are avidly captured several hours after intravenous injection by extrahepatic cells with phagocytic activity that include blood circulating monocytes and resident macrophages that are present in most of tissues.

Several models of experimental nephropathies in rats were used to demonstrate the detectability of intrarenal macrophagic activity in vivo: a model of nephrotic syndrome (69) with a diffuse decrease of SI predominating within the outer medulla; a model of acute graft rejection, with a diffuse homogenous decrease of SI in the three renal compartments (70); a model of antiglomerular basement membrane glomerulonephritis, comparable to Goodpasture's syndrome in humans, with a drop of SI within the cortex only (Fig. 12) (71); a model of ischemia–reperfusion, with a drop of signal within the medulla (72). The degree of decrease of SI was always correlated with the number of macrophages within each renal compartment and to the severity of disease.

The results of the first clinical study were recently reported (73), based on 12 patients. MRI was performed three days after USPIO injection (Sinerem[R], Guerbet Group) to ensure getting rid of signal changes from vascular blood volume, knowing that the blood half-life of USPIO is 36 hours. All patients but one, with an inflammatory component on cortical biopsy, showed a significant decrease of SI after USPIO injection. MR images of a patient with renal transplant in acute rejection are shown in Figure 13. Patients with chronic and fibrotic disease, without inflammatory components on biopsy, did not show any significant change. Three patients with

(A)   **(B)**

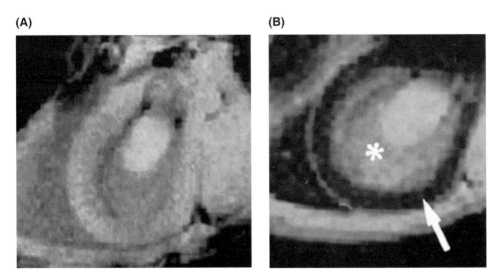

Figure 12   Accelerated nephrotoxic glomerulonephritis in rat, **(A)** before and **(B)** 24 hours after injection of USPIO. In **B**, there is a notable decrease in SI in the renal cortex (*arrow*) after injection, due to the superparamagnetic effect of USPIO, whereas no SI change is observed in any part of the medulla (*star*). *Abbreviations*: USPIO, ultrasmall particles iron oxide; SI, signal intensity. *Source*: From Ref. 71.

(A)   (B)

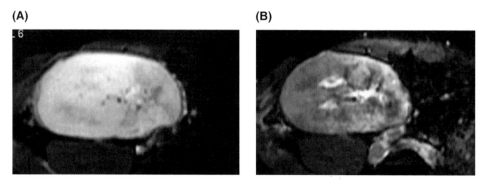

Figure 13 Patient with renal transplant and acute rejection. $T2^*$-weighted MRI (**A**) before and (**B**) 72 hours after intravenous injection of USPIO shows a decrease of signal related to inflammatory cellular infiltration in all renal compartments. *Abbreviations*: MRI, magnetic resonance imaging; USPIO, ultrasmall particles iron oxide.

acute tubular necrosis (two transplanted kidneys and one native kidney) showed a significant decrease of SI within the medulla. These preliminary clinical findings seem to corroborate experimental results and call for larger multicenter clinical trials and evaluation of imaging at two days after injection to reduce delay in the diagnosis.

Prognostic Factors in Chronic Renal Diseases

Medullary Hypoxia

Outer medulla is particularly sensitive to hypoxia because the active reabsorption process within the thick ascending loop of Henle requires high level of oxygen consumption (74). Therefore, decrease of medullary blood flow or increase in tubular reabsorption, as in diabetic nephropathy at the stage of hyperfiltration, may induce medullary hypoxia and secondary ischemia.

This blood oxygen level—dependent (BOLD)-sensitive MR approach has been already covered in a recent review (75). Using a multiecho gradient-echo sequence, $R2^*$ maps can be obtained showing a higher $R2^*$ within the medulla (i.e., lower pO_2) (Fig. 14A). This effect is better detected with 3 T magnets, which offer higher signal-to-noise ratio and greater sensitivity to magnetic susceptibility (Fig. 14B) (76). BOLD technique does not measure pO_2 directly but allows intrarenal $R2^*$ ($1/T2^*$) measurements, which are closely related to the concentration in deoxyhemoglobin (77,78). Therefore, absolute $R2^*$ values cannot be used in practice. If the disease is asymmetric, as in RAS, static comparison of both kidneys may identify hypoxia on one side. In parenchymal renal diseases, only dynamic changes following physiological or pharmacological manipulation can identify the kidney response. For example, Prasad et al. (79) demonstrated the medullary hypoxic effect of injection of radio-contrast agents in rats (known to induce acute medullary hypoperfusion). On the contrary, furosemide and water load increase medullary oxygenation (at least in young individuals) (80). These changes can be documented with dynamic BOLD imaging.

Interestingly, diabetic subjects are unable to increase the medullary oxygenation during water diuresis. In a comparative study with a matched control group, diabetic patients without microalbuminuria, hypertension, or renal insufficiency did not show any significant improvement of medullary oxygenation after water load (81), reflecting a probable deficiency in medullary vasodilatation, perhaps due to

(A)

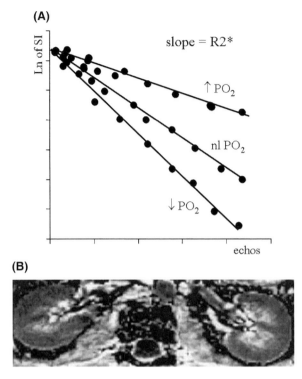

(B)

Figure 14   Principle of BOLD acquisition in the kidney. (**A**) The $R2^*$ is greater when the tissue pO_2 is low and lower when it is high. (**B**) A $T2^*$-weighted multiecho gradient-echo sequence allows to calculate a $R2^*$ map showing a higher $R2^*$ value within medulla, here obtained at 3 T. *Abbreviation*: BOLD, blood oxygen level—dependent. *Source*: From Ref. 76 (Part B).

reduction of local synthesis of prostaglandins, nitric oxide, or other vasoactive substances. Wider applications of this technique to clinical ischemic conditions of the medulla have still to be established.

MRI and Development of Intrarenal Fibrosis

Exaggeration of extracellular matrix synthesis, with excessive fibrillar collagens, characterizes the development of fibrotic lesions in the glomerular, interstitial, and vascular compartments (82), leading progressively to end-stage renal failure. Systems participating in these processes are better identified and various therapeutic interventions have been shown to prevent or favor regression of fibrosis in several experimental models (82). Therefore, development of new noninvasive methods for identification and quantification of fibrosis would also be worthwhile. Two approaches can be proposed with MRI: diffusion-weighted sequences or MR elastography.

With diffusion imaging, the ADC values would be reduced due to a restriction of the diffusion space in proportion with the development of fibrosis. Indeed, the first clinical trials on chronic renal diseases, including RAS and ureteral obstruction, showed a decrease of ADC values (83), which were highly correlated with serum creatinine levels. However, none of these studies presented correlation with the pathological quantification of fibrosis.

Fibrotic process altering the renal tissue structure changes the biomechanical properties of the kidney (84). Quantification of these tissue changes is now possible with ultrasonic or MR elastography. This method requires applying shear waves by means of a mechanical device, producing tissue displacements on the order of nanometers to micrometers. Propagation of these waves being dependent on viscoelastic properties of the tissue, its elastic characteristics can be quantified and/or mapped as parametric images. In the liver, the ultrasonic elastography has already been validated and is now used in clinical routine for follow-up of chronic liver diseases

(A)

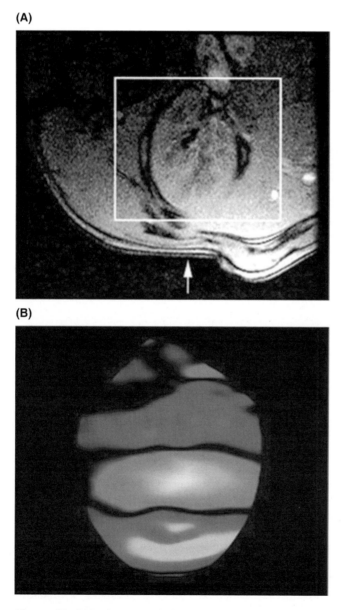

(B)

Figure 15 MR elastographic image of a human kidney in vivo. (**A**) Axial MRI through the left kidney of a normal volunteer. Mechanical shearing waves are applied with an oscillating plate at the body surface (*arrow*). (**B**) Corresponding wave image for the region included in the white outline. *Abbreviation*: MRI, magnetic resonance imaging. *Source*: From Ref. 84.

and preliminary results in kidney transplants have been reported (85). Using MR elastography, based on a phase-contrast technique utilizing cyclic motion–sensitized gradients to image mechanically applied propagating acoustic shear waves, Shah et al. (84) validated the method in vivo on rat models of nephrocalcinosis and obtained the first elastographic images of native human kidneys (Fig. 15). These extremely encouraging results still need clinical validation.

(A)   **(B)**

(C)

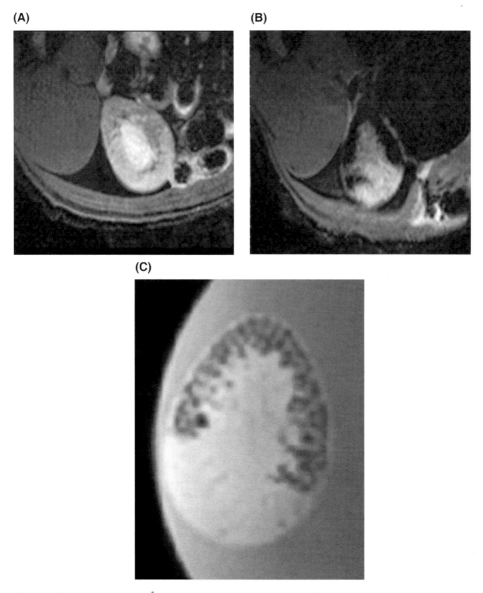

Figure 16 Transverse $T2^*$-weighted MR image of a rat kidney obtained (**A**) in vivo before and (**B**) in vivo and (**C**) ex vivo seven days after intra-arterial injection of magnetically labeled mesenchymal stem cells. The cells are still visible within the cortex and histology found the cells into glomeruli. *Abbreviation*: MR, magnetic resonance. *Source*: From Ref. 93.

CELL LABELING FOR FOLLOW-UP OF RENAL CELL THERAPY

Recovery of renal function after acute nephrotoxic or ischemic insult is dependent on the replacement of necrotic tubular cells with functional tubular epithelium (86). This cellular regeneration originates from resident cells or from extrarenal cells. Recently, the possibility of differentiation of bone-marrow-derived mesenchymal stem cells (MSC) into mesangial cells (87,88) and of hematopoietic stem cells into tubular cells was demonstrated in vivo (89), bringing great therapeutic promise for the future. Noninvasive imaging techniques allowing in vivo assessment of the location of stem cells could be of great value for experimental studies in which these cells are transplanted. It provides a tool to immediately verify if the grafted cells have reached the target organ, to estimate the number of cells that were seeded, and to assess the permanence of these cells over time with sequential imaging. Using SPIO preparations to magnetically label the cells, several groups have demonstrated the feasibility of grafting and subsequent visualization of progenitor different organs (90–92). The renal distribution of SPIO-labeled MSC following intravascular administration has been investigated recently. Labeled MSC were observed in vivo within the kidney cortex as long as seven days after injection into the renal artery, with 1.5 T MRI (Fig. 16) (93). In a model of acute glomerulopathy, with an intravenous administration of magnetically labeled mesenchymal stem cells, no renal uptake could be observed in vivo at 4.7 T, but imaging at very high field strength (9 T) showed that the cells had reached the diseased areas of the cortex (specific homing effect) (Fig. 17) (94).

CONCLUSION

MRI has now a huge potential for evaluation of volumetric or intrarenal contrast changes due to medical renal diseases. Noninvasive functional techniques already

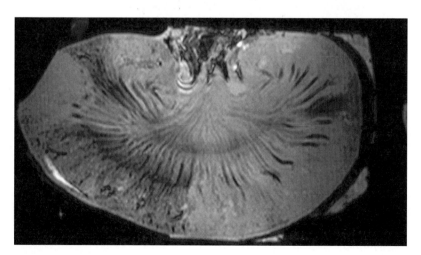

Figure 17   Longitudinal ex vivo $T2^{*}$-weighted MR image of a rat kidney at very high field strength (9 T) showing cortical low signal intensity areas related to magnetically labeled mesenchymal stem cells targeting the diseased areas of the kidney (homing effect) after intravenous administration. *Abbreviation*: MR, magnetic resonance.

provide semiquantitative parameters with similar performances to scintigraphic techniques. They could also in the near future provide absolute values of perfusion and GFR, as well as specific criteria for characterization of nephropathies or pertinent information for prognosis, which could have an impact on new therapies. Labeling progenitors for in vivo follow-up of cell therapy could help in recognizing the homing sites and in evaluating efficacy of cell therapies.

ACKNOWLEDGMENTS

Acknowledgments for collaborations in many experimental studies and for fruitful discussions to: C. Bos, J. Bulte, M. Claudon, C. Combe, Y. Delmas, C. Deminière, B. Denis de Senneville, P. Desbarat, J. Frøkier, I. Gordon, R. Jones, CTW. Moonen, M. Ries, and J. Ripoche.

REFERENCES

1. Semelka RC, Corrigan K, Ascher SM, Brown JJ, Colindres RE. Renal corticomedullary differentiation: observation in patients with differing serum creatinine levels. Radiology 1994; 190(1):149–152.
2. Chung JJ, Semelka RC, Martin DR. Acute renal failure: common occurrence of preservation of corticomedullary differentiation on MR images. Magn Reson Imaging 2001; 19(6):789–793.
3. Jeong JY, Kim SH, Lee HJ, Sim JS. Atypical low-signal-intensity renal parenchyma: causes and patterns. Radiographics 2002; 22(4):833–846.
4. Saxena AB, Busque S, Arjane P, Myers BD, Tan JC. Preoperative renal volumes as a predictor of graft function in living donor transplantation. Am J Kidney Dis 2004; 44(5):877–885.
5. Bakker J, Olree M, Kaatee R, et al. Renal volume measurements: accuracy and repeatability of US compared with that of MR imaging. Radiology 1999; 211(3):623–628.
6. Cost GA, Merguerian PA, Cheerasarn SP, Shortliffe LM. Sonographic renal parenchymal and pelvicaliceal areas: new quantitative parameters for renal sonographic followup. J Urol 1996; 156(2 Pt 2):725–729.
7. Roger SD, Beale AM, Cattell WR, Webb JA. What is the value of measuring renal parenchymal thickness before renal biopsy? Clin Radiol 1994; 49(1):45–49.
8. Mounier-Vehier C, Lions C, Devos P, et al. Cortical thickness: an early morphological marker of atherosclerotic renal disease. Kidney Int 2002; 61(2):591–598.
9. Coulam CH, Bouley DM, Sommer FG. Measurement of renal volumes with contrast-enhanced MRI. J Magn Reson Imaging 2002; 15(2):174–179.
10. Torres VE, Wang X, Qian Q, Somlo S, Harris PC, Gattone VH II. Effective treatment of an orthologous model of autosomal dominant polycystic kidney disease. Nat Med 2004; 10(4):363–364.
11. Chapman AB, Guay-Woodford LM, Grantham JJ, et al. Renal structure in early autosomal-dominant polycystic kidney disease (ADPKD): The Consortium for Radiologic Imaging Studies of Polycystic Kidney Disease (CRISP) cohort. Kidney Int 2003; 64(3):1035–1045.
12. King BF, Reed JE, Bergstralh EJ, Sheedy PF II, Torres VE. Quantification and longitudinal trends of kidney, renal cyst, and renal parenchyma volumes in autosomal dominant polycystic kidney disease. J Am Soc Nephrol 2000; 11(8):1505–1511.
13. Huang AJ, Lee VS, Rusinek H. MR imaging of renal function. Radiol Clin North Am 2003; 41(5):1001–1017.

14. Grenier N, Pedersen M, Hauger O. Functional and cellular MRI of the kidney. In: Prigent A, Piepsz A, eds. Functional Imaging in Nephron-Urology. Oxon, UK: Taylor & Francis Medical Books, 2006:173–196.

15. Pedersen M, Frokier J, Grenier N. Quantitative measurement of renal function using contrast enhanced MRI: an initial experience. Int Scientific Meeting Radionucl Nephr-Urol, ISCORN, La Baule, 2004, Poster presentation, M15.

16. Pedersen M, Shi Y, Anderson P, et al. Quantitation of differential renal blood flow and renal function using dynamic contrast-enhanced MRI in rats. Magn Reson Med 2004; 51(3):510–517.

17. Rusinek H, Lee VS, Johnson G. Optimal dose of Gd-DTPA in dynamic MR studies. Magn Reson Med 2001; 46(2):312–316.

18. Chen Z, Prato FS, McKenzie C. T1 fast acquisition relaxation mapping (T1-FARM): an optimized reconstruction. IEEE Trans Med Imaging 1998; 17(2):155–160.

19. Zheng J, Venkatesan R, Haacke EM, Cavagna FM, Finn PJ, Li D. Accuracy of T1 measurements at high temporal resolution: feasibility of dynamic measurement of blood T1 after contrast administration. J Magn Reson Imaging 1999; 10(4):576–581.

20. McKenzie CA, Pereira RS, Prato FS, Chen Z, Drost DJ. Improved contrast agent bolus tracking using T1 FARM. Magn Reson Med 1999; 41(3):429–435.

21. Pedersen M, Dissing T, Deding D, Grenier N, Yang Q, Frokier J. MR renography based on contrast-enhanced T1-mapping. In: ISfMRi Medicine, ed. International Society for Magnetic Resonance in Medicine, Miami, 7–13 May, 2005:526.

22. Schoenberg SO, Rieger J, Johannson LO, et al. Diagnosis of renal artery stenosis with magnetic resonance angiography: update 2003. Nephrol Dial Transplant 2003; 18(7):1252–1256.

23. Debatin JF, Ting RH, Wegmuller H, et al. Renal artery blood flow: quantitation with phase-contrast MR imaging with and without breath holding. Radiology 1994; 190(2):371–378.

24. Schoenberg SO, Just A, Bock M, Knopp MV, Persson PB, Kirchheim HR. Noninvasive analysis of renal artery blood flow dynamics with MR cine phase-contrast flow measurements. Am J Physiol 1997; 272(5 Pt 2):H2477–H2484.

25. Schoenberg SO, Knopp MV, Bock M, et al. Renal artery stenosis: grading of hemodynamic changes with cine phase-contrast MR blood flow measurements. Radiology 1997; 203(1):45–53.

26. Schoenberg SO, Knopp MV, Londy F, et al. Morphologic and functional magnetic resonance imaging of renal artery stenosis: a multireader tricenter study. J Am Soc Nephrol 2002; 13(1):158–169.

27. Trillaud H, Grenier N, Degreze P, Louail C, Chambon C, Franconi JM. First-pass evaluation of renal perfusion with TurboFLASH MR imaging and superparamagnetic iron oxide particles. J Magn Reson Imaging 1993; 3(1):83–91.

28. Prasad PV, Cannillo J, Chavez DR, et al. First-pass renal perfusion imaging using MS-325, an albumin-targeted MRI contrast agent. Invest Radiol 1999; 34(9):566–571.

29. Aumann S, Schoenberg SO, Just A, et al. Quantification of renal perfusion using an intravascular contrast agent (part 1): results in a canine model. Magn Reson Med 2003; 49(2):276–287.

30. Weisskoff RM, Chesler D, Boxerman JL, Rosen BR. Pitfalls in MR measurement of tissue blood flow with intravascular tracers: which mean transit time? Magn Reson Med 1993; 29(4):553–558.

31. Schoenberg SO, Aumann S, Just A, et al. Quantification of renal perfusion abnormalities using an intravascular contrast agent (part 2): results in animals and humans with renal artery stenosis. Magn Reson Med 2003; 49(2):288–298.

32. Vallee JP, Lazeyras F, Khan HG, Terrier F. Absolute renal blood flow quantification by dynamic MRI and Gd-DTPA. Eur Radiol 2000; 10(8):1245–1252.

33. Peters AM, Brown J, Hartnell GG, Myers MJ, Haskell C, Lavender JP. Non-invasive measurement of renal blood flow with 99mTc DTPA: comparison with radiolabelled microspheres. Cardiovasc Res 1987; 21(11):830–834.

34. Golay X, Hendrikse J, Lim TC. Perfusion imaging using arterial spin labeling. Top Magn Reson Imaging 2004; 15(1):10–27.

35. Calamante F, Thomas DL, Pell GS, Wiersma J, Turner R. Measuring cerebral blood flow using magnetic resonance imaging techniques. J Cereb Blood Flow Metab 1999; 19(7):701–735.

36. Prasad PV, Kim D, Kaiser AM, et al. Noninvasive comprehensive characterization of renal artery stenosis by combination of STAR angiography and EPISTAR perfusion imaging. Magn Reson Med 1997; 38(5):776–787.

37. Michaely HJ, Schoenberg SO, Ittrich C, Dikow R, Bock M, Guenther M. Renal disease: value of functional magnetic resonance imaging with flow and perfusion measurements. Invest Radiol 2004; 39(11):698–705.

38. Martirosian P, Klose U, Mader I, Schick F. FAIR true-FISP perfusion imaging of the kidneys. Magn Reson Med 2004; 51(2):353–361.

39. Rohrschneider WK, Haufe S, Wiesel M, et al. Functional and morphologic evaluation of congenital urinary tract dilatation by using combined static-dynamic MR urography: findings in kidneys with a single collecting system. Radiology 2002; 224(3):683–694.

40. Laissy JP, Faraggi M, Lebtahi R, et al. Functional evaluation of normal and ischemic kidney by means of gadolinium-DOTA enhanced TurboFLASH MR imaging: a preliminary comparison with 99Tc-MAG3 dynamic scintigraphy. Magn Reson Imaging 1994; 12(3):413–419.

41. Ros PR, Gauger J, Stoupis C, et al. Diagnosis of renal artery stenosis: feasibility of combining MR angiography, MR renography, and gadopentetate-based measurements of glomerular filtration rate. AJR Am J Roentgenol 1995; 165(6):1447–1451.

42. Rohrschneider WK, Hoffend J, Becker K, et al. Combined static-dynamic MR urography for the simultaneous evaluation of morphology and function in urinary tract obstruction. I. Evaluation of the normal status in an animal model. Pediatr Radiol 2000; 30(8):511–522.

43. Rohrschneider WK, Becker K, Hoffend J, et al. Combined static-dynamic MR urography for the simultaneous evaluation of morphology and function in urinary tract obstruction. II. Findings in experimentally induced ureteric stenosis. Pediatr Radiol 2000; 30(8):523–532.

44. Rohrschneider WK, Haufe S, Clorius JH, Troger J. MR to assess renal function in children. Eur Radiol 2003; 13(5):1033–1045.

45. Lee VS, Rusinek H, Noz ME, Lee P, Raghavan M, Kramer EL. Dynamic three-dimensional MR renography for the measurement of single kidney function: initial experience. Radiology 2003; 227(1):289–294.

46. Skov AR, Toubro S, Bulow J, Krabbe K, Parving HH, Astrup A. Changes in renal function during weight loss induced by high vs low-protein low-fat diets in overweight subjects. Int J Obes Relat Metab Disord 1999; 23(11):1170–1177.

47. K/DOQI clinical practice guidelines for chronic kidney disease: evaluation, classification, and stratification. Am J Kidney Dis 2002; 39(2 suppl 1):S1–S266.

48. Hackstein N, Heckrodt J, Rau WS. Measurement of single-kidney glomerular filtration rate using a contrast-enhanced dynamic gradient-echo sequence and the Rutland-Patlak plot technique. J Magn Reson Imaging 2003; 18(6):714–725.

49. Hermoye L, Annet L, Lemmerling P, et al. Calculation of the renal perfusion and glomerular filtration rate from the renal impulse response obtained with MRI. Magn Reson Med 2004; 51(5):1017–1025.

50. Annet L, Hermoye L, Peeters F, Jamar F, Dehoux JP, Van Beers BE. Glomerular filtration rate: assessment with dynamic contrast-enhanced MRI and a cortical-compartment model in the rabbit kidney. J Magn Reson Imaging 2004; 20(5):843–849.

51. Dumoulin CL, Buonocore MH, Opsahl LR, et al. Noninvasive measurement of renal hemodynamic functions using gadolinium enhanced magnetic resonance imaging. Magn Reson Med 1994; 32(3):370–378.

52. Niendorf ER, Santyr GE, Brazy PC, Grist TM. Measurement of Gd-DTPA dialysis clearance rates by using a Look-Locker imaging technique. Magn Reson Med 1996; 36(4):571–578.

53. Niendorf ER, Grist TM, Frayne R, Brazy PC, Santyr GE. Rapid measurement of Gd-DTPA extraction fraction in a dialysis system using echo-planar imaging. Med Phys 1997; 24(12):1907–1913.

54. Niendorf ER, Grist TM, Lee FT Jr, Brazy PC, Santyr GE. Rapid in vivo measurement of single-kidney extraction fraction and glomerular filtration rate with MR imaging. Radiology 1998; 206(3):791–798.

55. Schaefer PW, Grant PE, Gonzalez RG. Diffusion-weighted MR imaging of the brain. Radiology 2000; 217(2):331–345.

56. Murtz P, Flacke S, Traber F, van den Brink JS, Gieseke J, Schild HH. Abdomen: diffusion-weighted MR imaging with pulse-triggered single-shot sequences. Radiology 2002; 224(1):258–264.

57. Ries M, Jones RA, Basseau F, Moonen CT, Grenier N. Diffusion tensor MRI of the human kidney. J Magn Reson Imaging 2001; 14(1):42–49.

58. Ries M, Basseau F, Tyndal B, et al. Renal diffusion and BOLD MRI in experimental diabetic nephropathy. Blood oxygen level-dependent. J Magn Reson Imaging 2003; 17(1):104–113.

59. Ortiz A, Justo P, Sanz A, Lorz C, Egido J. Targeting apoptosis in acute tubular injury. Biochem Pharmacol 2003; 66(8):1589–1594.

60. Rana A, Sathyanarayana P, Lieberthal W. Role of apoptosis of renal tubular cells in acute renal failure: therapeutic implications. Apoptosis 2001; 6(1–2):83–102.

61. Hakumaki JM, Brindle KM. Techniques: visualizing apoptosis using nuclear magnetic resonance. Trends Pharmacol Sci 2003; 24(3):146–149.

62. Dagher PC, Herget-Rosenthal S, Ruehm SG, et al. Newly developed techniques to study and diagnose acute renal failure. J Am Soc Nephrol 2003; 14(8):2188–2198.

63. Kobayashi H, Kawamoto S, Jo SK, et al. Renal tubular damage detected by dynamic micro-MRI with a dendrimer-based magnetic resonance contrast agent. Kidney Int 2002; 61(6):1980–1985.

64. Cattell V. Macrophages in acute glomerular inflammation. Kidney Int 1994; 45(4): 945–952.

65. Grau V, Herbst B, Steiniger B. Dynamics of monocytes/macrophages and T lymphocytes in acutely rejecting rat renal allografts. Cell Tissue Res 1998; 291(1): 117–126.

66. Ysebaert DK, De Greef KE, Vercauteren SR, et al. Identification and kinetics of leukocytes after severe ischaemia/reperfusion renal injury. Nephrol Dial Transplant 2000; 15(10):1562–1574.

67. Schreiner GF, Harris KP, Purkerson ML, Klahr S. Immunological aspects of acute ureteral obstruction: immune cell infiltrate in the kidney. Kidney Int 1988; 34(4):487–493.

68. Erwig LP, Kluth DC, Rees AJ. Macrophages in renal inflammation. Curr Opin Nephrol Hypertens 2001; 10(3):341–347.

69. Hauger O, Delalande C, Trillaud H, et al. MR imaging of intrarenal macrophage infiltration in an experimental model of nephrotic syndrome. Magn Reson Med 1999; 41(1):156–162.

70. Ye Q, Yang D, Williams M, et al. In vivo detection of acute rat renal allograft rejection by MRI with USPIO particles. Kidney Int 2002; 61(3):1124–1135.

71. Hauger O, Delalande C, Deminiere C, et al. Nephrotoxic nephritis and obstructive nephropathy: evaluation with MR imaging enhanced with ultrasmall superparamagnetic iron oxide-preliminary findings in a rat model. Radiology 2000; 217(3):819–826.

72. Jo SK, Hu X, Kobayashi H, et al. Detection of inflammation following renal ischemia by magnetic resonance imaging. Kidney Int 2003; 64(1):43–51.

73. Hauger O, Grenier N, Deminière C, Delmas Y, Combe C. Late Sinerem®-enhanced MR imaging of Renal Diseases: a pilot study. In: Radiological Society of North America. Chicago: Radiological Society of North America, 2004:512.

74. Brezis M, Rosen S. Hypoxia of the renal medulla—its implications for disease. N Engl J Med 1995; 332(10):647–655.

75. Grenier N, Basseau F, Ries M, Tyndal B, Jones R, Moonen C. Functional MRI of the kidney. Abdom Imaging 2003; 28(2):164–175.

76. Li LP, Vu AT, Li BS, Dunkle E, Prasad PV. Evaluation of intrarenal oxygenation by BOLD MRI at 3.0 T. J Magn Reson Imaging 2004; 20(5):901–904.

77. Prasad PV, Chen Q, Goldfarb JW, Epstein FH, Edelman RR. Breath-hold R2* mapping with a multiple gradient-recalled echo sequence: application to the evaluation of intra-renal oxygenation. J Magn Reson Imaging 1997; 7(6):1163–1165.

78. Prasad PV, Edelman RR, Epstein FH. Noninvasive evaluation of intrarenal oxygenation with BOLD MRI. Circulation 1996; 94(12):3271–3275.

79. Prasad PV, Priatna A, Spokes K, Epstein FH. Changes in intrarenal oxygenation as evaluated by BOLD MRI in a rat kidney model for radiocontrast nephropathy. J Magn Reson Imaging 2001; 13(5):744–747.

80. Prasad PV, Epstein FH. Changes in renal medullary pO2 during water diuresis as evaluated by blood oxygenation level-dependent magnetic resonance imaging: effects of aging and cyclooxygenase inhibition. Kidney Int 1999; 55(1):294–298.

81. Economides PA, Caselli A, Zuo CS, et al. Kidney oxygenation during water diuresis and endothelial function in patients with type 2 diabetes and subjects at risk to develop diabetes. Metabolism 2004; 53(2):222–227.

82. Chatziantoniou C, Boffa JJ, Tharaux PL, Flamant M, Ronco P, Dussaule JC. Progression and regression in renal vascular and glomerular fibrosis. Int J Exp Pathol 2004; 85(1):1–11.

83. Namimoto T, Yamashita Y, Mitsuzaki K, Nakayama Y, Tang Y, Takahashi M. Measurement of the apparent diffusion coefficient in diffuse renal disease by diffusion-weighted echo-planar MR imaging. J Magn Reson Imaging 1999; 9(6):832–837.

84. Shah NS, Kruse SA, Lager DJ, et al. Evaluation of renal parenchymal disease in a rat model with magnetic resonance elastography. Magn Reson Med 2004; 52(1):56–64.

85. Weitzel WF, Kim K, Rubin JM, et al. Feasibility of applying ultrasound strain imaging to detect renal transplant chronic allograft nephropathy. Kidney Int 2004; 65(2):733–736.

86. Gupta S, Verfaillie C, Chmielewski D, Kim Y, Rosenberg ME. A role for extrarenal cells in the regeneration following acute renal failure. Kidney Int 2002; 62(4):1285–1290.

87. Imasawa T, Utsunomiya Y, Kawamura T, et al. The potential of bone marrow-derived cells to differentiate to glomerular mesangial cells. J Am Soc Nephrol 2001; 12(7):1401–1409.

88. Ito T, Suzuki A, Imai E, Okabe M, Hori M. Bone marrow is a reservoir of repopulating mesangial cells during glomerular remodeling. J Am Soc Nephrol 2001; 12(12):2625–2635.

89. Lin F, Cordes K, Li L, et al. Hematopoietic stem cells contribute to the regeneration of renal tubules after renal ischemia-reperfusion injury in mice. J Am Soc Nephrol 2003; 14(5):1188–1199.

90. Bulte JW, Zhang S, van Gelderen P, et al. Neurotransplantation of magnetically labeled oligodendrocyte progenitors: magnetic resonance tracking of cell migration and myelination. Proc Natl Acad Sci USA 1999; 96(26):15256–15261.

91. Hoehn M, Kustermann E, Blunk J, et al. Monitoring of implanted stem cell migration in vivo: a highly resolved in vivo magnetic resonance imaging investigation of experimental stroke in rat. Proc Natl Acad Sci USA 2002; 99(25):16267–16272.

92. Kraitchman DL, Heldman AW, Atalar E, et al. In vivo magnetic resonance imaging of mesenchymal stem cells in myocardial infarction. Circulation 2003; 107(18):2290–2293.

93. Bos C, Delmas Y, Desmouliere A, et al. In vivo MR imaging of intravascularly injected magnetically labeled mesenchymal stem cells in rat kidney and liver. Radiology 2004; 233(3):781–789.

94. Hauger O, Frost EE, Deminière C, et al. MR evaluation of the glomerular homing of magnetically labeled mesenchymal stem cells in a rat model of nephropathy. Radiology 2006; 238:200–210.

11

Magnetic Resonance Imaging of the Prostate Gland

Saroja Adusumilli
Division of Abdominal Imaging, Department of Radiology, Section of Magnetic Resonance Imaging, University of Michigan Health System, Ann Arbor, Michigan, U.S.A.

E. Scott Pretorius
Department of Radiology, Section of Magnetic Resonance Imaging, Hospital of the University of Pennsylvania, Philadelphia, Pennsylvania, U.S.A.

INTRODUCTION

Due to its excellent soft tissue contrast and direct multiplanar capabilities, magnetic resonance imaging (MRI) is well suited for evaluation of the prostate gland. Currently, most prostate magnetic resonance (MR) examinations are performed for staging of biopsy-proven prostate malignancies. However, prostate MRI can also be used to assess response to tumor therapy, to evaluate Müllerian abnormalities, and to diagnose complications of prostatitis. Applications of MRI in management of prostate disease will likely evolve with improvements in MR spectroscopic techniques, increased availability of 3 T scanners, and increased availability of MR scanners designed to permit MR-guided interventions.

MR TECHNIQUE

Endorectal MR technique

The endorectal coil is an intracavitary surface coil that provides high spatial resolution images with high signal-to-noise ratio (SNR) due to its ability to acquire thin slices at small fields of view (1–7). Disposable endorectal coils (Medrad, Pittsburgh, Pennysylvania) are commercially available for use on 1.0 and 1.5 T MRI scanners and are combined with a pelvic, phased-array coil for improved imaging of the anterior and superior aspects of the prostate gland as well for the remainder of the pelvis (Fig. 1) (5,7–11). The coil is placed in the rectum and an attached balloon is inflated with 60 to 100 cc of air to prevent movement of the coil. Antiperistaltic medications, such as glucagon (1 mg intramuscular; Glucagen, Bedford Laboratories, Bedford, Ohio), scopolamine butylbromide (20 mg intramuscular or intravenous; Buscopan,

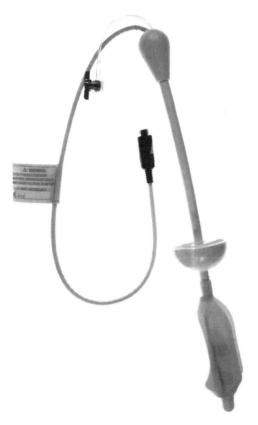

Figure 1 Endorectal coil. A disposable endorectal coil such as the one shown here (with permission by MedRad, Pittsburgh, Pennysylvania) provides high spatial resolution images of the prostate due to its ability to acquire thin slices at a small field-of-view.

Boehringer Ingelheim, New Zealand) or dicyclomine hydrochloride (10–20 mg oral; Bentyl; Aventis Pharmaceutricals, Bedford, New Jersey), are routinely administered to reduce motion artifacts and blurring that result from bowel peristalsis or the passage of gas into or out of the rectum during the MRI examination (11–13).

Imaging Protocol

Although diagnostic studies can be obtained on 0.5 to 1.0 T scanners, endorectal imaging of the prostate is usually performed on a 1.5 T field strength system to ensure good image quality and staging accuracy (14–19). A large field-of-view sagittal localizer sequence is used to ensure correct coil placement within the rectum and to prescribe subsequent sequences. Standard imaging includes a T1-weighted spin-echo sequence obtained in the axial plane and T2-weighted fast spin-echo sequences obtained in the axial, coronal, and sagittal planes. Endorectal coil images are obtained from the top of the seminal vesicles through the apex of the prostate gland. Sagittal and coronal planes are helpful in assessing the relationship of the prostate gland to the seminal vesicles and bladder base and in detecting tumors in the prostatic base and apex (11). Finally, larger field-of-view axial images are obtained through the entire pelvis using a phased-array pelvic surface coil to detect lymph node enlargement and osseous metastatic disease.

Endorectal coil imaging employs a small field-of-view (10–14 cm), thin slices (3–4 mm skip 0–1 mm), and high matrix (256×256 or 256×192). Although fat suppression is known to improve tissue contrast by increasing the dynamic range for signal intensity throughout the body, it has not been shown to improve the diagnosis of prostatic neoplasm or extracapsular extension (20). Therefore, fat suppression is generally not used for prostatic imaging because it decreases SNR, which limits visualization of anatomic detail, such as the prostatic capsule, and reduces contrast between low signal intensity extraprostatic tumor and high signal intensity periprostatic fat and definition of periprostatic anatomic planes and intra-prostatic tumor (20–24).

Role of Intravenous Gadolinium

Intravenous contrast is not routinely used for endorectal prostate MRI because of conflicting results in the literature. Several studies have suggested that dynamic, contrast-enhanced T1-weighted imaging during the early phase of enhancement improves the depiction of tumor margins, extracapsular tumor, and seminal vesicle or neurovascular bundle invasion (25,26). Gadolinium has also been shown to differentiate between benign and malignant low T2-signal intensity foci in the peripheral gland of the prostate gland (27–29). However, other investigators have failed to demonstrate any improvement in staging accuracy and tumor localization with dynamic contrast administration when compared to unenhanced T2-weighted imaging, and these researchers have concluded that the routine use of contrast is not warranted (19,27,30–33).

There is, however, consensus in the literature with respect to special circum-stances that may warrant the use of intravenous contrast. For example, equivocal cases of seminal vesicle invasion can benefit from gadolinium administration because enhancement of the lumen of the seminal vesicle (which ordinarily does not enhance) has been observed with tumor invasion and is occasionally superior to T2-weighted imaging (26,30,31). Gadolinium-enhanced MRI is also useful in determining the location and extent of necrosis in the prostate caused by such minimally invasive treatments as cryosurgery and high-intensity focused ultrasound (34). Cryosurgery results in destruction of the internal architecture of the gland with loss of normal zonal differentiation. Cryonecrotic tissue is avascular and demonstrates absent enhancement, which can be used as a sign of successful treatment (35).

Three Tesla Scanners

Endorectal coils are generally used for prostate imaging because a strong signal can be received from the posterior aspect of the prostate where 70% of cancers occur (Fig. 1) (36). However, at the apex of the prostate gland, the peripheral gland wraps all the way around the urethra and extends anterior to it, a location where there is only weak signal from the coil (36). Additional pitfalls of an endorectal coil include signal hyperintensity immediately surrounding the coil (near-field artifact) and struc-tural deformation of the peripheral zone of the prostate gland, which makes image interpretation difficult (37). Also, use of an endorectal coil is not possible in patients who have had an abdominoperineal resection and is contraindicated in patients with active inflammatory bowel disease. Additionally, it is not well tolerated by patients with severe hemorrhoidal disease or radiation-induced proctitis.

Imaging the prostate using a 3 T scanner and an external phased-array coil are being investigated as methods of improving SNR, thereby providing standard anatomic information and spectroscopy data without the use of an endorectal coil (36). Preliminary studies have shown that the zonal anatomy of the prostate is clearly visualized on a 3-T system and that the SNR is improved relative to a 1.5 T scanner (37). Limitations of higher field strength scanners include decreased penetration of the radio-frequency pulse and increased energy deposition into the body (37).

NORMAL PROSTATE GLAND

Anatomy

The prostate gland is an accessory exocrine gland of the male reproductive system, composed of glandular and fibromuscular tissue. The ejaculatory ducts course through the prostate gland to enter the prostatic urethra at the verumontanum, allowing prostatic secretions to liquefy semen.

From a radiologic standpoint, the prostate is divided into two important components: the central gland and the peripheral gland. The central gland is further divided into the transitional and central zones (38). The central zone surrounds the proximal urethra and ejaculatory ducts and encloses the transitional zone and periurethral glands. It is shaped like a funnel with its widest portion comprising the majority of the base of the prostate (39). In young men, the central gland is predominantly composed of the central zone, whereas, in older men with benign prostatic hypertrophy (BPH), the central gland is made largely of transitional zone. Ultimately, the central zone is no longer visible on MRI because it is compressed by the transitional zone, which assumes a progressively greater proportion of the prostatic volume (due to BPH) as the prostate gland ages (38,39).

The peripheral gland surrounds the distal prostatic urethra and is the major glandular component of the prostate, comprising the majority of the prostatic apex. It also extends superiorly along the posterolateral aspect of the prostate to surround the central zone (like a waffle cone around a scoop of ice cream) (38,39). Prostate carcinoma and prostatitis are more likely to occur in the peripheral gland (39).

The lymphatic drainage of the prostate gland includes the obturator, internal iliac, external iliac, common iliac, and presacral lymph node chains. Prostatic veins form a periprostatic venous plexus around the lateral and anterior aspects of the prostate, receive blood from the prostate and deep dorsal vein of the penis, and ultimately drain into the internal iliac veins (40). The anterior aspect of the plexus is known as the venous plexus of Santorini. Prominence of the anterior and posterior periprostatic veins near the apex has been associated with greater intraoperative blood loss during radical prostatectomy (41).

MR Appearance of the Normal Prostate

The prostate gland is of homogeneous, intermediate signal intensity on T1-weighted images, with poor differentiation of the zonal anatomy of the gland on this sequence (11,42,43). On T2-weighted sequences, zonal anatomy is better delineated because mucin-producing glands in the peripheral gland result in high signal intensity with respect to muscle (Fig. 2A and B) (11,42,43). A collagenous network can occasionally be seen as curvilinear low signal intensity structures against the background of normal high signal intensity peripheral gland (44). In patients with prostate cancer,

(A)

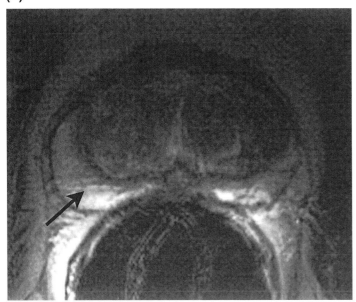

(B)

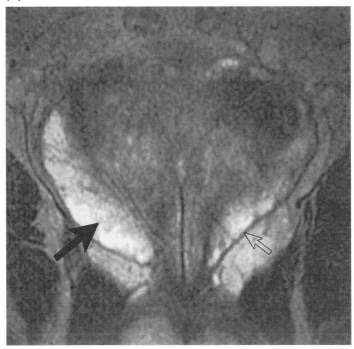

Figure 2 Normal prostate gland anatomy demonstrated in a 65-year-old man. (**A**) Axial and (**B**) coronal T2-weighted images demonstrate the normal high signal intensity of the peripheral gland (*black arrow*). The peripheral gland largely lies posterior and inferior to the central gland. The prostatic capsule (*open arrow*) appears as a thin rim of low signal intensity on T2-weighted imaging.

preservation of this collagenous network in a given region of the gland implies that this region is spared of neoplasm (44).

Relative to the peripheral gland, the central and transitional zones of the central gland are of lower T2-signal intensity, due to the presence of fewer glandular elements and larger amounts of stromal tissue and compact smooth muscle. The central gland is often heterogeneous on T2-weighted imaging because of variable hyperplasia of glandular elements, fibrous tissue, smooth muscle, and stroma (42,45). The prostate is surrounded by a 2 to 3 mm layer of fibromuscular capsule that lies between the glandular component of the periprostatic structures and appears as a thin rim of low signal intensity on T2-weighted imaging (Fig. 2B) (38,39).

The neurovascular bundles are paired structures that course along the postero-lateral aspect of the prostate and contain sympathetic nerves and veins. They are best depicted on T1-weighted imaging as hypointense structures at the posterolateral margins of the prostate gland surrounded by high signal intensity periprostatic fat (39,46,47). Various branches pierce the prostatic capsule and create sites of capsular weakness at the base and apex of the prostate. Due to slow venous flow, the peripro-static venous plexus appears as a high T2-signal intensity periprostatic rim in the lat-eral, posterolateral, and anterior periprostatic tissue (Fig. 3) (39,41,42). Periprostatic veins are not found in the space between the prostate and rectum. The periprostatic venous plexi are prominent in young patients with small prostates but become less prominent with advancing age (48).

The seminal vesicles are located posterior to the bladder base near the ureterove-sical junction and are located lateral to the ipsilateral vas deferens. Just proximal to the entry of the vas deferens into the prostate, the vas enlarges to form the ampulla (38,39).

On T2-weighted imaging, the seminal vesicles are surrounded by thin, low signal intensity walls and are internally T2-hyperintense to muscle due to their fluid content (Fig. 4A and B) (49). The ampullae of the vas deferens have thick,

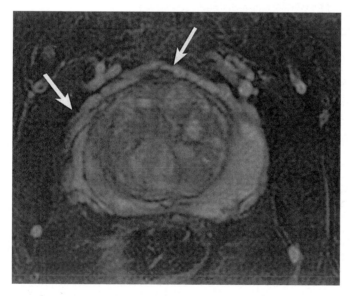

Figure 3 Normal prostate gland anatomy demonstrated in a 63-year-old man with BPH. Axial T2-weighted image with fat saturation demonstrates the periprostatic venous plexus as a high signal intensity periprostatic rim in the lateral and anterior periprostatic tissue (*white arrows*).

(A)

(B)

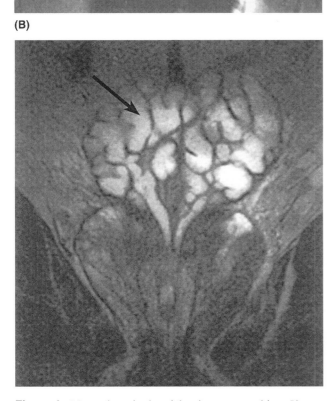

Figure 4   Normal seminal vesicles demonstrated in a 53-year-old man. (**A**) Axial and (**B**) coronal T2-weighted images demonstrate normal, thin-walled seminal vesicles that are of high signal intensity reflecting fluid content (*black arrow*). The axial image depicts the medial, thick-walled tubular vas deferens (*white arrows*).

low T2-signal intensity muscular walls that should not be confused with tumor invasion, because they are readily identified on MR imaging due to their characteristic medial location with respect to the seminal vesicles (Fig. 4B).

On gadolinium-enhanced imaging, the normal peripheral gland demonstrates uniform enhancement, which is usually less intense than that seen in the central gland. Central gland enhancement is often inhomogeneous in older patients due to the presence of benign prostatic hyperplasia (25,28,31,33,50).

MR IMAGING APPEARANCE OF PROSTATE PATHOLOGY

Hemorrhage

The peripheral gland of the prostate contains large amounts of the anticoagulant citrate, which is likely responsible for the frequent detection of significant hemorrhage following transrectal biopsy (4). Postbiopsy hemorrhage (methemoglobin) appears as an area of high signal intensity on T1-weighted imaging and of low signal intensity on T2-weighted imaging (51–53). The low T2-signal intensity of blood can mimic prostate adenocarcinoma. Therefore, it is recommended that MRI be performed at least three weeks following biopsy to improve accuracy in image interpretation (51–54). Even so, T1- and T2-weighted images should always be correlated in prostate MR examinations to minimize the risk of making a false-positive diagnosis of cancer, because blood can persist for an indeterminate amount of time following biopsy (20,54). Prostate malignancies tend to be hypointense to normal prostate on both T1- and T2-weighted imaging, whereas hemorrhage tends to be T1-hyperintense and T2-hypointense (Fig. 5) (52).

In patients who have undergone biopsy, hemorrhage may outline prostatic tumor—a phenomenon that has been termed the "halo" appearance (55). Hemorrhage may also assume a wedge-shaped and striated appearance on T2-weighted imaging in contrast to the round, masslike morphology more typical of tumor (52,53). When large amounts of hemorrhage are present, small foci of malignancy can be obscured.

Low signal intensity hemorrhage on T2-weighted imaging can also simulate tumor invasion to the seminal vesicles (51,53). Again, correlation with T1-weighted images, on which tumor is relatively hypointense and which hemorrhage is hyperintense, is frequently useful. Sources of hemorrhage in the seminal vesicles include retrograde spread of blood from the site of biopsy via the ejaculatory ducts, direct biopsy of the seminal vesicles, orchitis, prostatitis, and bleeding disorders (51).

Tumor invasion of the seminal vesicles can be associated with hemorrhage and is differentiated from postbiopsy blood by understanding the pattern of progression of tumor spread (51). Tumor first infiltrates the proximal (or medial) portions of one or both seminal vesicles and then extends to the middle or distal portions. Tumor invasion also tends to be more extensive in the seminal vesicle on the same side as the main bulk of the prostate cancer. Therefore, if low signal intensity material predominates in the periphery of the seminal vesicle or in the seminal vesicle opposite to the tumor, it is less likely to be neoplasm (51).

Benign Prostatic Hypertrophy

Nearly 80% of men develop BPH and as many as 30% require treatment to relieve symptoms of obstructed voiding, such as hesitancy, urgency, and nocturia (56).

(A)

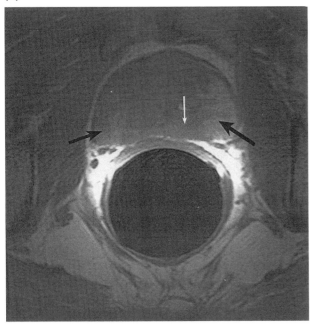

(B)

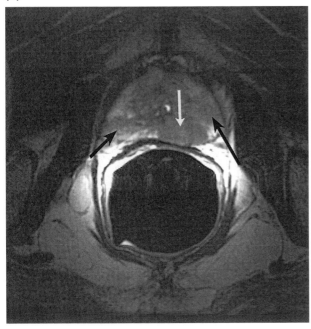

Figure 5 Sixty-two-year-old man with prostate cancer and postbiopsy hemorrhage. (**A**) Axial T1-weighted and (**B**) axial T2-weighted images reveal a low T1- and low T2-signal intensity cancer (*thin white arrow*) in the left paramedian region of the midgland. Postbiopsy hemorrhage manifests as high T1- and low T2-signal intensity methemoglobin (*black arrows*) in the left and right lateral aspects of the midgland.

Although prostatic enlargement is not required for these symptoms to be manifested, glandular enlargement, increased smooth muscle tone, and decreased prostatic compliance have been implicated as etiologies leading to clinical presentation (56). Treatment options include surgery, minimally invasive procedures (laser surgery), and such medications as alpha-adrenergic blockers and androgen blockade (56,57).

MRI features associated with BPH include marked enlargement of the central gland and "median lobe" hyperplasia. The MR appearance of BPH is dependent on the ratio of glandular and stromal tissue in the central gland, resulting in nodules of varying sizes and varying signal intensities in the transitional zone or periurethral glands (56). Sclerotic or fibromuscular BPH has low T2-signal intensity nodules because of a high concentration of collagen and smooth muscle, whereas glandular hyperplasia is characterized by high T2-signal intensity nodules due to dilated glandular elements (Fig. 6A) (56,58–60). The most common type of BPH actually contains both mixed glandular and stromal tissue (Fig. 6B). Although the majority of prostate cancers occur in the peripheral gland, a small percentage of tumors can coexist with BPH in the central gland. These tumors are very difficult or even impossible to diagnose on MRI, because they are surrounded by the mixed signal intensities of the prostatic tissue in the adjacent central gland.

Although MRI is not routinely used in evaluating patients with BPH, it has two potentially important roles in the management of these patients. Treatment decisions are partly based on prostate size and type of hyperplasia. For surgical intervention, a large prostate size may direct a patient to open prostatectomy rather than transurethral resection (TURP) (56). MR estimates of prostatic volume can be used in the selection of treatment and in determining response to treatments, such as androgen deprivation. MRI has been shown to be more accurate than transrectal ultrasound (TRUS) for volume determinations when using the formula for a prolate ellipse [volume = (AP × TRV × CC) × 0.52] (61–63). MRI may also be valuable in determining which patients will respond to a specific medication regimen based on the morphologic composition of the BPH. Alpha blockers are more effective in patients who have smaller prostates and more smooth muscle hyperplasia, whereas androgen deprivation using 5-alpha reductase inhibitors is more effective in patients who have larger prostate glands and more glandular hyperplasia (56,57). A recent study showed that MRI performed in patients who failed to respond to alpha blockers helped determine whether a patient would sufficiently respond to antiandrogen therapy based on the presence of high T2-signal intensity nodules (reflecting a greater percentage of glandular elements) (57).

Inflammatory Disease of the Prostate Gland

Acute bacterial prostatitis can be mistaken for prostate carcinoma on MRI because of similarities in the appearance of both entities. Acute bacterial prostatitis is rare but can result in either a low signal intensity lesion in the peripheral zone on T2-weighted images or ground glass homogeneous low T2-signal intensity in the central gland (64–66).

Chronic bacterial or nonbacterial prostatitis (which is more common than bacterial prostatitis) can be associated with an atrophic seminal vesicle. This condition results either in a diffuse striated area of low T2-signal intensity or in patchy curvilinear regions of alternating high and low T2- signal intensity (Fig. 7). Patients with chronic infection are less likely to be misdiagnosed with cancer because of the diffuse extent of disease and lack of mass effect (66).

(A)

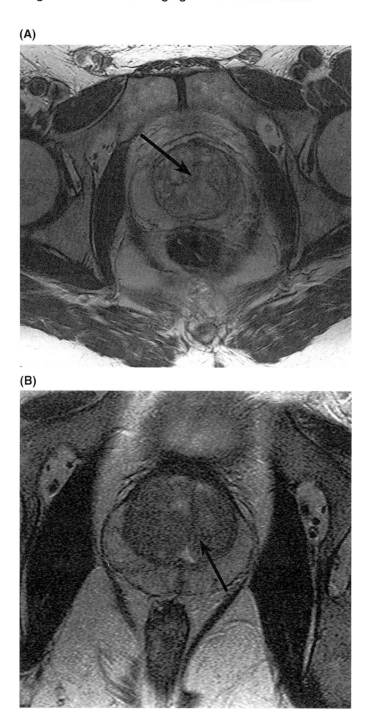

(B)

Figure 6 Two different patients with (**A**) glandular BPH and (**B**) mixed glandular and stromal BPH. (**A**) Demonstrates cystic or glandular hyperplasia, which is characterized by high
signal intensity nodules (*black arrow*) on this axial T2-weighted image. Stromal hyperplasia
depicted in (**B**) has low signal intensity areas on this axial T2-weighted image because of a high
concentration of collagen and smooth muscle (*black arrow*) as well as glandular hyperplasia.
Abbreviation: BPH, benign prostatic hypertrophy.

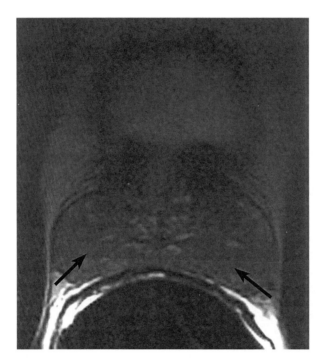

Figure 7 Prostatitis in a 20-year-old man. Axial T2-weighted image demonstrates abnormal diffuse low signal intensity throughout the entire peripheral gland (*black arrow*), representing prostatitis.

Abscesses of the prostate gland are rare, are found in elderly men, and usually result from inadequately treated acute bacterial prostatitis caused by *Escherichia coli*. Physical examination may reveal the diagnosis if there is fluctuation of the prostate on rectal examination. On MR imaging, an abscess is of low signal intensity on T1-weighted imaging and high signal intensity on T2-weighted imaging, occasionally mimicking a cyst (65,67).

Granulomatous prostatitis is an uncommon inflammatory disease of the prostate gland, which may also be mistaken for carcinoma because it manifests as nonspecific low T2-signal intensity lesions in the peripheral zone. Although the etiology is unclear, granulomatous prostatitis can be due to infection (hematogenous spread of mycobacterial tuberculosis) or surgery (TURP) or can be a local manifestation of a systemic granulomatous disease. Due to the lack of specificity on imaging, definitive diagnosis requires biopsy (68).

Prostatic and Periprostatic Cysts

Cysts of the prostate gland are uncommon and are classified into either congenital or acquired subtypes. The congenital cysts that will be discussed include Müllerian cysts, utricle cysts, and seminal vesicle cysts (Wolffian duct anomalies), whereas acquired lesions include cysts of BPH, prostatic retention cysts, ejaculatory duct cysts, and rarely cystic carcinoma or infection (69,70).

Two of the most widely described congenital cysts in the literature are utricular and Müllerian duct cysts, both of which are midline structures located posterior to the upper half of the prostatic urethra. The utricular cyst is the most common congenital cyst and occurs secondary to dilation of the prostatic utricle. It is usually 8 to 9 mm in size, does not extend above the base of the prostate gland, and communicates freely with the prostatic urethra (Fig. 8A and B). A utricular cyst is often

(A)

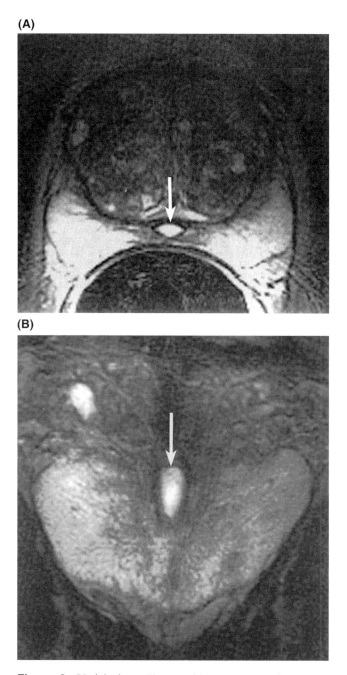

(B)

Figure 8 Utricle in a 70-year-old man. (**A**) Axial and (**B**) coronal T2-weighted images demonstrate a midline, benign utricular cyst of high signal intensity (*white arrow*).

diagnosed in childhood because of its association with hypospadias, cryptorchidism, and ipsilateral renal agenesis (69–71).

Müllerian duct cysts arise from the Müllerian duct remnants, which should regress in utero. These are a common cause of obstruction of the ejaculatory duct. They are spherical in shape and, if large in size, can lie superior to the prostate. They are connected to the verumontanum but do not communicate with the urethra. Müllerian duct cysts can contain hemorrhage and calculi and are associated with an increased risk of prostate carcinoma. Surgical correction of the cysts can relieve genital duct obstruction in men with infertility (69–71).

Seminal vesicle or Wolffian duct cysts result from congenital atresia of the ejaculatory duct and are often associated with ipsilateral renal agenesis. The cysts are unilateral, located laterally in the seminal vesicle, commonly protrude into the bladder, and may present with symptoms of hematospermia, hematuria, and epididymitis. Wall irregularity or a mass associated with the cyst is suggestive of underlying adenocarcinoma. If large enough, seminal vesicle cysts can cause extrinsic compression on the ejaculatory ductal system and contribute to male infertility (69,70,72,73).

Prostate Malignancies

MR Appearance of Prostate Cancer

Adenocarcinoma of the prostate is most commonly located in the peripheral gland and may be unifocal or multifocal. Lesions are of low signal intensity on T1- and T2-weighted imaging due to an increase in cell density and replacement of prostatic ducts (Fig. 9A and B) (4). However, it is the low T2-signal intensity that contributes to the decreased specificity in detection of cancerous lesions. Other etiologies of low T2-signal intensity include hemorrhage, prostatitis, posttherapy changes, and scar (51,52,65,66). On T1-weighted images, identification of high signal intensity blood surrounding low signal intensity tumor (halo sign) can help distinguish which components are related to hemorrhage and which to tumor, because these two abnormalities are sometimes identical in appearance on T2-weighted imaging (55).

If intravenous contrast is administered, prostate cancer shows early and rapid enhancement relative to surrounding peripheral gland and rapid wash-out on delayed images (74,75). Therefore, early dynamic images provide the best contrast between tumor and normal tissue (25,28,33).

The detection of central gland carcinoma, which is also of low T1- and T2-signal intensity, is difficult in the presence of nodular-appearing benign prostatic hyperplasia. Most central gland tumors are found incidentally during TURP of the prostate, but aggressive cancers can spread beyond the prostate. Endorectal MR can occasionally depict central tumors not detectable by digital rectal exam (DRE) or TRUS and may provide an alternative to random biopsies in patients with an elevated prostate specific antigen (PSA) and negative palpation and TRUS.

More unusual tumors of the prostate gland have unique imaging features on MRI. Mucinous adenocarcinoma of the prostate is a rare cancer that accounts for 2% of prostate neoplasms and requires that at least 25% of the tumor consist of pools of extracellular mucin (76–78). The mucin results in a different MR appearance than that of typical adenocarcinoma (76). Mucinous tumors show T2-signal intensity equal to or greater than that of normal peripheral gland and can therefore be

(A)

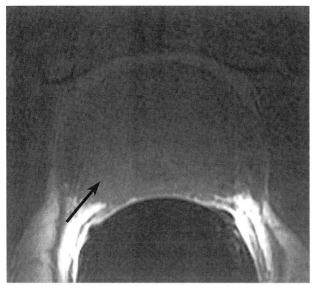

(B)

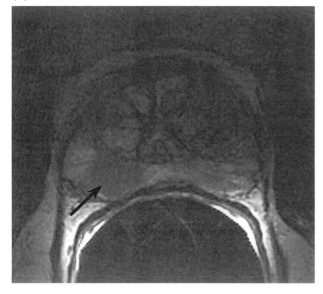

Figure 9 Sixty-two-year-old man with carcinoma confined to the prostate. (**A**) Axial T1-weighted and (**B**) axial T2-weighted images demonstrate a focal low T1-and low T2-signal intensity mass (*black arrow*) in the right posterior peripheral gland.

confused with normal prostate, dilated periprostatic veins, or other conditions, such as cysts or abscesses (76,77).

Prostate sarcomas account for less than 0.1% of prostate malignancies and carry a poor prognosis due to their aggressive natural history (79). Leiomyosarcoma is the most common cell type in adults, whereas rhabdomyosarcoma is more common in children (80,81). Prostate sarcomas tend to be large and lobulated at presentation and often invade the bladder, rectum, and other pelvic soft tissues (82).

Staging of Prostate Carcinoma

Staging assists in treatment planning because stage T1–T2 disease can be treated with radical prostatectomy, brachytherapy, or radiation therapy, whereas patients with diseases that are stage T3 or more advanced are not surgical candidates and may be more appropriately treated with hormonal therapy or palliative radiation (83). Clinical staging of prostate cancer using DRE, serum PSA level, and biopsy specimen tumor grade (Gleason score) is the most universally available method and is fairly specific for advanced disease (stage T3–T4) (83–85). However, the realization that this method understages early extracapsular spread of tumor has led to the development of such imaging techniques as endorectal MRI (83–85).

The tumor-node-metastasis (TNM) staging classification for prostate cancer includes evaluation of both local and distant extent of disease (Table 1) (86). The role

Table 1 TNM Staging Classification of Prostate Carcinoma

Stage	Description
Primary tumor (T)	
Tx	Tumor cannot be assessed
T0	No evidence of primary tumor
T1	Tumor not clinically palpable or visible by imaging, but
T1a	found incidentally during surgery, in 5% or less of tissue
T1b	found incidentally during surgery, in 5% or more of tissue
T1c	identified by needle biopsy performed because of elevated PSA
T2	Tumor confined within the prostate, involving
T2a	less than half a lobe of the prostate
T2b	half a lobe of the prostate, but not both lobes
T2c	both lobes of the prostate
T3	Tumor extending through the prostate capsule
T3a	Extracapsular extension through one lobe
T3b	Extracapsular extension through both lobes
T3c	Extracapsular extension into the seminal vesicles
T4	Tumor fixed, invading structures other than the seminal vesicles
T4a	Invasion of bladder neck, external sphincter, or rectum
T4b	Invasion of muscles and/or pelvic wall
Regional lymph nodes (N)	
Nx	Nodes cannot be assessed
N0	No regional node metastasis
N1	Single node metastasis, ≤2 cm in greatest dimension
N2	Single node metastasis; 2–5 cm in greatest dimension or multiple nodes, none larger than 5 cm
N3	Metastasis larger than 5 cm in any node
Distant metastasis (M)	
Mx	Presence of metastasis cannot be assessed
M0	No distant metastasis
M1	Distant metastasis
M1a	Nonregional lymph nodes involved
M1b	Bone(s) involved
M1c	Other site(s) involved

Abbreviations: PSA, prostate specific antigen; TNM, tumor-node-metastasis.
Source: From Ref. 86.

of MRI in prostate cancer is to differentiate patients with organ-confined disease (stage T1–T2) from patients with locally invasive disease that has extended beyond the capsule into the periprostatic fat, lymphatics, and seminal vesicles (stage T3), or into adjacent organs (stage T4).

The common pathways of prostate cancer spread, including capsular penetration, neurovascular bundle invasion, invasion of adjacent organs, regional lymph node metastases, and osseous metastases can all be assessed with MRI. When evaluating MR examinations for all these features, it must be remembered that high specificity (minimization of false-positive diagnoses) for the diagnosis of stage T3 disease is strongly desirable. This is because a false-positive diagnosis of tumor spread could deprive a patient of potentially curative surgery (87). For this reason, some radiologists classify a patient as suffering from stage T3 disease only if there is gross extracapsular tumor beyond the capsule or into the seminal vesicles (83).

Pathways of Spread

Capsular Penetration. Stage T1–T2 disease (cancer confined to the prostate) is established on MRI if one of the following three criteria is met: (i) if normal high T2-signal intensity peripheral gland is seen between the tumor and the prostatic capsule, (ii) if there is clear delineation of the capsule despite broad contact between the tumor and capsule, or (iii) if tumor causes only a smooth capsular bulge (9,43).

Five imaging features that are suspicious for capsular penetration include (i) irregularity of the gland contour, (ii) an irregular bulge of the capsule, (iii) frank disruption of the capsule, (iv) hypointense focal thickening of the capsule, or (v) retraction of the capsule adjacent to the tumor (Fig. 10) (9,15,44).

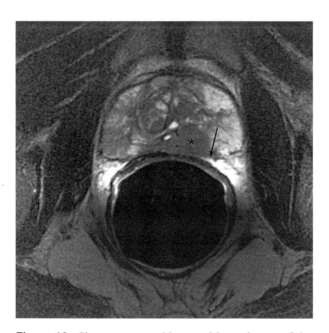

Figure 10 Sixty-two-year-old man with carcinoma of the prostate. Axial T2-weighted image demonstrate low signal intensity tumor (∗) in the mid–peripheral gland of the prostate. Irregularity of the gland contour and disruption of the thin black low signal intensity capsule (*thin black arrow*) reflects capsular penetration.

Extraprostatic spread of tumor is diagnosed if one of the three following imaging findings is present: (i) hypointense stranding in the periprostatic fat, (ii) obliteration of the fat plane between the posterior prostate and anterior rectum, or (iii) presence of clear-cut extracapsular tumor (9,15).

Differing sensitivities and specificities for endorectal MR diagnosis of capsular penetration (13% to 97% and 47% to 97%, respectively) have been reported (15,24). The lower sensitivities may reflect reader inexperience or use of very strict criteria for establishing the presence or absence of capsular penetration (24,87). However, reduced sensitivity may not have great clinical impact, because microscopic extracapsular tumor extension has been shown not to affect surgical cure rates or overall patient survival (15,88–90).

Neurovascular Bundle Invasion. The neurovascular bundles create a potential pathway for tumor spread because they course along the posterolateral aspect of the gland and pierce the capsule, resulting in areas of capsular weakness, particularly at the apex (39,43). Invasion of the neurovascular bundle may be better appreciated on T1-weighted imaging and can manifest as asymmetric enlargement of the bundle or as gross extracapsular extension of tumor at the posterolateral aspect of the prostate. Tumor infiltration into the neurovascular bundle may preclude treatment with nerve-sparing prostatectomy.

Seminal Vesicle Invasion. There are three possible pathways of seminal vesicle invasion: (i) direct spread along the ejaculatory ducts, (ii) direct extension of tumor from the base of the prostate, or (iii) skip metastases (91). Five MR findings that suggest seminal vesicle invasion are (i) asymmetry of the seminal vesicles caused by abnormal low T2-signal intensity, (ii) loss of the normal fat plane between the base of the prostate and inferior aspect of the seminal vesicles, (iii) low T2-signal intensity mass, (iv) focal or diffuse wall thickening, or (v) nonvisualization of the ejaculatory ducts or walls of the seminal vesicles (Fig. 11) (8,18,83,92).

Invasion of the wall of the seminal vesicle is classified as stage T3c disease and carries a worse prognosis than do capsular penetration or invasion of the soft tissue surrounding the seminal vesicle (T3a) (93). Invasion of the seminal vesicle is associated with microscopic lymph node metastases in 80% of cases, which increases the risk of recurrence after prostatectomy (94). Although early studies had demonstrated high specificity and low sensitivity of MRI in diagnosing seminal vesicle invasion, advancements in MRI imaging techniques have resulted in improved sensitivities (59–80%) and specificities (83–93%) (15,24,95). Some potential mimickers of invasion include (i) extrinsic compression of the seminal vesicle by BPH (83), (ii) inflammatory changes (43), (iii) postbiopsy hemorrhage (Fig. 12A and B) (51,52), (iv) prior radiation or hormonal therapy (96,97), and (v) amyloid deposition (98–100).

Regional Lymph Node Metastases. The likelihood of lymph node metastases is related to grade and stage of the primary mass. For example, a patient with a well-differentiated stage T1a tumor has a 0% chance of lymph node metastasis, whereas a patient with a poorly differentiated stage T3 tumor has 68% to 93% chance of metastases (101). The prognosis of patients with bilateral lymphadenopathy is poorer than for patients with a single ipsilateral lymph node (88).

Imaging the entire pelvis is important in staging prostate cancer because the lymphatic drainage of the prostate gland involves the obturator, internal iliac, external iliac, common iliac, and presacral lymph node chains (43). Lymphatic spread appears to be a stepwise process from the pelvis to the retroperitoneum in patients with newly diagnosed prostate cancer (102). However, lymph node metastases can

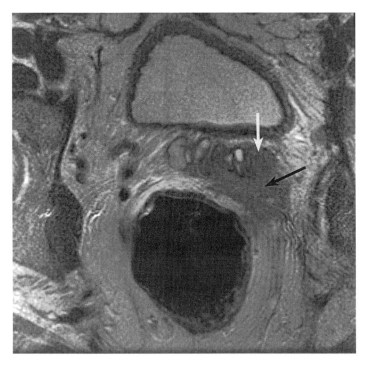

Figure 11 Forty-seven-year-old man with widespread prostate carcinoma. Axial T2-weighted image depicts low signal intensity tumor (*black arrow*) extending from the base of the prostate gland to invade nearly the entire left seminal vesicle and vas deferens (*white arrow*).

"skip" pelvic lymph nodes and appear in the retroperitoneum in men who have received radiotherapy with extended pelvic fields. Therefore, it is insufficient to image only the pelvis in patients with suspected disease recurrence (102).

Axial T1-weighted MR images have been shown to be at least equal to that of computed tomography (CT) in accuracy for the detection of nodal metastases (Fig. 13A and B). However, even normal-sized lymph nodes (usually defined as measuring < 1 cm in short-axis diameter) can contain metastatic cancer, which limits the overall sensitivity of CT and MRI in diagnosing metastases (101,103). Recent investigations using lymphotropic superparamagnetic iron oxide particles that target the reticuloendothelial system have improved the diagnosis of metastases by detecting metastatic foci in normal-sized lymph nodes (104–107). Whereas normal lymph node tissue takes up this agent and becomes low in T2-signal intensity, malignant tissue does not, but, instead, remains of higher T2-signal intensity, thereby permitting its detection (104). This technique may also overcome the known limitations of standard surgical pelvic lymphadenectomy, which may miss skip metastases to the common and internal iliac lymph node chains (104).

Invasion into Adjacent Organs. Stage T4 carcinoma of the prostate is defined as gross extraprostatic extension of tumor into adjacent tissues, such as the bladder, rectum, and levator ani muscles. Because of its proximity to the bladder base, direct cranial extension by tumor into the bladder is not uncommon (83). Findings indicative of bladder invasion include loss of the normal fat plane between the bladder and

(A)

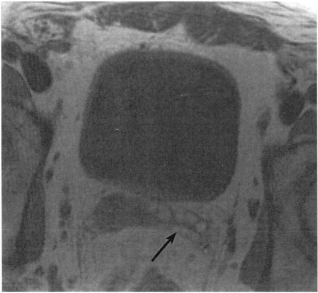

(B)

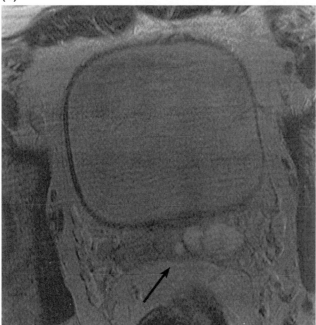

Figure 12 Left seminal vesicle hemorrhage in a 71-year-old man. (**A**) Axial T1-weighted and (**B**) axial T2-weighted images demonstrate high T1 and low T2-signal intensity methemoglobin (*black arrow*) in the left seminal vesicle, representing postbiopsy hemorrhage.

base of the prostate and discontinuity of the low signal intensity muscular bladder wall (83). Similar criteria are used to diagnose rectal wall invasion, although direct spread to the rectum is rare because Denonvilliers' fascia separates the anterior rectal wall from the posterior aspect of the prostate gland (83).

(A)

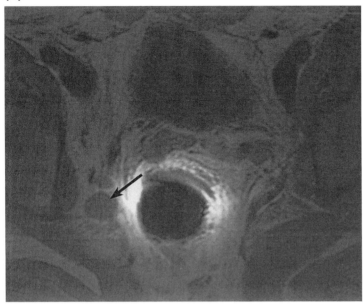

(B)

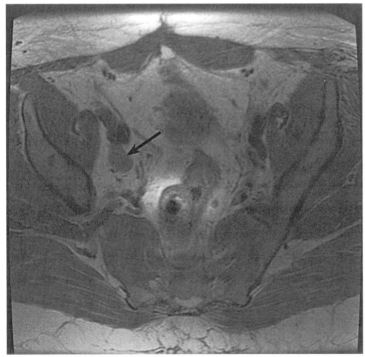

Figure 13 Forty-seven-year-old man with locoregional lymph node metastases from prostate carcinoma. Axial T1-weighted images demonstrate an enlarged periprostatic lymph node (*black arrow*) in (**A**) and an enlarged right external iliac lymph node (*black arrow*) in (**B**), representing metastatic disease.

Osseous Metastases. Hematogenous spread of prostate carcinoma usually results in osseous metastases. The periprostatic venous plexus drains into a venous plexus anterior to the sacrum, a plexus that communicates with the veins of the spine. This anatomy may explain the frequency of osseous metastases to the lumbo-sacral spine (38). Focal metastatic lesions appear as low signal intensity lesions within normal, high T1-signal intensity fatty marrow (Fig. 14) (108,109) and as high signal intensity lesions on fat-suppressed T2-weighted and short tau inversion recovery images (108,110). Routine MR imaging of the entire pelvis with T1- and T2-weighted sequences during the initial staging evaluation of patients with newly diagnosed prostate cancer may by useful in detecting osseous metastases. MRI is also helpful in the diagnosis of metastatic prostate cancer in the setting of inconclusive X-rays or suspected spinal cord compression (111,112).

Efficacy of Endorectal MRI in Staging Prostate Cancer

Variable results have been reported for detection of extracapsular tumor spread by endorectal MRI, with accuracies ranging from 54% to 88% (7,15,16,18,30,32,90,113). Reader experience is felt to be a major determinant of diagnostic accuracy and can result in a 30% variation among readers (18). Accuracy and reproducibility of MR image interpretation may be improved with computer-aided analysis, MR spectroscopy, and better training of readers (9,114–116). The role of MRI in staging prostate cancer continues to be controversial, and some argue that the diagnostic accuracy is insufficiently great to recommend its routine use (117). Studies have shown that physicians overuse MRI when staging newly diagnosed prostate cancer in patients at low risk for lymph node metastases (118,119). Other investigators

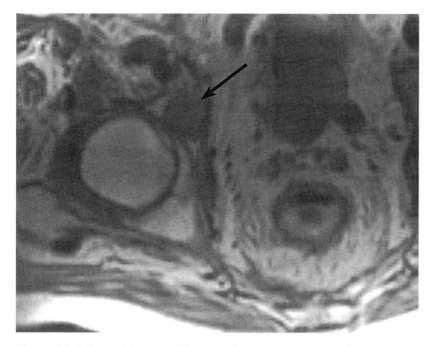

Figure 14 Ninety-eight-year-old man with osseous metastases from prostate cancer. Axial T1-weighted image demonstrates a focal low T1-signal intensity metastasis in the anterior column of the right acetabulum.

suggest that MRI is most beneficial and cost effective when reserved for patients at intermediate risk for extracapsular spread as defined by a PSA level of 10 to 20 ng/mL, biopsy Gleason score of 5 to 7, and DRE findings of stage T1–T2 (83).

EVOLVING TECHNOLOGIES IN IMAGING OF THE PROSTATE GLAND

The emergence of disease-targeted ablative therapies, such as cryosurgery, brachytherapy, high-intensity focused ultrasound, and intensity-modulated radiation therapy, has necessitated accurate pretreatment tumor localization and staging. These techniques also require a means by which to assess posttreatment tumor response. Although standard endorectal coil MRI provides excellent anatomic detail of the prostate, it is limited by decreased specificity with regards to tumor detection and localization. As has been seen, a large number of false-positive diagnoses can occur due to hemorrhage, prostatitis, and therapeutic effects, causing low signal intensity on T2-weighted imaging (116,120). A number of emerging approaches have shown promise in improving upon these limitations in MRI specificity.

Magnetic Resonance Spectroscopy

General Principles of MRS

Magnetic resonance spectroscopy (MRS) provides metabolic information from multiple contiguous voxels within the prostate and has been shown to improve tumor localization (121), prediction of extracapsular spread of tumor (122), and response to therapy (123–126).

MR spectroscopy of the prostate is based on the relative concentrations of metabolites that exist in prostate cells and extracellular ducts. Healthy prostate gland cells produce and secrete large amounts of citrate, due to high levels of zinc in the prostate, which inhibit the enzyme aconitase and thereby prevent oxidation of citrate in the Krebs cycle (Fig. 15A and B). In comparison, in prostate cancer cells, zinc levels decrease significantly, citrate metabolism increases, and prostate epithelial cells lose their ability to produce large amounts of citrate. The transformation of prostate gland cells into citrate-oxidizing cells increases energy production, which promotes accelerated proliferation of malignant tissue (127,128). Decreased citrate in prostate cancer cells is also attributed to changes in the organization of the tissue because there is loss of normal ductal morphology (123). There is also an elevation of choline-containing compounds in carcinoma cells relative to normal peripheral gland tissue. This is a less understood mechanism but is attributed to altered metabolism of phospholipids in growing malignant cells (123,129,130).

The three metabolites—citrate, choline, creatine (the last remaining relatively constant in both normal and abnormal prostatic tissue)—produce distinct frequencies in the resonance spectrum and can be detected when spectroscopy is added to a routine clinical endorectal MR examination. Both studies use the same scanner and coil. The ability of MRS to detect elevated choline and decreased citrate levels in tumor cells depends on adequate suppression of adjacent water and lipid signal that exist in the prostate and periprostatic tissue (Fig. 16A and B) (120).

Three-dimensional MRS imaging is a methodology that can assess citrate and other metabolites in the entire prostate with a voxel size of 0.24 cc (129). The data may be subsequently overlaid on a corresponding T2-weighted MR image. The

(A)

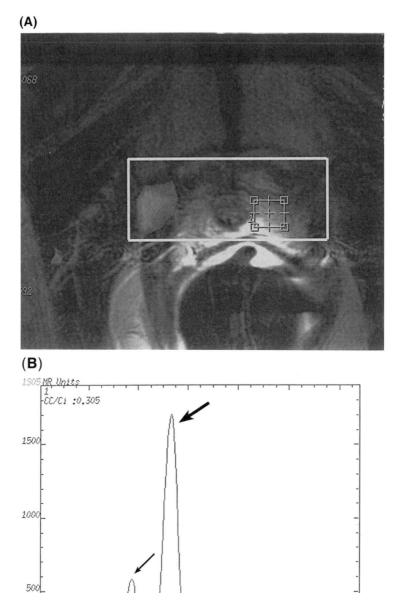

(B)

Figure 15 Sixty-four-year-old with a normal metabolic profile of the prostate gland. (**A**) Axial T2-weighted image demonstrates a normal region of peripheral zone of the left prostate gland demarcated by the cursor. (**B**) The NMR spectra of this same tissue reveal a normal pattern of a high citrate peak (*thick black arrow*) and a low choline peak (*thin black arrow*). *Abbreviation*: NMR, nuclear magnetic resonance.

(A)

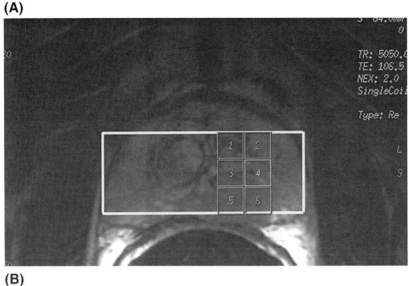

(B)

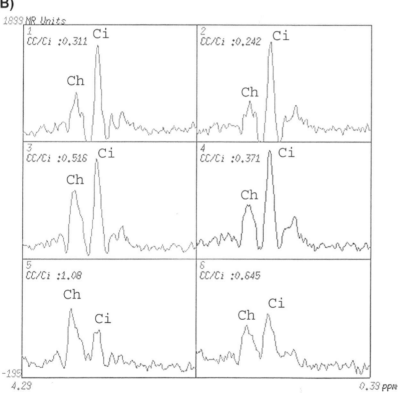

Figure 16 Sixty-two-year-old man with prostate cancer and abnormal MR spectroscopy. (**A**) Axial T2-weighted image reveals a box (numbered 1–6) that demarcates normal tissue (boxes 1 and 2), indeterminate tissue (boxes 3 and 4), and low signal intensity cancerous tissue (boxes 5 and 6). (**B**) The corresponding MR spectra reveal a normal pattern of high citrate and relatively low choline levels in boxes 1 to 4 and an abnormal pattern of a suppressed citrate peak and relatively elevated choline peak reflecting cancer in boxes 5 and 6 (Ci = citrate and Ch = choline). *Abbreviation*: MR, magnetic resonance.

3D acquisition allows the dataset to be viewed in any plane and the spectroscopic voxel position to be changed to better match an abnormality on T2-weighted imaging (128,129). The concordance of MRI and MRS leads to a more confident diagnosis of cancer and extracapsular tumor spread, which helps minimize the interreader variability that can result in the reported wide range of accuracies (56% to 93%) (120,122).

Localization of Tumor and Assessment of Extracapsular Spread of Tumor

Accurate tumor localization can help target TRUS-guided biopsies in patients with elevated PSA levels but negative previous biopsies, guide targeted therapies, and monitor the progress of patients who have chosen watchful waiting as a treatment option (83). Combined MRI–MRS has an accuracy rate similar to biopsy for localization of tumor in a specific sextant of the prostate and at the apex of the gland, is better than biopsy. The addition of MRS to standard MRI provides better detection of cancer than MRI alone and increases the specificity of tumor diagnosis from 46% to 61% up to 94% (121). Postbiopsy hemorrhage may hinder the interpretation of standard T2-weighted images because blood products can persist as long as four months and mimic low T2-signal intensity tumor (52). Kaji et al. showed that adding MRS to conventional endorectal MRI significantly improves the accuracy (from 52% to 75%) and specificity (from 26% to 66%) of tumor detection in the background of postprocedural hemorrhage (54).

Attempts have been made to use MRS to evaluate the central gland for tumors. As many as 30% of cancers occur in the transitional zone. These are often missed on routine endorectal MRI because they cannot be distinguished from the heterogeneous appearance of coexisting, surrounding, or adjacent BPH. Unfortunately, decreased citrate and elevated choline levels have been found in stromal BPH. Therefore, the broad range of metabolite ratios precludes the use of a single ratio to distinguish cancers from benign tissue (131).

The presence and extent of extracapsular spread of tumor greatly affects the choice of tumor therapy and has been the focus of recent MRS investigations. Although endorectal coil imaging with T2-weighted sequences has improved the detection of tumor spread, men are being diagnosed at earlier stages with microscopic spread that is not visible on MR images (8). Prostate cancer volume has been shown to be a good predictor of extracapsular spread on histopathologic studies (132). Tumor volume, as estimated by MRS, is higher in patients with extracapsular spread than in patients without spread and has improved the diagnostic accuracy of staging (9,120).

Assessment of Cancer Therapy

Local recurrence of cancer after treatment is often suspected due to rising or detectable PSA levels. However, PSA is not specific for tumor, can take one to two years to reach a nadir after treatment, and can be difficult to interpret in the setting of hormonal deprivation. The only way to definitively diagnose recurrent disease is by biopsy, but this method is subject to sampling errors. Because treatments with radiation, cryosurgery, and hormonal therapy result in necrosis of both normal glandular tissue and cancer cells, they can produce diffuse low T2-signal intensity and loss of zonal anatomy (35,96,97,124,133,134), making tumor detection difficult. Standard MRI may have difficulty in distinguishing benign prostatic tissue, inflammatory cells, and necrotic tissue from cancer cells. MRS can be extremely helpful in this setting. MRS shows histologically necrotic tissue to have no discernible citrate or choline. Although citrate is uniformly suppressed in areas of both necrosis and tumor and cannot be used for assessment, elevation of choline in a particular voxel raises the suspicion that recurrent or residual cancer is present (134).

Following radiotherapy, accurate early measurement of tumor response is important in assessing dose escalation and treatment failures that may require salvage therapy (124). When cryosurgery has been performed, MRS increases the sensitivity in detecting local recurrence in patients who still have elevated PSA after the procedure. MRI–MRS can also help identify lesions for repeat biopsy or cryosurgery (125,126).

Recently, hormonal ablation (or deprivation) therapy has been used as a primary or adjuvant therapy for patients with localized disease (123,135,136). Hormonal therapy deprives both healthy and malignant cells of androgen, which results in tissue atrophy and a decrease in overall gland and tumor volume. The marked glandular shrinkage and increased periglandular fibrous tissue results in a small prostate with poor zonal differentiation and diffuse low T2-signal intensity throughout the peripheral gland, which makes it difficult to identify tumor (97,137,138). The low T2-signal intensity results in an overestimation of tumor presence and extracapsular spread. A time-dependent loss of all metabolites (metabolic atrophy) occurs in a certain percentage of patients on long-term therapy and is greater in regions of cancer when compared to healthy peripheral glandular tissue. Citrate levels decrease faster than that of other metabolites because of hormonal control of citrate production and secretion (137). Recent studies have shown that residual choline may be used as a substitute marker for cancer after prolonged hormonal ablation therapy and that the combination of MRI and MRS can provide better localization of tumor (139).

Diffusion-Weighted Imaging

Diffusion-weighted MR imaging (DWI) is a technique that relates image intensities to the relative mobility of endogenous tissue water molecules. The microenvironment of the water molecules influences the freedom of diffusion and is reflected in the measurement of the apparent diffusion coefficient (ADC). Preliminary work on DWI in the prostate gland has shown that the mean ADC is lower in malignant peripheral zone tissue than in benign or normal peripheral zone tissue (140,141). This significant reduction of the mobility of water molecules observed in tumors may be secondary to replacement of water-rich acinar cells by numerous, closely packed cancerous cells and to an increased nuclear-to-cytoplasmic ratio. ADC values are higher in normal peripheral zone relative to the central gland, which again reflect the higher mobile water content in the luminal spaces of the peripheral gland relative to the compact central gland (140,141). DWI of the prostate gland is in its infancy, even as a research tool, but may establish a role in the future as a noninvasive marker for treatment response of prostate cancer.

Role of MRI in Radiotherapy Treatment

Radiation therapy of prostate cancer has more recently focused on conformal radiotherapy (CRT), which delivers high radiation doses to the target volume while sparing normal tissue and intensity-modulated radiotherapy, which customizes the dose

(A)

(B)

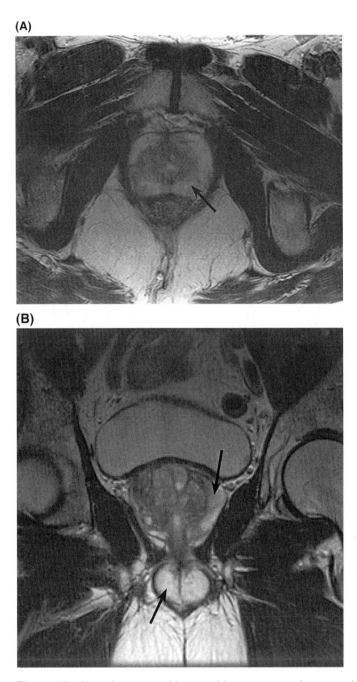

Figure 17 Sixty-three-year-old man with prostate carcinoma undergoing radiation therapy. (**A**) Axial T2-weighted image demonstrates the peripheral gland of the prostatic apex (*black arrow*). (**B**) A coronal T2-weighted image also clearly delineates the peripheral gland of the prostate (*long black arrow*) and the penile bulb (*short black arrow*) which will aid in customizing the delivered dose to the tumor.

distribution and delivers a nonuniform dose to the target (142,143). A higher level of accuracy is needed for localization of tumor and for delineating the prostate and other structures in the pelvis, such as the penile bulb, rectum, and bladder. CT over-estimates prostate volume and cannot clearly separate the prostate from the bladder base, seminal vesicles, rectal wall, and neurovascular bundle (142,144,145). Using axial and coronal MRI images to delineate the prostatic apex and other structures has allowed for a reduction in dose to the rectum and penile bulb, thereby minimizing rectal and urologic complications of treatment (Fig. 17A and B) (142,145,146). Fusion of the CT and MRI data currently provides valuable anatomic information for radiation treatment planning (147) and in the future will also integrate functional imaging, such as MRS, to more accurately define the spatial extent of the cancer (148).

MR-Guided Intervention in Prostate Cancer

Patients are now able to undergo MR-guided procedures of the prostate gland due to the development of real-time intraoperative MR systems (149). A transperineal prostate biopsy has been successfully performed on an open configuration, 0.5-T MRI scanner in patients who are unable to undergo transrectal ultrasound-guided biopsies because of prior rectal surgery (150–152).

Brachytherapy, which is a form of radiation therapy in which the radiation is delivered to the target site by the temporary or permanent insertion of radioactive seeds, can also be performed under MR guidance via the transperineal approach (153). A growing number of patients are choosing brachytherapy as their primary treatment modality, with the seeds traditionally placed into the prostate under ultrasound guidance (153–155). This technique can sometimes result in suboptimal placement of radioactive material leading to rectal bleeding, urinary incontinence, and fistula formation (156). Until recently, the primary role of MRI in brachytherapy had been to evaluate the distribution of seeds in the prostate, as well as to detect any extraprostatic seeds and treatment-related changes in the prostate (157–161).

Research on real-time 3D MR–guided seed implantation using an open configuration double-magnet scanner is on going. This scanner configuration allows the perineum to be accessed for seed placement, while the patient's head is accessible for anesthesia (150,153,162). The seed number, strength, and catheter trajectory can be checked for accuracy and modified within seconds (153).

Recently, a more sophisticated method of real-time dosimetric feedback has allowed for more effective delivery of radiation dose to the target volume. These techniques can provide high dose coverage within the prostate without exceeding the maximal dose allowed for surrounding normal tissue, which ultimately may improve treatment options for localized cancer because of reduced morbidity (163).

CONCLUSION

MRI has emerged as a useful tool to improve staging of men with biopsy-proven prostate carcinoma. MRI can also be used to evaluate complications of prostatitis and Müllerian abnormalities and assess response to tumor therapies. New advances in MR spectroscopy and greater availability of interventional MR scanners will likely expand the role of MR in management of prostatic diseases in the near future.

REFERENCES

1. D'Amico AV, Whittington R, Schnall M, et al. The impact of the inclusion of endorectal coil magnetic resonance imaging in a multivariate analysis to predict clinically unsuspected extraprostatic cancer. Cancer 1995; 75:2368–2372.
2. Huch Boni RA, Meyenberger C, Pok Lundquist J, Trinkler F, Lutolf U, Krestin GP. Value of endorectal coil versus body coil MRI for diagnosis of recurrent pelvic malignancies. Abdom Imaging 1996; 21:345–352.
3. Martin JF, Hajek P, Baker L, Gylys-Morin V, Fitzmorris-Glass R, Mattrey RR. Inflatable surface coil for MR imaging of the prostate. Radiology 1988; 167:268–270.
4. Schiebler ML, Schnall MD, Pollack HM, et al. Current role of MR imaging in the staging of adenocarcinoma of the prostate. Radiology 1993; 189:339–352.
5. Schnall MD, Lenkinski RE, Pollack HM, Imai Y, Kressel HY. Prostate: MR imaging with an endorectal surface coil. Radiology 1989; 172:570–574.
6. Cheng DTC. MR imaging of the prostate and bladder. Semin Ultrasound CT MRI 1998; 19:67–89.
7. Schnall MD, Imai Y, Tomaszewski J, Pollack HM, Lenkinski RE, Kressel HY. Prostate cancer: local staging with endorectal surface coil MR imaging. Radiology 1991; 178:797–802.
8. Hricak H, White S, Vigneron D, et al. Carcinoma of the prostate gland: MR imaging with pelvic phased-array coils versus integrated endorectal—pelvic phased-array coils. Radiology 1994; 193:703–709.
9. Yu KK, Hricak H, Alagappan R, Chernoff DM, Bacchetti P, Zaloudek CJ. Detection of extracapsular extension of prostate carcinoma with endorectal and phased-array coil MR imaging: multivariate feature analysis. Radiology 1997; 202:697–702.
10. Schnall MD, Connick T, Hayes CE, Lenkinski RE, Kressel HY. MR imaging of the pelvis with an endorectal-external multicoil array. J Magn Reson Imaging 1992; 2:229–232.
11. Siegelman ES. Magnetic resonance imaging of the prostate. Semin Roentgenol 1999; 34:295–312.
12. Kier R, Wain S, Troiano R. Fast spin-echo MR images of the pelvis obtained with a phased-array coil: value in localizing and staging prostatic carcinoma. Am J Roentgenol 1993; 161:601–606.
13. Marti-Bonmati L, Graells M, Ronchera-Oms CL. Reduction of peristaltic artifacts on magnetic resonance imaging of the abdomen: a comparative evaluation of three drugs. Abdom Imaging 1996; 21:309–313.
14. Bezzi M, Kressel HY, Allen KS, et al. Prostatic carcinoma: staging with MR imaging at 1.5 T. Radiology 1988; 169:339–346.
15. Bartolozzi C, Menchi I, Lencioni R, et al. Local staging of prostate carcinoma with endorectal coil MRI: correlation with whole-mount radical prostatectomy specimens. Eur Radiol 1996; 6:339–345.
16. Huch Boni RA, Boner JA, Debatin JF, et al. Optimization of prostate carcinoma staging: comparison of imaging and clinical methods. Clin Radiol 1995; 50:593–600.
17. Bates TS, Cavanagh PM, Speakman M, Gillatt DA. Endorectal MRI using a 0.5 T midfield system in the staging of localized prostate cancer. Clin Radiol 1996; 51:550–553.
18. Tempany CM, Zhou X, Zerhouni EA, et al. Staging of prostate cancer: results of Radiology Diagnostic Oncology Group project comparison of three MR imaging techniques. Radiology 1994; 192:47–54.
19. Bates TS, Gillatt DA, Cavanagh PM, Speakman M. A comparison of endorectal magnetic resonance imaging and transrectal ultrasonography in the local staging of prostate cancer with histopathological correlation. Br J Urol 1997; 79:927–932.
20. Ikonen S, Karkkainen P, Kivisaari L, et al. Endorectal magnetic resonance imaging of prostatic cancer: comparison between fat-suppressed T2-weighted fast spin echo and three-dimensional dual-echo, steady-state sequences. Eur Radiol 2001; 11:236–241.

21. Tsuda K, Yu KK, Coakley FV, Srivastav SK, Scheidler JE, Hricak H. Detection of extracapsular extension of prostate cancer: role of fat suppression endorectal MRI. J Comput Assist Tomogr 1999; 23:74–78.

22. Parivar F, Rajanayagam V, Waluch V, Eto RT, Jones LW, Ross BD. Endorectal surface coil MR imaging of prostatic carcinoma with the inversion-recovery sequence. J Magn Reson Imaging 1991; 1:657–664.

23. Mirowitz SA, Heiken JP, Brown JJ. Evaluation of fat saturation technique for T2-weighted endorectal coil MRI of the prostate. Magn Reson Imaging 1994; 12: 743–747.

24. Ikonen S, Karkkainen P, Kivisaari L, et al. Magnetic resonance imaging of clinically localized prostatic cancer. J Urol 1998; 159:915–919.

25. Brown G, Macvicar DA, Ayton V, Husband JE. The role of intravenous contrast enhancement in magnetic resonance imaging of prostatic carcinoma. Clin Radiol 1995; 50:601–606.

26. Ogura K, Maekawa S, Okubo K, et al. Dynamic endorectal magnetic resonance imaging for local staging and detection of neurovascular bundle involvement of prostate cancer: correlation with histopathologic results. Urology 2001; 57:721–726.

27. Padhani AR, Gapinski CJ, Macvicar DA, et al. Dynamic contrast enhanced MRI of prostate cancer: correlation with morphology and tumour stage, histological grade and PSA. Clin Radiol 2000; 55:99–109.

28. Namimoto T, Morishita S, Saitoh R, Kudoh J, Yamashita Y, Takahashi M. The value of dynamic MR imaging for hypointensity lesions of the peripheral zone of the prostate. Comput Med Imaging Graph 1998; 22:239–245.

29. Turnbull LW, Buckley DL, Turnbull LS, Liney GP, Knowles AJ. Differentiation of prostatic carcinoma and benign prostatic hyperplasia: correlation between dynamic Gd-DTPA-enhanced MR imaging and histopathology. J Magn Reson Imaging 1999; 9:311–316.

30. Huch Boni RA, Boner JA, Lutolf UM, Trinkler F, Pestalozzi DM, Krestin GP. Contrast-enhanced endorectal coil MRI in local staging of prostate carcinoma. J Comput Assist Tomogr 1995; 19:232–237.

31. Mirowitz SA, Brown JJ, Heiken JP. Evaluation of the prostate and prostatic carcinoma with gadolinium-enhanced endorectal coil MR imaging. Radiology 1993; 186:153–157.

32. Quinn SF, Franzini DA, Demlow TA, et al. MR imaging of prostate cancer with an endorectal surface coil technique: correlation with whole-mount specimens. Radiology 1994; 190:323–327.

33. Jager GJ, Ruijter ET, van de Kaa CA, et al. Dynamic TurboFLASH subtraction technique for contrast-enhanced MR imaging of the prostate: correlation with histo-pathologic results. Radiology 1997; 203:645–652.

34. Larson BT, Collins JM, Huidobro C, Corica A, Vallejo S, Bostwick DG. Gadolinium-enhanced MRI in the evaluation of minimally invasive treatments of the prostate: correlation with histopathologic findings. Urology 2003; 62:900–904.

35. Vellet AD, Saliken J, Donnelly B, et al. Prostatic cryosurgery: use of MR imaging in evaluation of success and technical modifications. Radiology 1997; 203:653–659.

36. Kaji Y, Wada A, Imaoka I, et al. Proton two-dimensional chemical shift imaging for evaluation of prostate cancer: external surface coil vs. endorectal surface coil. J Magn Reson Imaging 2002; 16:697–706.

37. Kim HW, Buckley DL, Peterson DM, et al. In vivo prostate magnetic resonance imaging and magnetic resonance spectroscopy at 3 Tesla using a transceive pelvic phased array coil: preliminary results. Invest Radiol 2003; 38:443–451.

38. Coakley FV, Hricak H. Radiologic anatomy of the prostate gland: a clinical approach. Radiol Clin North Am 2000; 38:15–30.

39. Nunes LW, Schiebler MS, Rauschning W, et al. The normal prostate and periprostatic structures: correlation between MR images made with an endorectal coil and cadaveric microtome sections. AJR Am J Roentgenol 1995; 164:923–927.

40. Poon PY, Bronskill MJ, Poon CS, McCallum RW, Bruce AW, Henkelman RM. Identification of the periprostatic venous plexus by MR imaging. J Comput Assist Tomogr 1991; 15:265–268.

41. Coakley FV, Eberhardt S, Wei DC, et al. Blood loss during radical retropubic prostatectomy: relationship to morphologic features on preoperative endorectal magnetic resonance imaging. Urology 2002; 59:884–888.

42. Gevenois PA, Salmon I, Stallenberg B, van Sinoy ML, van Regemorter G, Struyven J. Magnetic resonance imaging of the normal prostate at 1.5 T. Br J Radiol 1990; 63:101–107.

43. Bartolozzi C, Crocetti L, Menchi I, Ortori S, Lencioni R. Endorectal magnetic resonance imaging in local staging of prostate carcinoma. Abdom Imaging 2001; 26:111–122.

44. Outwater EK, Petersen RO, Siegelman ES, Gomella LG, Chernesky CE, Mitchell DG. Prostate carcinoma: assessment of diagnostic criteria for capsular penetration on endorectal coil MR images. Radiology 1994; 193:333–339.

45. Ishida J, Sugimura K, Okizuka H, et al. Benign prostatic hyperplasia: value of MR imaging for determining histologic type. Radiology 1994; 190:329–331.

46. Hricak H, Dooms GC, McNeal JE, et al. MR imaging of the prostate gland: normal anatomy. AJR Am J Roentgenol 1987; 148:51–58.

47. Tempany CM, Rahmouni AD, Epstein JI, Walsh PC, Zerhouni EA. Invasion of the neurovascular bundle by prostate cancer: evaluation with MR imaging. Radiology 1991; 181:107–112.

48. Allen KS, Kressel HY, Arger PH, Pollack HM. Age-related changes of the prostate: evaluation by MR imaging. AJR Am J Roentgenol 1989; 152:77–81.

49. Phillips ME, Kressel HY, Spritzer CE, et al. Normal prostate and adjacent structures: MR imaging at 1.5 T. Radiology 1987; 164:381–385.

50. Siegelman ES, Schnall MD. Contrast-enhanced MR imaging of the bladder and prostate. Magn Reson Imaging Clin N Am 1996; 4:153–169.

51. Mirowitz SA. Seminal vesicles: biopsy-related hemorrhage simulating tumor invasion at endorectal MR imaging. Radiology 1992; 185:373–376.

52. White S, Hricak H, Forstner R, et al. Prostate cancer: effect of postbiopsy hemorrhage on interpretation of MR images. Radiology 1995; 195:385–390.

53. Ikonen S, Kivisaari L, Vehmas T, et al. Optimal timing of post-biopsy MR imaging of the prostate. Acta Radiol 2001; 42:70–73.

54. Kaji Y, Kurhanewicz J, Hricak H, et al. Localizing prostate cancer in the presence of postbiopsy changes on MR images: role of proton MR spectroscopic imaging. Radiology 1998; 206:785–790.

55. Adusumilli S, Pretorius ES. Magnetic resonance imaging of prostate cancer. Semin Urol Oncol 2002; 20:192–210.

56. Grossfeld GD, Coakley FV. Benign prostatic hyperplasia: clinical overview and value of diagnostic imaging. Radiol Clin North Am 2000; 38:31–47.

57. Mimata H, Nomura Y, Kasagi Y, et al. Prediction of alpha-blocker response in men with benign prostatic hyperplasia by magnetic resonance imaging. Urology 1999; 54:829–833.

58. Kahn T, Burrig K, Schmitz-Drager B, Lewin JS, Furst G, Modder U. Prostatic carcinoma and benign prostatic hyperplasia: MR imaging with histopathologic correlation. Radiology 1989; 173:847–851.

59. Hruban RH, Zerhouni EA, Dagher AP, Pessar ML, Hutchins GM. Morphologic basis of MR imaging of benign prostatic hyperplasia. J Comput Assist Tomogr 1987; 11:1035–1041.

60. Schiebler ML, Tomaszewski JE, Bezzi M, et al. Prostatic carcinoma and benign prostatic hyperplasia: correlation of high-resolution MR and histopathologic findings. Radiology 1989; 172:131–137.

61. al-Rimawi M, Griffiths DJ, Boake RC, Mador DR, Johnson MA. Transrectal ultrasound versus magnetic resonance imaging in the estimation of prostatic volume. Br J Urol 1994; 74:596–600.

62. Sosna J, Rofsky NM, Gaston SM, DeWolf WC, Lenkinski RE. Determinations of prostate volume at 3-Tesla using an external phased array coil: comparison to pathologic specimens. Acad Radiol 2003; 10:846–853.
63. Rahmouni A, Yang A, Tempany CM, et al. Accuracy of in-vivo assessment of prostatic volume by MRI and transrectal ultrasonography. J Comput Assist Tomogr 1992; 16:935–940.
64. Lovett K, Rifkin MD, McCue PA, Choi H. MR imaging characteristics of noncancerous lesions of the prostate. J Magn Reson Imaging 1992; 2:35–39.
65. Ikonen S, Kivisaari L, Tervahartiala P, Vehmas T, Taari K, Rannikko S. Prostatic MR imaging. Accuracy in differentiating cancer from other prostatic disorders. Acta Radiol 2001; 42:348–354.
66. Cruz M, Tsuda K, Narumi Y, et al. Characterization of low-intensity lesions in the peripheral zone of prostate on pre-biopsy endorectal coil MR imaging. Eur Radiol 2002; 12:357–365.
67. Papanicolaou N, Pfister RC, Stafford SA, Parkhurst EC. Prostatic abscess: imaging with transrectal sonography and MR. AJR Am J Roentgenol 1987; 149:981–982.
68. Naik KS, Carey BM. The transrectal ultrasound and MRI appearances of granulomatous prostatitis and its differentiation from carcinoma. Clin Radiol 1999; 54:173–175.
69. McDermott VG, Meakem TJ 3rd, Stolpen AH, Schnall MD. Prostatic and periprostatic cysts: findings on MR imaging. AJR Am J Roentgenol 1995; 164:123–127.
70. Parsons RB, Fisher AM, Bar-Chama N, Mitty HA. MR imaging in male infertility. Radiographics 1997; 17:627–637.
71. Gevenois PA, Van Sinoy ML, Sintzoff SA Jr, et al. Cysts of the prostate and seminal vesicles: MR imaging findings in 11 cases. AJR Am J Roentgenol 1990; 155:1021–1024.
72. Honig SC. New diagnostic techniques in the evaluation of anatomic abnormalities of the infertile male. Urol Clin North Am 1994; 21:417–432.
73. Schnall MD, Pollack HM, Van Arsdalen K, Kressel HY. The seminal tract in patients with ejaculatory dysfunction: MR imaging with an endorectal surface coil. AJR Am J Roentgenol 1992; 159:337–341.
74. Rouviere O, Raudrant A, Ecochard R, et al. Characterization of time-enhancement curves of benign and malignant prostate tissue at dynamic MR imaging. Eur Radiol 2003; 13:931–942.
75. Engelbrecht MR, Huisman HJ, Laheij RJ, et al. Discrimination of prostate cancer from normal peripheral zone and central gland tissue by using dynamic contrast-enhanced MR imaging. Radiology 2003; 229:248–254.
76. Outwater E, Schiebler ML, Tomaszewski JE, Schnall MD, Kressel HY. Mucinous carcinomas involving the prostate: atypical findings at MR imaging. J Magn Reson Imaging 1992; 2:597–600.
77. Schiebler ML, Schnall MD, Outwater E. MR imaging of mucinous adenocarcinoma of the prostate. J Comput Assist Tomogr 1992; 16:493–494.
78. Elbadawi A, Craig W, Linke CA, Cooper RA Jr. Prostatic mucinous carcinoma. Urology 1979; 13:658–666.
79. Sexton WJ, Lance RE, Reyes AO, Pisters PW, Tu SM, Pisters LL. Adult prostate sarcoma: the M. D. Anderson Cancer Center Experience. J Urol 2001; 166:521–525.
80. Mansouri H, Kanouni L, Kebdani T, Hassouni K, Sifat H, Gueddari BE. Primary prostatic leiomyosarcoma. J Urol 2001; 165:1676.
81. Cheville JC, Dundore PA, Nascimento AG, et al. Leiomyosarcoma of the prostate. Report of 23 cases. Cancer 1995; 76:1422–1427.
82. Russo P, Demas B, Reuter V. Adult prostatic sarcoma. Abdom Imaging 1993; 18:399–401.
83. Yu KK, Hawkins RA. The prostate: diagnostic evaluation of metastatic disease. Radiol Clin North Am 2000; 38:139–157, ix.
84. D'Amico AV, Whittington R, Malkowicz SB, et al. Critical analysis of the ability of the endorectal coil magnetic resonance imaging scan to predict pathologic stage, margin

status, and postoperative prostate-specific antigen failure in patients with clinically organ-confined prostate cancer. J Clin Oncol 1996; 14:1770–1777.

85. Mukamel E, Hanna J, deKernion JB. Pitfalls in preoperative staging in prostate cancer. Urology 1987; 30:318–321.

86. Fleming I. AJCC (American Joint Committee on Cancer) Cancer Staging Manual. Philadelphia, PA: Lippincott-Raven, 1997.

87. Langlotz C, Schnall M, Pollack H. Staging of prostatic cancer: accuracy of MR imaging. Radiology 1995; 194:645–646; discussion 647–648.

88. Hering F, Rist M, Roth J, Mihatsch M, Rutishauser G. Does microinvasion of the capsule and/or micrometastases in regional lymph nodes influence disease-free survival after radical prostatectomy? Br J Urol 1990; 66:177–181.

89. Epstein JI, Carmichael MJ, Pizov G, Walsh PC. Influence of capsular penetration on progression following radical prostatectomy: a study of 196 cases with long-term followup. J Urol 1993; 150:135–141.

90. Jager GJ, Ruijter ET, van de Kaa CA, et al. Local staging of prostate cancer with endorectal MR imaging: correlation with histopathology. AJR Am J Roentgenol 1996; 166:845–852.

91. Wheeler TM. Anatomic considerations in carcinoma of the prostate. Urol Clin North Am 1989; 16:623–634.

92. Chelsky MJ, Schnall MD, Seidmon EJ, Pollack HM. Use of endorectal surface coil magnetic resonance imaging for local staging of prostate cancer. J Urol 1993; 150:391–395.

93. Epstein JI, Carmichael M, Partin AW, Walsh PC. Is tumor volume an independent predictor of progression following radical prostatectomy? A multivariate analysis of 185 clinical stage B adenocarcinomas of the prostate with 5 years of followup. J Urol 1993; 149:1478–1481.

94. Lange PH, Narayan P. Understaging and undergrading of prostate cancer. Argument for postoperative radiation as adjuvant therapy. Urology 1983; 21:113–118.

95. Rorvik J, Halvorsen OJ, Albrektsen G, Ersland L, Daehlin L, Haukaas S. MRI with an endorectal coil for staging of clinically localised prostate cancer prior to radical prostatectomy. Eur Radiol 1999; 9:29–34.

96. Chan TW, Kressel HY. Prostate and seminal vesicles after irradiation: MR appearance. J Magn Reson Imaging 1991; 1:503–511.

97. Chen M, Hricak H, Kalbhen CL, et al. Hormonal ablation of prostatic cancer: effects on prostate morphology, tumor detection, and staging by endorectal coil MR imaging. AJR Am J Roentgenol 1996; 166:1157–1163.

98. Jager GJ, Ruijter ET, de la Rosette JJ, van de Kaa CA. Amyloidosis of the seminal vesicles simulating tumor invasion of prostatic carcinoma on endorectal MR images. Eur Radiol 1997; 7:552–554.

99. Kaji Y, Sugimura K, Nagaoka S, Ishida T. Amyloid deposition in seminal vesicles mimicking tumor invasion from bladder cancer: MR findings. J Comput Assist Tomogr 1992; 16:989–991.

100. Ramchandani P, Schnall MD, LiVolsi VA, Tomaszewski JE, Pollack HM. Senile amyloidosis of the seminal vesicles mimicking metastatic spread of prostatic carcinoma on MR images. AJR Am J Roentgenol 1993; 161:99–100.

101. Jager GJ, Barentsz JO, Oosterhof GO, Witjes JA, Ruijs SJ. Pelvic adenopathy in prostatic and urinary bladder carcinoma: MR imaging with a three-dimensional TI-weighted magnetization-prepared-rapid gradient-echo sequence. AJR Am J Roentgenol 1996; 167:1503–1507.

102. Spencer JA, Golding SJ. Patterns of lymphatic metastases at recurrence of prostate cancer: CT findings. Clin Radiol 1994; 49:404–407.

103. Oyen RH, Van Poppel HP, Ameye FE, Van de Voorde WA, Baert AL, Baert LV. Lymph node staging of localized prostatic carcinoma with CT and CT-guided fine-needle aspiration biopsy: prospective study of 285 patients. Radiology 1994; 190:315–322.

104. Harisinghani MG, Barentsz J, Hahn PF, et al. Noninvasive detection of clinically occult lymph-node metastases in prostate cancer. N Engl J Med 2003; 348:2491–2499.

105. Harisinghani MG, Barentsz JO, Hahn PF, et al. MR lymphangiography for detection of minimal nodal disease in patients with prostate cancer. Acad Radiol 2002; 9(suppl 2):S312–S313.

106. Bellin MF, Roy C, Kinkel K, et al. Lymph node metastases: safety and effectiveness of MR imaging with ultrasmall superparamagnetic iron oxide particles—initial clinical experience. Radiology 1998; 207:799–808.

107. Vassallo P, Matei C, Heston WD, McLachlan SJ, Koutcher JA, Castellino RA. AMI-227-enhanced MR lymphography: usefulness for differentiating reactive from tumor-bearing lymph nodes. Radiology 1994; 193:501–506.

108. Avrahami E, Tadmor R, Dally O, Hadar H. Early MR demonstration of spinal metastases in patients with normal radiographs and CT and radionuclide bone scans. J Comput Assist Tomogr 1989; 13:598–602.

109. Freedman GM, Negendank WG, Hudes GR, Shaer AH, Hanks GE. Preliminary results of a bone marrow magnetic resonance imaging protocol for patients with high-risk prostate cancer. Urology 1999; 54:118–123.

110. Heshiki A. Bone marrow MRI in prostate cancer. Adv Exp Med Biol 1992; 324: 209–215.

111. Fujii Y, Higashi Y, Owada F, Okuno T, Mizuno H. Magnetic resonance imaging for the diagnosis of prostate cancer metastatic to bone. Br J Urol 1995; 75:54–58.

112. Turner JW, Hawes DR, Williams RD. Magnetic resonance imaging for detection of prostate cancer metastatic to bone. J Urol 1993; 149:1482–1484.

113. D'Amico AV, Schnall M, Whittington R, et al. Endorectal coil magnetic resonance imaging identifies locally advanced prostate cancer in select patients with clinically localized disease. Urology 1998; 51:449–454.

114. Harris RD, Schned AR, Heaney JA. Staging of prostate cancer with endorectal MR imaging: lessons from a learning curve. Radiographics 1995; 15:813–829; discussion 829–832.

115. Seltzer SE, Getty DJ, Tempany CM, et al. Staging prostate cancer with MR imaging: a combined radiologist-computer system. Radiology 1997; 202:219–226.

116. Dhingsa R, Qayyum A, Coakley FV, et al. Prostate cancer localization with endorectal MR imaging and MR spectroscopic imaging: effect of clinical data on reader accuracy. Radiology 2004; 230:215–220.

117. Perrotti M, Kaufman RP Jr, Jennings TA, et al. Endo-rectal coil magnetic resonance imaging in clinically localized prostate cancer: is it accurate? J Urol 1996; 156: 106–109.

118. Kindrick AV, Grossfeld GD, Stier DM, Flanders SC, Henning JM, Carroll PR. Use of imaging tests for staging newly diagnosed prostate cancer: trends from the CaPSURE database. J Urol 1998; 160:2102–2106.

119. O'Dowd GJ, Veltri RW, Orozco R, Miller MC, Oesterling JE. Update on the appropriate staging evaluation for newly diagnosed prostate cancer. J Urol 1997; 158: 687–698.

120. Kurhanewicz J, Swanson MG, Nelson SJ, Vigneron DB. Combined magnetic resonance imaging and spectroscopic imaging approach to molecular imaging of prostate cancer. J Magn Reson Imaging 2002; 16:451–463.

121. Scheidler J, Hricak H, Vigneron DB, et al. Prostate cancer: localization with three-dimensional proton MR spectroscopic imaging—clinicopathologic study. Radiology 1999; 213:473–480.

122. Yu KK, Scheidler J, Hricak H, et al. Prostate cancer: prediction of extracapsular extension with endorectal MR imaging and three-dimensional proton MR spectroscopic imaging. Radiology 1999; 213:481–488.

123. Swanson MG, Vigneron DB, Tran TK, Kurhanewicz J. Magnetic resonance imaging and spectroscopic imaging of prostate cancer. Cancer Invest 2001; 19:510–523.

124. Menard C, Smith IC, Somorjai RL, et al. Magnetic resonance spectroscopy of the malignant prostate gland after radiotherapy: a histopathologic study of diagnostic validity. Int J Radiat Oncol Biol Phys 2001; 50:317–323.

125. Parivar F, Hricak H, Shinohara K, et al. Detection of locally recurrent prostate cancer after cryosurgery: evaluation by transrectal ultrasound, magnetic resonance imaging, and three-dimensional proton magnetic resonance spectroscopy. Urology 1996; 48:594–599.

126. Kurhanewicz J, Vigneron DB, Hricak H, et al. Prostate cancer: metabolic response to cryosurgery as detected with 3D H-1 MR spectroscopic imaging. Radiology 1996; 200:489–496.

127. Swanson MG, Vigneron DB, Tabatabai ZL, et al. Proton HR-MAS spectroscopy and quantitative pathologic analysis of MRI/3D-MRSI-targeted postsurgical prostate tissues. Magn Reson Med 2003; 50:944–954.

128. Kurhanewicz J, Vigneron DB, Nelson SJ, et al. Citrate as an in vivo marker to discriminate prostate cancer from benign prostatic hyperplasia and normal prostate peripheral zone: detection via localized proton spectroscopy. Urology 1995; 45:459–466.

129. Kurhanewicz J, Vigneron DB, Hricak H, Narayan P, Carroll P, Nelson SJ. Three-dimensional H-1 MR spectroscopic imaging of the in situ human prostate with high (0.24–0.7-cm³) spatial resolution. Radiology 1996; 198:795–805.

130. Ackerstaff E, Pflug BR, Nelson JB, Bhujwalla ZM. Detection of increased choline compounds with proton nuclear magnetic resonance spectroscopy subsequent to malignant transformation of human prostatic epithelial cells. Cancer Res 2001; 61:3599–3603.

131. Zakian KL, Eberhardt S, Hricak H, et al. Transition zone prostate cancer: metabolic characteristics at 1H MR spectroscopic imaging—initial results. Radiology 2003; 229:241–247.

132. Bostwick DG, Graham SD Jr, Napalkov P, et al. Staging of early prostate cancer: a proposed tumor volume-based prognostic index. Urology 1993; 41:403–411.

133. Kalbhen CL, Hricak H, Shinohara K, et al. Prostate carcinoma: MR imaging findings after cryosurgery. Radiology 1996; 198:807–811.

134. Hricak H, Schoder H, Pucar D, et al. Advances in imaging in the postoperative patient with a rising prostate-specific antigen level. Semin Oncol 2003; 30:616–634.

135. Fair WR, Aprikian A, Sogani P, Reuter V, Whitmore WF Jr. The role of neoadjuvant hormonal manipulation in localized prostatic cancer. Cancer 1993; 71:1031–1038.

136. Meyer F, Bairati I, Bedard C, Lacombe L, Tetu B, Fradet Y. Duration of neoadjuvant androgen deprivation therapy before radical prostatectomy and disease-free survival in men with prostate cancer. Urology 2001; 58:71–77.

137. Mueller-Lisse UG, Swanson MG, Vigneron DB, et al. Time-dependent effects of hormone-deprivation therapy on prostate metabolism as detected by combined magnetic resonance imaging and 3D magnetic resonance spectroscopic imaging. Magn Reson Med 2001; 46:49–57.

138. Padhani AR, MacVicar AD, Gapinski CJ, et al. Effects of androgen deprivation on prostatic morphology and vascular permeability evaluated with MR imaging. Radiology 2001; 218:365–374.

139. Mueller-Lisse UG, Vigneron DB, Hricak H, et al. Localized prostate cancer: effect of hormone deprivation therapy measured by using combined three-dimensional 1H MR spectroscopy and MR imaging: clinicopathologic case-controlled study. Radiology 2001; 221:380–390.

140. Gibbs P, Tozer DJ, Liney GP, Turnbull LW. Comparison of quantitative T2 mapping and diffusion-weighted imaging in the normal and pathologic prostate. Magn Reson Med 2001; 46:1054–1058.

141. Issa B. In vivo measurement of the apparent diffusion coefficient in normal and malignant prostatic tissues using echo-planar imaging. J Magn Reson Imaging 2002; 16:196–200.

142. Steenbakkers RJ, Deurloo KE, Nowak PJ, Lebesque JV, van Herk M, Rasch CR. Reduction of dose delivered to the rectum and bulb of the penis using MRI delineation for radiotherapy of the prostate. Int J Radiat Oncol Biol Phys 2003; 57:1269–1279.

143. Ling CC, Humm J, Larson S, et al. Towards multidimensional radiotherapy (MD-CRT): biological imaging and biological conformality. Int J Radiat Oncol Biol Phys 2000; 47:551–560.

144. Gossmann A, Okuhata Y, Shames DM, et al. Prostate cancer tumor grade differentiation with dynamic contrast-enhanced MR imaging in the rat: comparison of macromolecular and small-molecular contrast media—preliminary experience. Radiology 1999; 213:265–272.

145. Rasch C, Barillot I, Remeijer P, Touw A, van Herk M, Lebesque JV. Definition of the prostate in CT and MRI: a multi-observer study. Int J Radiat Oncol Biol Phys 1999; 43:57–66.

146. Debois M, Oyen R, Maes F, et al. The contribution of magnetic resonance imaging to the three-dimensional treatment planning of localized prostate cancer. Int J Radiat Oncol Biol Phys 1999; 45:857–865.

147. Kagawa K, Lee WR, Schultheiss TE, Hunt MA, Shaer AH, Hanks GE. Initial clinical assessment of CT-MRI image fusion software in localization of the prostate for 3D conformal radiation therapy. Int J Radiat Oncol Biol Phys 1997; 38:319–325.

148. Mizowaki T, Cohen GN, Fung AY, Zaider M. Towards integrating functional imaging in the treatment of prostate cancer with radiation: the registration of the MR spectroscopy imaging to ultrasound/CT images and its implementation in treatment planning. Int J Radiat Oncol Biol Phys 2002; 54:1558–1564.

149. Jolesz FA. 1996 RSNA Eugene P. Pendergrass New Horizons Lecture. Image-guided procedures and the operating room of the future. Radiology 1997; 204:601–612.

150. Cormack RA, D'Amico AV, Hata N, Silverman S, Weinstein M, Tempany CM. Feasibility of transperineal prostate biopsy under interventional magnetic resonance guidance. Urology 2000; 56:663–664.

151. D'Amico AV, Tempany CM, Cormack R, et al. Transperineal magnetic resonance image guided prostate biopsy. J Urol 2000; 164:385–387.

152. Hata N, Jinzaki M, Kacher D, et al. MR imaging-guided prostate biopsy with surgical navigation software: device validation and feasibility. Radiology 2001; 220:263–268.

153. D'Amico AV, Cormack R, Tempany CM, et al. Real-time magnetic resonance image-guided interstitial brachytherapy in the treatment of select patients with clinically localized prostate cancer. Int J Radiat Oncol Biol Phys 1998; 42:507–515.

154. D'Amico AV, Vogelzang NJ. Prostate brachytherapy: increasing demand for the procedure despite the lack of standardized quality assurance and long term outcome data. Cancer 1999; 86:1632–1634.

155. Ragde H, Blasko JC, Grimm PD, et al. Interstitial iodine-125 radiation without adjuvant therapy in the treatment of clinically localized prostate carcinoma. Cancer 1997; 80:442–453.

156. Wallner K, Roy J, Zelefsky M, Fuks Z, Harrison L. Short-term freedom from disease progression after I-125 prostate implantation. Int J Radiat Oncol Biol Phys 1994; 30:405–409.

157. Dubois DF, Prestidge BR, Hotchkiss LA, Bice WS Jr, Prete JJ. Source localization following permanent transperineal prostate interstitial brachytherapy using magnetic resonance imaging. Int J Radiat Oncol Biol Phys 1997; 39:1037–1041.

158. Amdur RJ, Gladstone D, Leopold KA, Harris RD. Prostate seed implant quality assessment using MR and CT image fusion. Int J Radiat Oncol Biol Phys 1999; 43:67–72.

159. Coakley FV, Hricak H, Wefer AE, Speight JL, Kurhanewicz J, Roach M. Brachytherapy for prostate cancer: endorectal MR imaging of local treatment-related changes. Radiology 2001; 219:817–821.

160. Dubois DF, Prestidge BR, Hotchkiss LA, Prete JJ, Bice WS Jr. Intraobserver and interobserver variability of MR imaging- and CT-derived prostate volumes after transperineal interstitial permanent prostate brachytherapy. Radiology 1998; 207:785–789.
161. Moerland MA, Wijrdeman HK, Beersma R, Bakker CJ, Battermann JJ. Evaluation of permanent I-125 prostate implants using radiography and magnetic resonance imaging. Int J Radiat Oncol Biol Phys 1997; 37:927–933.
162. D'Amico AV, Cormack RA, Tempany CM. MRI-guided diagnosis and treatment of prostate cancer. N Engl J Med 2001; 344:776–777.
163. Cormack RA, Kooy H, Tempany CM, D'Amico AV. A clinical method for real-time dosimetric guidance of transperineal 125I prostate implants using interventional magnetic resonance imaging. Int J Radiat Oncol Biol Phys 2000; 46:207–214.

12

Nuclear Medicine in Nephrourology

A. J. W. Hilson

Department of Nuclear Medicine, Royal Free Hospital, London, U.K.

INTRODUCTION

This chapter considers the present state of some areas of controversy in Nuclear Medicine as applied to the renal tract. It is based on the author's biases but also reflects the views presented by major authorities in the field at the 12th International Committee of Radionuclides in Nephro-Urology meeting on "The Role of Functional Imaging in Nephro-Urology" at La Baule, France, in May 2004, the Society of Nuclear Medicine Meeting in Philadelphia in June 2004, and the International Sentinel Lymph Node Congress in Los Angeles in December 2004. Unreferenced statements are either the author's opinion or based on presentations and discussions at these meetings.

URINARY TRACT INFECTION IN CHILDREN

The "classical" teaching is that acute pyelonephritis is a serious disease that needs treating urgently, not only because the child is sick but also because it may lead to permanent renal scarring and eventually to chronic renal disease. This, in turn, is thought to lead to raised blood pressure and renal failure. The argument is then that early detection and treatment will lead to a reduced incidence of these major complications.

Assuming that this hypothesis is correct, the consensus is that the technetium (Tc)-99m dimercaptosuccinic acid (DMSA) scan is the preferred method of identifying renal parenchymal abnormalities. This needs to be done to high quality, and this requires attention to technique, especially in very young children. The child should not be sedated but reassured by good handling. The equipment should be organized so that there is the minimum separation between the gamma camera and the child (if possible, the child should be actually on the collimator). Posterior and posterior oblique views should be obtained using a high-resolution collimator with a pixel size of 2 mm. There is no benefit in normally positioned kidneys in obtaining an anterior view. However, if only one kidney is visualized in the normal position, it is essential to record images of the entire abdomen.

Single photon emission computed tomography (SPECT) gives further information about the distribution of tracer in the kidney, but it may be misleading in children and should not be used routinely by inexperienced centers. (In adults, it is a useful method of displaying a three-dimensional (3-D) functional map of the kidneys.).

There is disagreement as to the correct timing of the study, and to some extent this depends on the reason for performing the study. In some units, it is felt that confirming the clinical diagnosis of acute pyelonephritis is important, and that, if a parenchymal defect is identified on an acute-phase DMSA study, then this is an indication for admission of the child and treatment with intravenous antibiotics. In this approach, the study should be performed on admission and then repeated later to confirm resolution of the parenchymal defect. It is known from animal studies that this functional defect may persist for several months after the acute infection.

Other units take a more pragmatic view and only perform a late study, arguing that, if this is normal, nothing else is indicated and that the decision as to whether to give intravenous antibiotics should be determined purely on clinical grounds.

Regardless, there is now good evidence that this late study should be performed at least five months after the acute episode, and most units now perform this late study at six months. If this study is abnormal, there is a consensus that the child is at risk of deterioration in renal function. Defects seen at this stage are traditionally referred to as "scars." This is based on animal studies, showing that in acute pyelonephritis produced by direct intrarenal injection of bacteria (or similar models), a permanent scar may be produced.

This takes us to the crux of the current controversy. It is probably only reasonable to refer to "scars" where we have evidence that the kidney was normal prior to the infection and that the defect in parenchymal function has appeared following the infection. This is obviously not a common situation, because very few children with their first apparent urinary tract infection have had a previous DMSA scan. Therefore, when a defect is seen following an infection, we do not know whether we are dealing with a scar that has developed in a previously normal kidney or whether we actually are dealing with a kidney that had an underlying abnormality, which has predisposed that kidney to the infection. There is now considerable evidence that this latter scenario is often correct and that many of these children have an abnormal urinary tract associated with a "dysplastic" or "dysmorphic" kidney. The corollary of this is that the hypothesis, at the start of section, that treatment will lead to a reduction in hypertension and renal failure is likely to be false, because the development of these sequelae is predetermined by the underlying nephrourological abnormality. Indeed, the review of Urinary Tract Infection by the American Academy of Pediatrics (1) specifically makes the point that there is no evidence. Further support comes from Scandinavia, where there has been a long tradition of intensive therapy of acute infection. However, figures from the European Dialysis and Transplant Registry clearly show that the prevalence of end-stage renal failure has not changed dramatically, and the prevalence is similar to that in other European countries.

Therefore, the rationale for DMSA scans is likely to change, and they will be done to identify the kidney at risk of progressive deterioration. In this scenario, my personal view is that we will then change to assessing the single kidney glomerular filtration rate (SKGFR), using the DMSA to look for further focal renal damage as well as the divided function, together with the total GFR from a single-sample Cr-51-ethylenediamine tetraacetic acid (Cr-51-EDTA) clearance performed at the same attendance. From the divided function and the total GFR, the SKGFR may be calculated. This is a practical combination (already used in some centers). The child attends, and is cannulated. The Cr-51-EDTA is injected, followed by the DMSA. The child returns three to four hours later; when the sample is taken for the GFR estimation, the cannula is removed, and the DMSA images are recorded.

VESICOURETERIC REFLUX

The consensus here is that the indirect radionuclide cystogram is the method of choice for follow-up of proven reflux in children who are old enough to cooperate. Because it cannot supply morphological imaging, it cannot exclude abnormal anatomy, especially posterior urethral valves in boys. Therefore it is felt that at least one structural study [micturating cystourethrography (MCUG), with or without urodynamics] should be performed at first presentation. The rationale for follow-up (often not clearly formulated) is that if there is persisting reflux-accompanied urinary tract infections, surgical correction is indicated and will prevent infections, scarring, and deterioration in renal function. It is also often felt necessary to give long-term antibiotic prophylaxis as long as reflux persists. This is based on the experimental work of Risdon and Ransley, which showed that pyelonephritis developed in the setting of reflux, infection, and compound calyces.

However, there are now several studies showing that there is no difference between the outcome, in terms of renal function, whether the children are treated medically or surgically. This has led to a view similar to that discussed above that vesicoureteric reflux is a marker of an abnormal nephrourological system, which may, in a small number of cases, progress to renal failure regardless of intervention. In this view, the demonstration of reflux identifies a urinary tract that is "at-risk."

OBSTRUCTION

This is another area of continuing discussion. Again, the underlying problem is that of the definition of obstruction. My view, which reflects the generality, is that it is important to differentiate acute obstruction from chronic and partial from total. (However, it must be acknowledged that at least one eminent authority feels that "this is rubbish—it's like pregnancy—you can't be a bit pregnant or a bit obstructed!")

The consensus opinion is that in acute total obstruction (such as that produced by occlusion of the ureter by a calculus), nuclear medicine methods have nothing to offer.

Similarly, in chronic obstruction in adults, there is no method available for predicting response to relief of the obstruction.

Where there is an element of consensus, is in chronic partial obstruction, the classical paradigm for which is pelviureteric junction obstruction. Here, the most widely accepted definition is that this condition exists where the outflow from the renal pelvis is unable to cope with the maximum input to which it may be exposed. This is best assessed using a furosemide-induced diuresis. There is considerable evidence that giving the diuretic 15 minutes before the tracer ("F-15") produces a better diuretic response and, therefore, stresses the system to a greater extent. Our experience is that a dose of 40 mgm of furosemide given to a well-hydrated patient may produce a diuresis of over 40 mL/min—more than enough to stress the system. There is now considerable evidence that giving the diuretic at the same time as the tracer gives very similar results and has the advantage that it reduces the number of venepunctures, because the diuretic may be given through the same cannula as the tracer—simplifying the procedure for children. Both give clearer results than the "traditional" approach of giving the diuretic 20 minutes into the study ("F + 20").

Another advance has been the acceptance of more objective measures for quantifying the response to diuresis. The model is the assessment of the "Output Efficiency" of the system (2). Basically, this looks at the output from the kidney as a percentage of the input. A normal kidney puts out over 76% of the activity that enters it within 20 minutes. This has been shown to be a robust parameter.

One area of uncertainty is the cause of the observation that, in neonates and young children, a partially obstructed kidney may show increased rather than decreased uptake of Tc-99m-mercaptoacetyltriglycine (Tc-99m-MAG3) and contribute more than 50% of the divided function. The cause for this is uncertain. The most likely explanation is that, in chronic partial obstruction, there is an increased extraction fraction for Tc-99m-MAG3. This phenomenon probably does not occur with Tc-99m-DMSA.

PET

One of the areas of growth in nuclear medicine is that of positron emission tomography (PET).

This is based on the concept that many biological tracers are difficult to prepare in a radiolabelled form using conventional isotopes, often because they are small molecules and the insertion of a large radioactive atom, such as Tc-99m, I-123, or I-131, changes its behavior significantly. However, there are several low-atomic-number isotopes of potential value, which share the characteristic that they decay by giving off a positron. This particle is a positively charged electron, which only travels a millimetre or so before it meets a (more conventional) negatively charged electron. The two fuse and give off annihilation radiation consisting of two 511 keV gamma rays. These two particles are given off at almost exactly 180° to each other. If these are detected in a suitable machine, it is possible to reconstruct the 3-D distribution of the original activity in the subject. Nowadays, the majority of new machines also have a computed tomography (CT) scanner incorporated (PET/CT), which gives two advantages. First, it allows for accurate correction of the PET images for the effect of attenuation by the body tissues, and the necessary data can be acquired in two minutes, rather than the 20 minutes necessary with older methods. Second because the two sets of images are intrinsically aligned, it allows for accurate localization of sites of increased uptake.

The most widely used tracer in applications of interest to urogenital imaging is F^{18}-fluorodeoxyglucose (FDG). This is a substituted sugar, which is taken into cells through glucose transporters (mainly glucose transporter type 1), then metabolized by hexokinase, but it cannot pass further along the metabolic chain. Its concentration therefore reflects the metabolic activity of the cells. Many tumors have increased glucose uptake and, therefore, concentrate FDG. Normal uptake is seen in tissues that predominantly rely on glucose for their metabolic activity—especially the brain and heart—and also in muscle. It is excreted via the kidneys into urine, which may present problems. The tracer has to be prepared at a center that has a cyclotron, but these are now relatively widespread, and there are networks for the distribution of the radiotracer that has a half-life of just under two hours.

In testicular cancer, there is usually avid uptake of FDG, more so with seminomas than nonseminomas, and it appears to be an accurate method of staging, although probably not more so than CT. However, it is considerably more accurate than CT in restaging after chemotherapy, although early imaging after chemotherapy (within two weeks) may produce some false positives as a result of increase in inflammation. If necessary, it can be used for targeting biopsy. It is also more accurate than CT in detecting recurrence.

In cervical cancer, FDG-PET seems to be more accurate than CT or magnetic resonance imaging (MRI) in detecting lymph node metastases; and in a multivariate analysis, the most significant determinant of progression-free survival is the presence of positive para-aortic lymph nodes on an FDG-PET scan. It also appears to be the most accurate method of detecting recurrent and metastatic disease.

In ovarian cancer, PET has been shown to be accurate in restaging for lesions more than 5 mm in size but may miss smaller lesions and disseminated disease.

FDG-PET has not yet been shown to be of value in prostate or bladder cancer, partially because of physiological excretion via the urinary tract and also because of relatively low uptake. Studies are in progress using labeled amino acids, which seem promising.

PROSTASCINT™

This is a monoclonal antibody (originally known as CYT-356) to the prostatic surface membrane antigen. It is labeled with In-111. The approved name is capromab pendetide.

This antigen is thought to occur only at the surface of "metabolically" prostate cells. Therefore, under normal conditions, localization should only occur in the prostate. Any accumulation outside the prostate must logically be in metastatic cancer deposits. The acquisition of the data is not simple. Because it is a large molecule, localization is slow, and imaging is performed at 72 or 96 hours, with repeat images 24 or 48 hours later, if the findings are uncertain. The analysis of the images is also complex, as there is considerable blood pool activity. Typically, this requires acquisition of a separate set of images of the blood pool using Tc-99m-red blood cells.

In a series of 181 studies in patients with a rising prostate-specific antigen (PSA) after radical prostatectomy, focal accumulation was seen localized to the prostatic fossa in 34% of the cases, to abdominal lymph nodes in 23%, and to pelvic nodes in 22%. Forty-two percent of these patients had localization outside the prostatic fossa. Half of the localizations in the prostatic fossa were confirmed by biopsy (3).

Obviously, it would be of value if this method could be used for initial staging of high-risk prostate cancer.

When compared with surgical lymphadenectomy specimens in a series of 31 patients, the sensitivity, specificity, positive predictive value (PPV), negative predictive value (NPV), and accuracy of the scan were 94%, 42%, 53%, 92%, and 65%, respectively, when analyzed by surgical site and 100%, 33%, 62%, 100%, and 68%, respectively, analyzed by patient (4).

In another study of 160 patients, in 152 evaluable patients, the sensitivity was 72%, the specificity 62%, the PPV 62%, and the NPV 72%. In the same patients, the sensitivity of CT and MRI was 4% and 15%, respectively (5).

In a series of 198 patients with clinical high-risk T2 or T3 disease, 39% had pelvic lymph node deposits on pathology. The Prostascint™ study had a PPV of 67% (6).

The same group have also reported (7), on a series of studies in high-risk patients prior to pelvic lymph node dissection, a PPV of 62%, an NPV of 72%, sensitivity of 62%, and a specificity of 72%; for prostatic bed recurrence, using needle biopsy as the reference, the figures were PPV of 50%, NPV of 70%, sensitivity of 49%, and specificity of 71%.

However, in a group of 22 patients with less extensive disease—lower PSA values and lower Gleason scores—who had bilateral pelvic and obturator node resections at the time of surgery, the accuracy was lower (8). Nine of the 88 node basins were positive on the Prostascint[TM] study, but only one (11%) was histologically involved. Of 79 scan-negative node groups, five were involved, giving a sensitivity of 17%, a specificity of 90%, NPV of 94%, and PPV of 11% (8).

It is this problem of identifying the accuracy of localization that is at the heart of trying to assess the value of this agent. There is some indirect evidence of accuracy of localization. In a group of 32 patients with prostate cancer who had a Prostascint[TM] study and then had salvage radiotherapy to the pelvis, sixteen out of 23 (70%) men with a normal scan outside the prostatic fossa achieved a durable complete response, compared to two of nine (22%) who had a positive scan outside the prostatic fossa and pelvis (9).

A potentially useful approach to improving accuracy has recently been reported (10). These authors used fusion of the Prostascint[TM] volume dataset with CT and MR datasets. Fifty-eight patients were studied. Seventy-four of 161 sites of reported uptake on the Prostascint[TM] study were found to be negative after fusion, corresponding to normal tissue, such as bowel, vessel, or bone marrow. In two patients, nodal disease was identified on the fused data only. Twenty-five patients previously thought to have nodal disease appeared to have only local disease after fusion. Obviously one problem is that there is no external verification of the results, but the numbers are compatible with the reported accuracy in other studies. This also reflects the experience in improved accuracy from fusion of datasets in PET (see below). These authors used CT and MRI datasets acquired separately, but it is of interest that the major manufacturers of nuclear medicine equipment are now producing gamma cameras with built-in CT systems.

For the moment, it appears that Prostascint[TM] is of moderate value in localizing recurrence but is not sufficiently reliable for initial staging prior to curative therapy.

SENTINEL NODE LOCALIZATION

The concept of the sentinel node is one that is becoming accepted as being valuable in several groups of cancers. The hypothesis is that lymphatic drainage of tumors occurs in an orderly manner. The first node draining any lymphatic pathway is regarded as the sentinel node, in that any tumor dissemination along this pathway will occur via this node. Therefore, if this node is not involved with metastatic tumor, then nodes more distal to the tumor along this pathway will not be involved. For instance, in carcinoma of the breast, if the sentinel node is identified and removed and if it shows no tumor, the probability of axillary recurrence of tumor in major series is only 5/1543, even without axillary clearance. This means that in these patients there is less surgery, markedly reduced morbidity, and less expense. Similarly, in malignant melanoma, the technique is used to identify the sentinel node, which is then sampled. Freedom from metastasis is strongly predictive of a longer recurrence-free period, again without the need to do a block lymph node dissection.

The usual technique uses a combination of a radioactive colloid and a blue dye. Prior to surgery, the radioactive colloid is injected adjacent to the tumor, and its pattern of drainage imaged with a gamma camera ("Lymphoscintigraphy"). The first node in the drainage pathway is identified and marked on the skin. The patient then goes for surgery, and at the start of the procedure, a blue dye is injected in or around the tumor. This tracks rapidly along lymphatic channels, making them easier for the surgeon to identify. Knowing where the sentinel node lies, the surgeon tracks the lymphatic channel to the node. This is identified using a radiation probe. In the jargon, the node must be "blue and hot." The imaging is necessary because the pattern of lymphatic drainage may be very variable.

The node(s) removed is subjected to more detailed histopathological examination, which is feasible because only a limited number of nodes are being examined. One area of uncertainty that this leads to is that, with the more detailed examination, more lymph node metastases are detected. Conventionally, these are separated into "macrometastases" that exceed 2 mm in diameter and correspond to those deposits found on traditional histological assessment; "micrometastases" less than 2 mm in diameter, which may be found on the multiple thinner sections found in this approach; and "isolated tumor cells."

In general surgery, the technique is now being assessed in head-and-neck cancer, upper gastrointestinal, and colorectal tumors.

The technique is being used in some urogenital tumors.

In cervical cancer, the technique has been applied, using an endoscopic gamma probe after injection of blue dye and colloid and followed by endoscopic lymphadenectomy at the time of surgery. The numbers are small, but the technique appears feasible.

In vulvar cancer, the approach appears to work, and data are awaited.

In penile cancer, a study of 121 T2-3N0 patients in whom regional lymph node dissection was only performed if the sentinel lymph node was positive, the five-year disease-specific survival was 96% in sentinel-node negative patients and 66% in sentinel-node positive patients. The sentinel-node status was the strongest independent prognostic factor for survival. In a separate study, a comparison of sentinel-node histology with the findings at radical inguinal lymphadenectomy showed a 100% NPV and 90% sensitivity. A refinement to this technique is to use fine needle aspiration cytology of the suspicious inguinal nodes under ultrasound control. If this is positive, then it is reasonable to proceed directly to inguinal dissection, reserving the sentinel-node procedure for the remainder.

In prostate cancer, the accuracy of the sentinel-node approach has been tested in a series of 41 patients, with extended pelvic lymph node dissection as the gold standard. Eight patients had macrometastases, and four had micrometastases. If only the sentinel-node had been examined, the sensitivity, specificity, and false-negative rate would have been 92%, 98%, and 8%, respectively. Recording the localization of the sentinel node in three dimensions using SPECT, then fusing the image to a CT scan allows better localization and permits the use of endoscopic minilaparotomy for the prostatic resection. This approach also looks promising in bladder cancer.

REFERENCES

1. Downs SM. Practice parameter: the diagnosis, treatment, and evaluation of the initial urinary tract infection in febrile infants and young children. American Academy of Pediatrics. Committee on Quality Improvement. Subcommittee on Urinary Tract Infection. Pediatrics 1999; 103(4 Pt 1):843–852.

2. Chaiwatanarat T, Padhy AK, Bomanji JB, Nimmon CC, Sonmezoglu K, Britton KE. Validation of renal output efficiency as an objective quantitative parameter in the evaluation of upper urinary tract obstruction. J Nucl Med 1993; 34:845–848.

3. Deb N, Goris M, Trisler K, et al. Treatment of hormone-refractory prostate cancer with 90Y-CYT-356 monoclonal antibody. Clin Cancer Res 1996; 2(8):1289–1297.

4. Bermejo CE, Coursey J, Basler J, Austenfeld M, Thompson I. Histologic confirmation of lesions identified by Prostascint scan following definitive treatment. Urol Oncol 2003; 21(5):349–352.

5. Manyak MJ, Hinkle GH, Olsen JO, et al. Immunoscintigraphy with indium-111-capromab pendetide: evaluation before definitive therapy in patients with prostate cancer. Urology 1999; 54(6):1058–1063.

6. Polascik TJ, Manyak MJ, Haseman MK, et al. Comparison of clinical staging algorithms and 111indium-capromab pendetide immunoscintigraphy in the prediction of lymph node involvement in high risk prostate carcinoma patients. Cancer 1999; 85(7): 1586–1592.

7. Rosenthal SA, Haseman MK, Polascik TJ. Utility of capromab pendetide (ProstaScint) imaging in the management of prostate cancer. Tech Urol 2001; 7(1):27–37.

8. Ponsky LE, Cherullo EE, Starkey R, Nelson D, Neumann D, Zippe CD. Evaluation of preoperative ProstaScint scans in the prediction of nodal disease. Prostate Cancer Prostatic Dis 2002; 5(2):132–135.

9. Kahn D, Williams RD, Haseman MK, Reed NL, Miller SJ, Gerstbrein J. Radioimmunoscintigraphy with In-111-labeled capromab pendetide predicts prostate cancer response to salvage radiotherapy after failed radical prostatectomy. J Clin Oncol 1998; 16(1):284–289.

10. Schettino CJ, Kramer EL, Noz ME, Taneja S, Padmanabhan P, Lepor H. Impact of fusion of indium-111 capromab pendetide volume data sets with those from MRI or CT in patients with recurrent prostate cancer. Am J Roentgenol 2004; 183(2): 519–524.

13

Percutaneous Interventions in the Urinary Tract

Parvati Ramchandani
Department of Radiology, University of Pennsylvania Medical Center, Philadelphia, Pennsylvania, U.S.A.

INTRODUCTION

Percutaneous interventional procedures are widely used in the upper urinary tract. This chapter addresses the most commonly performed procedures—percutaneous nephrostomy (PCN), ureteral stenting and dilation, interventions in obstructed renal transplants, and interventions for upper urinary tract stone disease.

PCN

First performed to relieve urinary obstruction half a century ago (1), PCN is currently also used to gain access to the collecting system for therapeutic and diagnostic procedures and to divert urine and allow the closure of a ureteral fistula or a dehiscent urinary tract anastomosis. The frequency with which the procedure is performed for these different indication varies in different institutions.

Drainage of Obstructed Urinary Tract

Radiologists perform the majority (nearly 74%) of upper urinary tract decompressions (2), even in this era of turf battles and attempts to increase market share by different specialties. The remainder of the decompressions are mostly performed by urologists. Although urologist-initiated renal access is often a prelude to stone removal [percutaneous nephrostolithotomy (PCNL)], the availability of C-arm fluoroscopy units in operating rooms and ultrasound machines in urology departments allows urologists to perform PCN for decompression of the collecting systems as well (3,4). However, Bird et al. found that only 11% of urologists performing PCNL created the PCN access themselves (5).

PCN is most often requested in patients after imaging studies demonstrate hydroureteronephrosis. These studies may indicate the etiology, as well as the anatomic level, of the obstruction. In one series that studied patients with urinary obstruction who underwent PCN (6), calculus disease was responsible for obstruction in 26% of patients and malignancy in 61%, with carcinoma of the bladder, cervix, and colon being the most common primary tumors to cause urinary obstruction. When ureteral obstruction results in renal impairment, noncontrast computed tomography (CT) appears to be the best imaging modality to identify a calculus as a cause of obstruction whereas magnetic resonance urography (MRU) is superior for identifying noncalculus causes of obstruction (Fig. 1A,B) (7,8). In patients with normal renal function, contrast-enhanced CT can identify the presence and cause of hydronephrosis in nearly all cases (9). MRU is particularly helpful in delineating the anatomy in patients with urinary diversion to bowel conduits (10).

In a chronically obstructed kidney that appears to be either nonfunctioning or poorly functioning, renal drainage by PCN may allow the assessment of residual recoverable function so that one can determine whether a kidney is worth salvaging. Kidneys that contribute 15% to 20% of overall renal function after relief of obstruction are usually deemed to be worth salvaging (11). The presence of renal parenchymal atrophy on CT or renal ultrasonography does not necessarily predict a poor potential for functional recovery after drainage with a PCN. In patients with bilateral obstruction due to an underlying malignancy, imaging studies can help determine which kidney is less obstructed and has a larger amount of residual renal parenchyma. If unilateral PCN is performed in such patients, drainage of the less affected kidney may be more effective in restoring renal function to baseline (Fig. 1D).

Technique of PCN

A drainage catheter placed through a retrograde approach, usually cystoscopy, is the preferred method to provide renal drainage in all patients, because it avoids the complications inherent in a PCN. The percutaneous route should ideally be reserved for patients in whom retrograde attempts are either unsuccessful or not feasible (11).

Preprocedural Evaluation

Preprocedural evaluation in patients being considered for PCN includes assessing the risk for bleeding and procedure-related infection. The surgical and medical literature does not support routine laboratory coagulation screening in all patients (12–14), but radiologists vary in their practices. Some advise routine testing of all patients undergoing invasive procedures (15), whereas others believe that it is sufficient to carefully question the patient for bleeding history, known liver disease, renal failure, use of antiplatelet drugs, and anticoagulant use to identify those with a potential increased risk for bleeding complications (16). Postponing an emergent PCN to wait for laboratory results is generally not believed to be necessary (17).

Correction of abnormal coagulation is needed if international normalized ratios (INR, which is used to standardize reporting of prothrombin time) and activated partial thromboplastin time (PTT) are greater than 1.5 times the normal range (13). Fresh frozen plasma (FFP) will correct congenital factor deficiency and acquired coagulopathy. The corrective effect lasts only six hours; hence the procedure has to be appropriately timed with the FFP infusion. If patients are on heparin, discontinuing the infusion and waiting two to three hours to perform the procedure is often sufficient because heparin has a half-life of 60 minutes (longer in patients with liver disease) (13). Abnormalities related to coumadin use can be corrected with

(A) (B)

(C) (D)

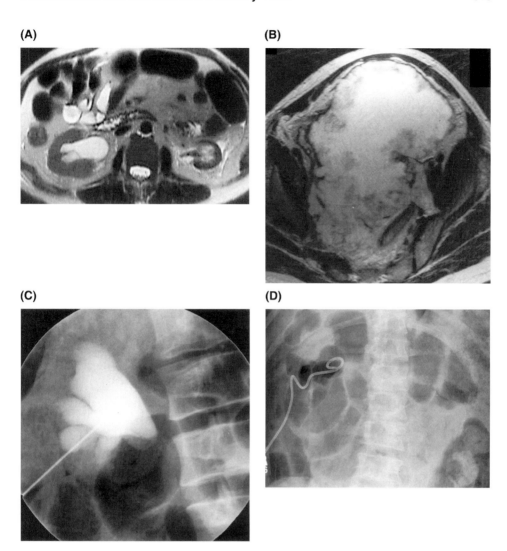

Figure 1 A 24-year-old man with renal insufficiency due to bilateral ureteral obstruction by a large pelvic mass. (**A**) Axial T2-weighted MRI image through the kidneys demonstrates hydronephrosis of the right collecting system. The left kidney is atrophic. Other images demonstrated a dilated left ureter, indicating that the left renal atrophy was likely due to hydronephrotic atrophy from obstruction. (**B**) Axial T2-weighted MRI image through the pelvis demonstrates a large pelvic sarcoma. Other images (not shown) demonstrated marked compression of the urinary bladder. The ureteral orifices could not be identified at cystoscopy. (**C**) Contrast injection through a needle placed for PCN demonstrates right hydronephrosis. The procedure was performed with ultrasound guidance (not shown). (**D**) A self-retaining loop nephrostomy catheter was placed to drain the right kidney. Because the patient's disease was unresectable, only a unilateral right nephrostomy was performed. There was subsequent improvement in renal function. *Abbreviations*: MRI, magnetic resonance imaging; PCN, percutaneous nephrostomy.

vitamin K1 or FFP administration (13). Most interventionalists do not postpone invasive procedures in patients who have taken aspirin or other drugs known to interfere with platelet function, such as nonsteroidal anti-inflammatory drugs and the newer betalactam antibiotics (13). Platelet transfusion will correct drug-induced

prolongation of the bleeding time, if needed. Farrell and Hicks reported that a platelet count less than $100,000/dL$ (6) was a significant risk factor for bleeding and was
associated with a higher transfusion rate after PCN. However a platelet count
greater than $50,000/dL$ is believed to be a safe value for most patients (13).

Septicemia is less common with genitourinary interventions than with biliary
procedures, but the risk of periprocedural sepsis is increased in the elderly, in dia-
betics, in patients with indwelling catheters, stones, or ureterointestinal anastomosis,
or in the clinical presence of infection (18,19). The organisms that commonly infect
the genitourinary tract are gram-negative rods, such as *Escherichia coli*, Proteus,
Klebsiella, and enterococcus. Antibiotic prophylaxis should ideally be based on culture results, but broad-spectrum antibiotics active against the common urinary
pathogens, such as aminoglycosidae (e.g., gentamycin) in conjunction with ampicil-
lin or cefazolin, or ceftriaxone (20), can be used in the absence of culture results.
Antibiotics are best administered immediately prior to or less than two hours before
the procedure (20). If given more than three hours prior to the procedure, the incidence of adverse infectious events increases fivefold (21). Antibiotic administration
should be continued till satisfactory renal drainage is assured (20,22,23). Cochran
et al. (22) reported that prophylactic antibiotics were beneficial in decreasing the
development of sepsis in patients at high or low risk for developing sepsis.

PCNs are often performed as an inpatient procedure. When performed on an
outpatient basis, 12% to 25% of patients may require admission to the hospital after
the procedure because of such complications as bleeding or sepsis (16). Patients who
may not be suitable candidates for outpatient PCN include those with hypertension,
untreated urinary tract infection, coagulopathy, and staghorn calculi (16,22).

Periprocedural Monitoring

Standard measures, such as continuous electrocardiogram monitoring during the
procedure, and large-bore and secure intravenous access are routinely used. Intravenous sedation combined with local anesthesia is sufficient to keep most patients
comfortable. Use of transcutaneous oximetry is also recommended.

Procedure

The patients are positioned in either a prone or a prone-oblique position with the
ipsilateral side elevated 20° to 30°; however, if the patient cannot lie prone, the procedure can be performed with the patient in a supine-oblique position. CT guidance
is particularly helpful in the latter situation, allowing the completion of the procedure in 81% of patients in one series where a hybrid CT–fluoroscopy unit was used
(24). In this study (24), the initial puncture was performed with CT guidance and the
subsequent manipulations for catheter placement were performed using fluoroscopic
guidance. Preprocedural CT or magnetic resonance (MR) scanning is highly recommended in patients with an aberrant anatomy (e.g., severe scoliosis or congenital
renal abnormalities such as a horseshoe kidney) so that the relationship of the kidney
to the liver, spleen, colon, gallbladder, and pleural space can be determined.

In most patients, the collecting system is localized using either fluoroscopy or
ultrasound (US) guidance. When the collecting system is moderately or severely
dilated, US guidance is successful in aiding entry into the collecting system in 85%
to 95% of patients. Conversely, in only mildly dilated collecting systems, the success
rate may be as low as 50% (25). Regardless of the degree of renal collecting system
dilatation, if renal function is poor (the usual case with obstruction) or if contrast

cannot be administered, US guidance, preferably real-time, is the preferred way to localize the collecting system.

Once the collecting system has been punctured, the remainder of the procedure is usually performed using fluoroscopic guidance alone, although there are reports of using sonography alone for the entire procedure (26).

Fluoroscopic guidance can be used to enter the collecting system if a prior urographic study is available for guidance, if there is an opaque calyceal calculus that can serve as the target for puncture (Fig. 2B,D), or if the collecting system can be opacified with contrast (either by excretion after intravenous administration or by means of a retrograde catheter) (Fig. 3A,B). Blind punctures of the kidney using anatomic landmarks, such as the "lumbar notch" (27,28), are apt to require multiple punctures for optimal entry in as many as 40% of cases, and should be measures of last resort in modern radiology departments where the availability of ultrasound can facilitate appropriate and safe puncture of the collecting system with the fewest number of attempts.

Numerous techniques have been described for PCN placement (6,15,16,27,29,30), all of which entail imaging and puncturing the collecting system, dilating the tract, and then placing a catheter. Planning the puncture site is a crucial step in the procedure. The skin puncture site is chosen so that the catheter enters the flank in the posterior axillary line and courses subcostally below the inferior margin of the 12th rib. This is done to minimize the chance of injury to the intercostal artery located on the inferior margin of the rib and also to decrease the chance of intercostal nerve irritation, which can be very painful. If the intercostal space between the 11th and 12th ribs must be used for the procedure, care should be taken to stay close to the superior aspect of the 12th rib to avoid the neurovascular bundle. The puncture and, therefore, the nephrostomy tract should traverse the renal parenchyma before entering the collecting system so that the parenchyma can provide a secure seal around the catheter.

Entry into the collecting system should ideally be into a posteriorly directed calyx through the relatively avascular posterolateral plane of the kidney, the so-called avascular plane/line of Brodel. This is the zone where the renal artery divides into its major ventral and dorsal branches and lies at the junction of the anterior two-thirds and posterior one-third of the kidney, just posterior to the lateral convex border of the kidney. The posterior calyces point to this plane and can be identified as the more medially positioned calyces. Entry into the posterior calyces minimizes the risk of entering the large vessels in the renal hilum. If PCN is being performed for drainage alone, virtually any posterior calyx can be suitable for access, although an interpolar or lower polar posterior calyx is usually chosen. However, if PCN is to be followed by ureteral stent insertion, an interpolar calyceal entry is preferable so that the vector of pushing forces can be directed toward the ureteropelvic junction. Access through the upper pole calyces may be required in patients with stones, in which case an intercostal tract may be needed.

Once the puncture site is chosen, local anesthesia is liberally administered into the skin site and throughout the proposed track to the level of the renal fascia.

A variety of puncture sets using coaxial needles and/or sheaths are commercially available for the procedure. After localization, the collecting system is initially punctured with thin-walled, flexible, 21- or 22-gauge needles. A sample of urine is withdrawn and sent for culture, if necessary. A small amount of contrast is then injected to confirm the needle position and to determine the calyceal entry site. In a dilated and obstructed collecting system, an attempt should be made to decompress the collecting system before contrast injection, to avoid overdistension and possible sepsis. If the initial entry point into the collecting system is not optimal, a second

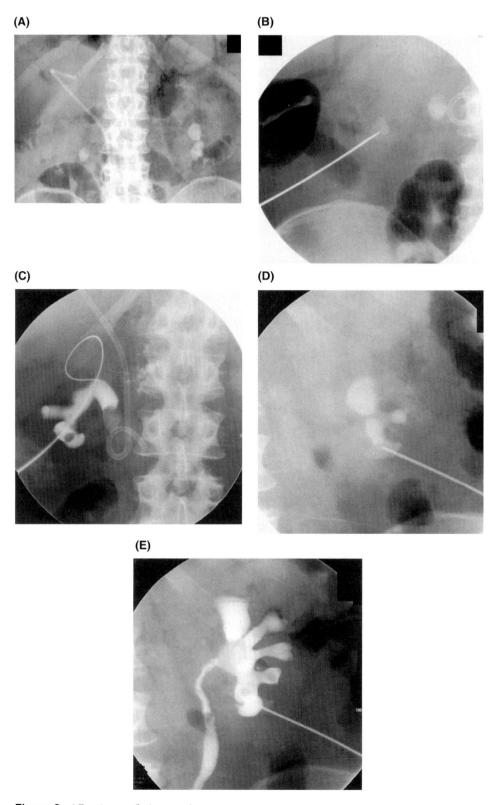

Figure 2 (*Caption on facing page*)

puncture is performed into the desired calyx; the first needle is not removed, to avoid decompression of the collecting system through the needle site and to provide a route for continuing opacification of the collecting system (Fig. 4).

In patients undergoing nephrostomy for subsequent stone removal, initial puncture with 18-gauge needles is preferable because they are less flexible and thus easier to direct into the desired calyx than smaller gauge needles. Puncture of the renal infundibula or pelvis should be avoided because there is a high risk of injury to the interlobar vessels and the major segmental branches of the renal artery and vein. Sampaio et al. found that punctures through the calyceal fornix were highly unlikely to cause renal arterial injury, whereas infundibular punctures lacerated interlobar or segmental arteries in 23% of cases and direct renal pelvic punctures caused injury to a large retropelvic vessel in 33% of cases (Fig. 4C) (31).

After advancing a guidewire through the needle, the nephrostomy track is dilated with fascial dilators to one size larger than the intended nephrostomy catheter, and the nephrostomy catheter is then placed. A self-retaining catheter is preferable, and these may be of a pigtail, accordion, Malecot, or Foley type. A "self-retaining" loop-type catheter (Cope loop catheter) in used in most cases because it is less prone to being inadvertently withdrawn than are the Malecot and Foley catheters (Fig. 1D).

Contraindications

The only absolute contraindication to PCN is the presence of an uncorrectable bleeding disorder; however, if the bleeding diathesis is due to a coagulopathy caused by urosepsis, urinary drainage will be necessary before the bleeding abnormality can be corrected. If there are severe electrolyte changes because of the obstructive uropathy (e.g., hyperkalemia with serum potassium levels above $7\,mEq/L$), emergency hemodialysis and/or ion exchange therapy should be considered before PCN to quickly correct the electrolyte abnormalities, because the cardioplegia associated with hyperkalemia can be refractory to all therapy.

Results

PCN catheter placement is successful in 98% to 99% of patients with obstructed dilated kidneys (6,17,30,32). Success rates are lower, in the range of 91% to 92%, when sonography alone is used for the procedure (26,33). In nondilated systems or in complex stone cases, 85% to 90% success rates have been reported (34,35).

Lee et al. (17) analyzed the outcomes of emergency nephrostomies performed by radiologists with different levels of experience. All operators performed a minimum of 10 PCNs a year. Although all the operators successfully placed drainage

---

Figure 2 (*Figure on facing page*) Bilateral renal calculi in a 65-year-old man. (**A**) Plain radiograph of the abdomen demonstrates bilateral renal calculi, with partial staghorn configuration on the left. (**B**) Fluoroscopic guidance was used to target the right lower pole stone-bearing calyx for puncture. Note the second stone adjacent to the spine, which was located in the proximal ureter. A pigtail catheter medial to the kidney is in the biliary system in this patient who has had a liver transplant. (**C**) Contrast injection demonstrates that the proximal ureteral stone is causing obstruction. The lower pole stone is seen as a filling defect in the opacified collecting system. (**D**) Fluoroscopic guidance was also used to puncture the lower pole stone-bearing calyx of the left kidney. (**E**) Nephrostogram demonstrates the left staghorn calculus as a filling defect in the opacified renal pelvis and the lower pole calyces and infundibula.

(A)

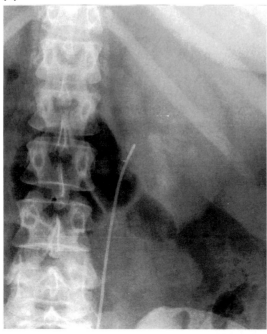

(B)

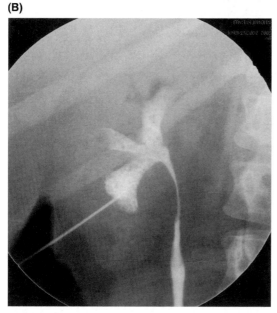

Figure 3 A 58-year-old woman who failed SWL for a left renal calculus. (**A**) Plain film demonstrates very faintly opaque calculus fragments coating the lower pole calyces and infundibulae. The patient had previously undergone SWL for a large left renal calculus (not shown). Note the retrograde catheter, which was placed so that contrast could be injected to facilitate the PCN placement. (**B**) Prone retrograde pyelogram shows innumerable stone fragments throughout the left pyelocalyceal system (patient is prone). PCN was performed through a lower pole calyx, and all fragments were successfully removed. *Abbreviations*: PCN, percutaneous nephrostomy; SWL, shock wave lithotripsy.

(A)

(B)

(C)

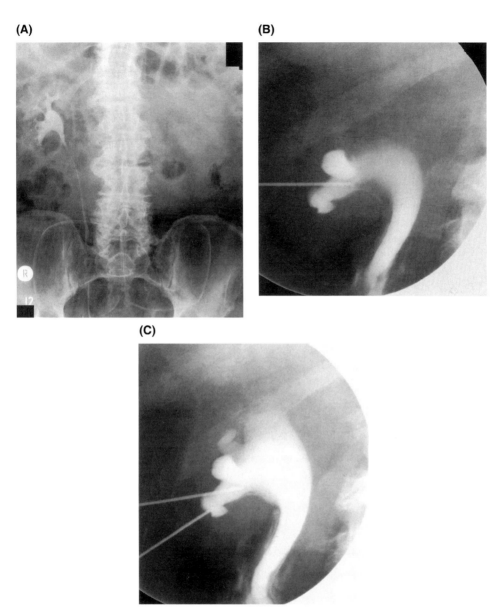

Figure 4 A 65-year-old man who had ureteroscopic removal of a distal left ureteral calculus. (**A**) IVU one month following ureteroscopy shows no excretion from left kidney due to high-grade obstruction. The patient was asymptomatic, and the IVU was a routine follow-up study after ureteroscopy. (**B**) Using ultrasound guidance, the collecting system was punctured. Contrast injection opacifies the hydronephrotic left collecting system (patient is prone). Note that the needle enters the collecting system in the lower pole infundibulum, a site that is unsuitable for catheter placement. (**C**) Fluoroscopic guidance was used to enter a lower pole calyx. Note that the initial needle is left in place to inject contrast and prevent decompression of the collecting system. The drainage catheter was placed through the lower pole entry site. *Abbreviation*: IVU, intravenous urogram.

catheters on an emergent basis, mean procedure and fluoroscopy times were significantly longer for the more inexperienced radiologists (fluoroscopy and procedure times of 2 and 25 minutes for experienced operators and 10 and 42 minutes for inexperienced operators). Further, 20% to 33% of the procedures performed by inexperienced operators were repeated the next day because of catheter dislodgment or malposition, and emergency PCNs by less experienced radiologists resulted in higher rates of postprocedure sepsis and transfusions.

Also, Lewis and Patel (36) found that proportionately more complications occurred when the procedures were performed after working hours rather than during regular working hours (5.7% vs. 1.8%). Because many patients who have nephrostomies after working hours may be sicker and have more complicated medical conditions than do those patients undergoing elective procedures, it is essential that appropriate staff and equipment be available at all hours to provide a consistently high level of care at all times (15,37).

When obstruction is complicated by urosepsis or azotemia, the response to renal decompression is often immediate, with fever and flank pain improving in 24 to 48 hours after PCN drainage (38). When obstruction and infection are due to ureteral calculi, retrograde ureteral catheterization and PCN are equally effective in relieving the obstruction and infection, with neither technique superior to the other in promoting rapid drainage or clinical defervescence (39). However, percutaneous manipulations themselves can precipitate septicemia (manifested as shaking chills and fever) in these patients. For this reason, it is important that these patients be treated with intravenous antibiotics before the attempted PCN. In addition, forceful opacification of the collecting system to visualize the site and cause of obstruction should be deferred until the collecting system has been adequately decompressed for 24 to 48 hours and the patient is afebrile. In patients with fungal urinary infections, topical antibiotics can be directly infused into the kidneys if systemic toxicity prevents achieving effective therapeutic levels by parenteral administration. Obstructing fungus balls can also be extracted through the nephrostomy tract (40).

In patients with azotemia secondary to obstruction, PCN can rapidly return renal function to normal or near normal levels. In one series (41) renal function normalized in 66% of patients in 15 days, and improved enough to obviate dialysis in 28%. The mean number of days needed for normalization of renal function was 7.7 ± 4.1 days. Patients with benign causes of obstruction or gynecologic malignancies showed the best improvement, whereas older patients and those with prostate cancer showed the least improvement in their renal function. PCN can also be a temporizing measure to improve or at least preserve renal function while other therapies, such as radiation or chemotherapy, are given time to reverse malignant causes of obstruction. PCN drainage may also be required to optimize renal function before definitive surgery or to allow the administration of nephrotoxic drugs such as cisplatin.

In patients with malignancies, the ureters can be obstructed by contiguous involvement or direct extrinsic compression. The need for external nephrostomy drainage is often permanent in such patients because ureteral stents often fail in adequately draining patients with extrinsic obstruction (42,43). Even with careful patient selection, 32% of patients are unable to achieve any improvement in the quality of life after PCN (44). Long-term survival after palliative diversion for malignant ureteral obstruction is poor. In one series (45), only 25% of patients were alive at one year, and in another series (46), patients with ureteral obstruction secondary to bladder cancer had a mean survival of only 4.9 months (1–14 months). If a PCN is performed in these circumstances, only unilateral drainage is usually required.

Bilateral nephrostomy usually confers no added benefit (41). In patients with bilateral obstruction due to malignancies, a reasonable approach is to drain the symptomatic side, if there is one, or to drain the kidney that appears to have more preserved renal parenchyma, as gauged by cross-sectional imaging (Fig. 1) (15). The contralateral kidney is then drained only if there is suspected infection or if unilateral drainage does not improve renal function enough to allow for administration of any necessary chemotherapy.

Complications

The Standards of Practice Document by the Society of Cardiovascular and Interventional Radiology and an American College of Radiology (ACR) practice guideline for the performance of PCN provide guidelines and thresholds for complications associated with PCN (47,48). The overall serious complication rate of PCN is low, with a mortality of 0.2% compared to a surgical mortality of 6.0% (6).

Complications related to PCN (6,30,32,47,48) can be divided into major, procedure-related complications (4% to 6% incidence) and minor complications (10% to 28% incidence). Major complications include hemorrhage and sepsis.

Major Complication: Hemorrhage. Hemorrhage requiring transfusion or other therapy occurs in 1.0% to 2.4% of patients (6,32,49) and is usually related to renal arterial pseudoaneurysms or arteriovenous fistulas due to laceration of lobar arteries. Using small-needle access systems (21- or 22-gauge needle) may be no safer than 18-gauge needle systems (50). However, avoiding puncture of the anteromedial renal vessels by accessing the kidney through its relatively avascular posterolateral aspect (Brodel's line) may decrease the incidence of this complication (27,51).

Most hemorrhages associated with nephrostomy placement are transient and self-limited. It is not uncommon to have pink or slightly bloody urine drainage for several days after a nephrostomy, and this is not considered a complication. Serious vascular trauma is suspected if the urine continues to be grossly bloody after three to five days, if new intrapelvic clots are observed on nephrostograms, or if there is a significant drop in the hematocrit. If the drop in the hematocrit is out of proportion to the urine blood loss, a retroperitoneal hematoma should be suspected and a CT scan obtained. Unsuspected retroperitoneal hematomas not requiring treatment have been reported in 13% of patients on CT scans performed after nephrostomy tube placement (52). Angiography and possible arterial embolization should be considered in patients who have significant continuous or recurrent bleeding for longer than four to five days after PCN placement (49).

Major Complication: Sepsis. The incidence of sepsis after nephrostomy tube placement has been reported to be 1.4% to 21.0% (6,15,22,38). This wide variation is likely due to the differing definitions of sepsis in different series. Farrell and Hicks (6) reported that 1.3% of their patients required observation in the intensive care unit for sepsis or hypotension. The use of antibiotic-bonded nephrostomy catheters appears to have no influence on the overall incidence of infective complications associated with nephrostomy drainage (53).

Air embolism has been reported in patients in whom air was injected through a retrograde catheter (pneumopyelogram) to visualize the collecting system (54). Using CO_2 rather than air as a negative contrast in the collecting system can avoid this complication.

Other Major Complications: Bowel and Splenic Injuries. Inadvertent injury of adjacent organs is uncommon, with no such complications observed in a series of 160 emergent procedures (17) and only one pneumothorax seen in Farrell and Hicks' series of 454 patients (6). Puncture of the gastrointestinal tract is a rare complication. The colon may lie posterior or posterolateral to the kidney and can be entered during a PCN (55,56). Retrorenal position of the colon is more common in patients who are thin and have little retrorenal fat, who have colonic dilation, or who have an abnormal anatomy, such as marked kyphosis or scoliosis (55). The colon was posterior to the medial 2/3 of the kidney in 4.7% of prone patients at the level of the lower poles and posterior to the lateral 1/3 of the kidney in 10% of patients in one report (57). When there is doubt about safe access, preprocedure CT to delineate the anatomy is prudent. A transcolonic nephrostomy tract was seen in 2 out of 1000 cases of PCNL in one series (55). The complication can often be managed conservatively, with drainage of both the kidney and the colon by separate catheters till the created nephrocolic fistula heals (55,56).

Duodenal injury is a rare complication (58). Inadvertent puncture of the spleen can cause severe hemorrhage or even a splenic abscess in patients, with infected urine (59).

Other Major Complications: Thoracic Injuries. An intercostal approach (often required for access to the upper poles of the kidneys) causes more thoracic complications than a subcostal puncture (60). In expiration, a posterior intercostal approach between the 11th and 12th ribs poses little risk of injury to the spleen and liver (57), but the lungs remain vulnerable to puncture in many patients. The right lung is in the path of the needle in 29% and the left lung in 14% of patients in expiration. During maximal inspiration, the lung would be in the needle path in most patients in whom an intercostal puncture is performed. Other thoracic complications include pleural effusion, pneumonia, atelectasis, hydrothorax, and pneumothorax.

Minor Complications. Minor complications that may occur are catheter dislodgment and urine extravasation. Catheter dislodgement in the early postplacement period occurs in less than 1% of patients but increases to 11% to 30% in the following months (6,17). Dislodgement in the first week after placement often necessitates a new PCN insertion and the creation of a new tract.

Radiation Dose

Nephrostomy tube placement is considered a low–radiation dose procedure (61), with peak skin doses usually less than 1 Gy; however, exposure can be higher in as many as 12% of cases (62,63). This is an important consideration in pregnant patients who present with obstruction and require percutaneous drainage.

Follow-Up

Most PCN drainage catheters are replaced every three to four months on an outpatient basis. An interval longer than three months is frequently associated with tube occlusion (15). Replacement of occluded nephrostomy tubes can pose a challenge as intraluminal encrustation may prevent passage of a guidewire (64). Furthermore, with Malecot catheters, tissue may occasionally grow through the wings of the catheter, making them resistant to removal (65). Because of this problem, Stewart et al. believe that if nephrostomy tube drainage is required for longer than a few weeks, Malecot-type winged catheters should not be used (65).

Catheter flushing at home between tube changes, whether by visiting nurses or the patient, does little to favorably influence the incidence of tube encrustation in most patients. In patients with rapid tube encrustation, a high fluid intake is the best way to keep catheters open.

The presence of a nephrostomy tube invariably causes bacteriuria, candiduria, or pyuria within nine weeks of initial nephrostomy tube drainage. Prophylactic antibiotics in patients with PCN tubes does not prevent bacteriuria and, instead, contributes to the emergence of organisms that are resistant to the antibiotics being administered (66).

Antibiotic prophylaxis is unnecessary in routine catheter exchanges when the catheters have been draining adequately and, in fact, fails to prevent bacteremia (66,67). Cronan et al. (66,67) found that asymptomatic bacteremia occurred in 11% of routine tube changes and that preprocedural antibiotics were unsuccessful in preventing bacteremia. This has implications for patients at risk for endocarditis, in whom routine tube changes should be preceded by antibiotic therapy with the aim of eradicating bacteriuria. Antibiotics should be chosen for activity against the organisms isolated in the urine, and after bacteriuria has been eliminated, an antibiotic regimen recommended in the American Heart Association guidelines for genitourinary procedures should be administered in conjunction with an elective nephrostomy tube change.

PCN for Urinary Diversion

PCN is often performed to allow the closure of a ureteral fistula, ureteral leak, or a dehiscent urinary tract anastomosis. In most cases, PCN drainage alone is unsuccessful in totally diverting the urine, and either ureteral stenting or ureteral occlusion (the latter in patients with intractable vesicovaginal fistulas) is additionally required. In Farrell and Hicks' large series of patients (6), urinary fistulae were the most common nonobstructive indication for PCN placement (although this series did not include patients undergoing PCN for removal of stones). Urinary diversion by PCN alone has been used with some success to treat patients with intractable hemorrhagic cystitis (68).

PCN to Gain Access to the Collecting System

This application of PCN is the most frequent indication for the procedure in many institutions, particularly where the urologists are active in endourologic therapy. Some examples of such procedures include the treatment of renal or ureteral calculi (stone fragmentation, removal, or chemolysis); ureteral interventions, such as stricture dilation or stent placement; retrieval of foreign bodies, such as fractured stent fragments; nephroscopic surgery, such as endopyelotomy for ureteropelvic junction (UPJ) obstruction; and brush biopsy or percutaneous therapy of urothelial tumors. Interventions can often be done in the same sitting as the PCN if the procedure is not complicated by excessive bleeding and if there is no infection. Ureteral interventions and PCN for urinary stone treatment are discussed in greater detail later in this chapter.

URETERAL STENTING

Ureteral intubation is essential in the management of patients with nephroureteral obstruction and with urinary fistulas, in patients undergoing open ureteral surgery, and prior to extracorporeal shock wave lithotripsy (ESWL).

Stent Materials

The ideal ureteral stent should be easy to insert and retrieve, be biocompatible, and resist encrustation, infection, and occlusion. It should also be biodurable and remain chemically stable in urine to resist breakage, be radio-opaque, resist migration, have good flow characteristics so that urine flow can be effectively restored and maintained in both intramural and extramural obstruction, and be comfortable for the patient. A number of materials have been used in the quest to produce a ureteral stent, but no such "ideal" material is available to date (69–72).

Urinary stents in current use are made of blends of synthetic polymers, such as polyurethane and silicone, as well as other materials (69,70). Initially, ureteral stents made of pure polyethylene and polyurethane were used, but these fell out of favor due to stent fractures in patients whose polyethylene stents were left indwelling beyond the maximum recommended six-month period (72–75) and to the poor biocompatibility of polyurethane stents, which resulted in epithelial erosions and ulcers in the ureter.

Ureteral stents made of silicone, C-Flex[®], and Percuflex[®] are also in wide clinical use and are offered by many manufacturers. Currently, stents made of C-Flex, and Percuflex appear to confer the most advantages with regard to patency, flexibility, resistance to migration, good urine flow rates, and resistance to fracturing. The manufacturers recommend stent exchange at three to six month intervals, although in certain clinical situations, such as terminal malignancy, stent replacement can be deferred for a longer period if the stent is functioning well. Coating stents with hydrogels—hydrophilic polymers that allow water to be trapped in their chemical structure—appears to improve biocompatibility by reducing frictional irritation and encrustation (70,73).

Percuflex is a proprietary biocompatible olefinic copolymer material from Boston Scientific Corporation (Medi-Tech, Microvasive, Natick, Massachusetts) that has a high tensile strength (and therefore the largest available inner lumen for a given outside diameter), an intrinsic low coefficient of friction, which facilitates stent placement, and long-term biodurability with resistance to fracture and migration (74). Although the manufacturer recommends replacing stents made with Percuflex every six months, Rackson et al. (74) found that these stents remain patent for a mean period of 10 months. Of all currently available stent materials, Percuflex may represent one of the most balanced stent materials available.

C-Flex is a proprietary silicone-modified copolymer from Consolidated Polymer Technologies (Clearwater, Florida) that was designed to be urine compatible. Although not as strong as Percuflex or polyurethane, the material has sufficient tensile strength to allow good flow rates and coil strength. The stent resists both migration and fracture (75) and demonstrates an overall patency rate of 80%. The external surface of the stent is slippery, a property that enhances resistance to stent encrustation and also makes stent placement easier.

Silicone stents are the gold standard owing to their tissue compatibility and inert nature. Silicone stents retain their softness, flexibility, and elasticity even 10 years after placement, but their inherently low tensile strength limits the inner diameter of the stents and the size of the side holes of the stents constructed from this material, thus reducing their functional efficacy. Silicone also has a high coefficient of surface friction, which makes stent insertion difficult and necessitates placement through a peel-away sheath. It is also poorly radio-opaque, making fluoroscopic monitoring during insertion difficult. For these reasons, silicone is not the preferred choice of material for stents, particularly for indwelling ureteral stents. Currently, silicone stents are usually placed intra-operatively.

Endoureteral implantation of self-expanding metal stents was a natural off-shoot of experience with metal stent use in the biliary tract and urethra. These stents have been used primarily in patients with malignant ureteral obstruction (76–79) as an alternative to conventional, double-pigtail ureteral stents, with the hope that ureteral patency could be maintained for a longer period without the need for stent exchange. The potential incorporation of the stent into the ureteric wall with covering by urothelium should theoretically avoid calcium encrustation, infection, and risk of migration. However, hyperplasia of the urothelium leading to stent occlusion, encrustation, and hematuria has been reported with metal stents such as Wallstents (Medinrent, Lausanne, Switzerland) (76–78), and therefore, the role of metal stents in the treatment of ureteral obstruction remains in evolution. Because the biocompatibility of metallic devices in the urinary tract is unknown, as are also the effects of the corrosive action of urine and extracellular fluids on the metal, researchers have been reluctant to use metal stents in ureteral obstruction from benign disease (71,80,81).

Recently, metal stents made of nickel-titanium alloy (Nitinol) have been used. Kulkarni et al. (82) reported on a thermoexpandable shape memory alloy Memokath 051 ureteral stent (Engineers and Doctors of Copenhagen, Denmark) that was placed in patients with malignant and benign ureteral strictures. They reported no encrustation or epithelial hyperplasia with a mean follow-up of 19.3 months. These stents can also be removed many weeks after placement by cooling to 10°C.

There has also been much interest in using biodegradable materials to obviate the necessity of stent removal in patients who require temporary stenting (70,83). Variation in the time to degradation is one of the problems with these materials. pH-sensitive stents that dissolve if the urine is alkalinized with oral bicarbonate administration are also being investigated for use in long-term stenting (84).

Technique

Ureteral stents can be inserted through a PCN tract or retrograde through the urethra or a urinary conduit. In difficult cases, a combined approach may be required. Successfully deployed ureteral stents allow for urine drainage and diversion without the inconvenience of a drainage bag.

Antegrade Ureteral Stenting

Percutaneous antegrade stent insertion is performed when retrograde insertion fails or is not possible. Antegrade ureteral stenting requires percutaneous access to the collecting system, preferably through an interpolar or upper pole calyx, because this approach allows the pushing forces to be directed toward the ureteropelvic junction (UPJ). A guidewire is then maneuvered across the ureteral obstruction using a combination of preshaped catheters (cobra, multipurpose) and guidewires. Hydrophilic-coated guidewires (glidewires) are particularly helpful in crossing tight strictures. The use of transrenal Teflon sheaths (peel-away or non-peel-away) also facilitates the placement of stents through an area of tight ureteral narrowing, by preventing buckling in the subcutaneous tissues and in the renal pelvis (85,86) as the stent encounters high resistance in the area of a tight stricture. In difficult cases, a guidewire can be passed antegrade through the urethra so that it can be grasped at both ends—the nephrostomy site and the urethra—and the stent can be advanced by pushing and pulling (87,88). If the urine draining from the nephrostomy is bloody or infected, stent placement should be deferred until the urine clears.

Two kinds of ureteral stents can be inserted in an antegrade fashion: an internal stent (double-J or double-pigtail) and an external–internal stent (nephroureteral) (Fig. 5A,B). External–internal stents (nephroureteral stents, Fig. 5A) are introduced percutaneously and advanced into the urinary bladder or bowel. A segment of the stent remains protruding from the flank and is capped externally to allow antegrade (internal) urine drainage. Side holes at the level of the renal pelvis allow urine to drain distally through the stent. External–internal stents can be easily exchanged percutaneously and also be irrigated to maintain patency. They are used in patients in whom the stent placement is only for a short period (as after stone removal or ureteral dilation) and in patients in whom retrograde stent exchange would be difficult because of bladder disease or distortion or because of neurologic or orthopedic problems that make cystoscopic exchange of a stent challenging.

Completely internalized ureteral stents (Fig. 5B) do not protrude from the flank, an obvious cosmetic and nursing advantage. A period of external drainage through a PCN for two to seven days prior to attempted ureteral stent placement

(A)   **(B)**

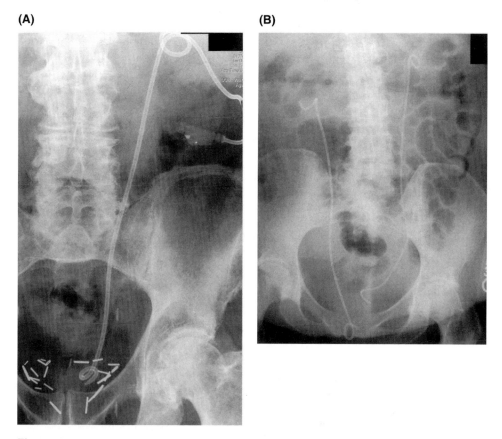

Figure 5 Types of ureteral stents. (**A**) Nephroureteral stent with proximal self-retaining pigtail in renal pelvis and distal pigtail end in urinary bladder. (**B**) Bilateral double-pigtail ureteral stents in a patient with bilateral obstruction due to an enlarged myomatous uterus. The right ureteral stent is a little too long and can potentially produce bladder symptoms, such as suprapubic pain or dysuria.

was the convention when the procedure first came into use but since has been found to be unnecessary in most cases (85,86,89,90). A nephrostomy tube is left in place for 24 to 48 hours after stent placement so that antegrade pyelography can be performed to confirm stent patency before the nephrostomy catheter is removed. It is important to use fluoroscopic guidance when removing the nephrostomy catheter in order to prevent inadvertent extraction of a double-pigtail ureteral stent that may be trapped by a portion of the nephrostomy catheter (91). If the urine is bloody, nephrostomy catheter drainage should be maintained until the urine clears.

Recently, Patel and Abubacker (90) reported on their experience in 41 patients in whom ureteral stents were placed without a postprocedural nephrostomy tube. Exclusion criteria were suspected pyonephrosis, coagulopathy, and emergency cases. After stent placement, the authors performed a nephrostogram, and if there was contrast flow into the bladder, a blood clot filling less than half the renal pelvis, and no bleeding around a wire left in the tract after stent placement, a nephrostomy tube was not placed. The procedure was technically successful in 36 of 41 patients (88%) and clinically successful in 34 of 41 (83%) patients. Two patients became septic and required repeat nephrostomy tube insertion. Based on their experience, the authors recommend that patients who have had genitourinary tract surgery or recent instrumentation, such as a failed attempt at retrograde stent insertion, should have nephrostomy tubes left in postprocedure for drainage, because such patients appear to have a predisposition to infection (90).

Per Urethral (Retrograde) Ureteral Stenting

The retrograde route for access to the kidneys or ureters is a familiar one to most urologists. When the endoscopic retrograde approach is unsuccessful in placing a stent or a guidewire, a PCN is usually requested by the urologists, followed by stent placement through the PCN tract. However, an unsuccessful or incomplete retrograde procedure can often be successfully completed with fluoroscopy and the use of guidewires and catheters (92,93) in an interventional radiology suite. Fostering a close working relationship with the urologists can facilitate referrals for such cases, and thus potentially avoid a nephrostomy.

Primary retrograde catheterization of the ureter without cystoscopic assistance has been reported (94–96). The procedure was successful in 70% of cases in a small series (94), with patients requiring only mild intravenous sedation and with fluoroscopy times averaging less than three minutes. The trigone is identified by cystography, and the ureteral orifice is cannulated using a combination of angled-tip glidewires and angled hockey-stick catheters. Replacement of ureteral stents using fluoroscopic control (as opposed to cystoscopy) has been reported, with successful exchange possible in 97% of cases (97,98). The bladder end of the stent is grasped with a snare or lasso, withdrawn through the urethra, and then replaced over a guidewire using the standard technique. The technique is easier in female patients, although it has also been used in a few male patients.

Choosing the Correct Length of Ureteral Stent

A ureteral stent of the correct length will ensure patient comfort, trouble-free drainage and prevent irritative voiding symptoms. Ureteral stents are available in lengths ranging from 20 to 28 cm (a further range of shorter stents are also available for renal transplant patients); a specific length has to be chosen for each patient.

Multilength or flexible-length ureteral stents are also available. They are made of a softer polymer that allows the pigtail to unfurl to the proper length, but these stents are less stable in position, and the proper positioning of the pigtails can be difficult (99). In a correctly positioned stent, the proximal pigtail should be formed within the renal pelvis, and the distal pigtail should project beyond the vesicoureteral junction (VUJ). Stents that are too short will retract into the ureter when the proximal pigtail forms in the renal pelvis, complicating stent retrieval. An overly long stent will be redundant within the bladder and may cause irritative voiding symptoms (Fig. 5B).

Accurately estimating stent length (85,99) can be difficult. In the technique called the kinked/bent wire technique, an attempt is made to directly measure ureteral length by kinking a wire when it is just beyond the VUJ in the urinary bladder and then kinking it again after withdrawing it into the renal pelvis. Patel and Abubacker found that this technique overestimated the ureteral length in 83% of patients (90). These authors also found that the patient height was the most reliable method to estimate stent length, with patients less than 5 ft 10 inch. in height receiving 22 cm–long stents, patients 5 ft 10 inch. to 6 ft 4 inch. in height 24 cm–long stents, and patients greater than 6 ft 4 inch. in height 26 cm–long stents. Other authors have also reported on using patient height as a guide for stent length (99,100).

Other methods to estimate ureteral length are using an endocatheter ruler, or calculating ureteral length from a previous imaging study, such as an intravenous urogram (101,102).

Results

Antegrade ureteral stenting is successful in 88% to 96% of cases, and more than 80% of obstructed ureters can be primarily stented without the need for prior nephrostomy (89,90,92). Failure of placement is usually related to marked ureteral angulation or encasement by tumor or fibrosis. Technical failures can be minimized by placing the nephrostomy in a favorable calyx so as to provide the best vector for stent advancement, using transrenal sheaths as a buttress and using appropriately stiff guidewires. Passing the wire through the urethra to gain control over both ends of the wire is also helpful in particularly difficult cases (86). Partial ureteral obstruction, where a guidewire can be passed across the stricture, does not necessarily equate with an easier attempt at stenting (89).

If stenting cannot be accomplished at the initial sitting, attempts following nephrostomy drainage for a few days are often successful because of a decrease in ureteral tortuosity and/or edema that may have developed as a result of the ureteral obstruction. In Patel and Abubacker's series (90), 5 of 41 patients could not be stented initially due to tight strictures. Four of these five patients were successfully stented eventually. In the same series, all patients who underwent a two-step procedure (nephrostomy drainage for some duration followed by attempted stenting) were successfully stented. The complication rate was slightly higher in the one-step patient group (6%) compared to the two-step group (2%) and consisted primarily of sepsis. Not surprisingly, the one-step procedure was significantly cheaper than the two-step procedure.

Ureteral stenting appears to be more effective in relieving intrinsic ureteral obstruction due to such causes as stones and strictures (103) and not to be as effective in relieving obstruction caused by extrinsic obstruction related to malignancies. Yosepowitch et al. (103) reported an initial success rate for retrograde stenting of 94% for intrinsic disease and 73% for extrinsic disease. After three months, all stents functioned in all patients with intrinsic disease, but only 56.4% of stents functioned in patients with extrinsic obstruction. These authors also found that stent diameter did not correlate with successful drainage. Similarly, Chung et al. (104) and Docimo and Dewolf (43) noted a 40% and 45% rate of stent failure in patients with extrinsic obstruction by malignant disease.

The etiology for the impaired stent function in patients with extrinsic obstruction is not completely clear. It is believed that urine drainage in a stented ureter is primarily due to ureteral peristalsis, which causes urine to flow around the stent. With extrinsic malignant ureteral compression, tumor encasement of the ureter may affect the muscular activity (and hence peristalsis) of the ureter and also prevent ureteral distension, both of which are necessary to maintain flow around the stent (105).

It has been found, however, that patients in whom 7 French internalized ureteral stents fail to drain the collecting system adequately can often be effectively drained antegrade by a large-bore (10 French) nephroureteral catheter. There is also a report of successful drainage with the placement of two ureteral stents when a single ureteral stent had failed (106). In this series, two 7 French stents or a combination of 6 and 8 French stents were used. Flank pain and hydronephrosis were alleviated, and the treated patients reported no discomfort associated with the presence of two stents.

There are also other situations besides extrinsic obstruction of the ureter where stents may not function well, or be poorly tolerated, necessitating PCN drainage. Patients with large pelvic tumors that compress the bladder or with high intraluminal pressures within the bladder (as can be caused by bladder outlet obstruction) may not drain well antegrade. Patients with small, irritable bladders (as with tuberculous cystitis or following radiation or chemotherapy) may not tolerate the presence of a stent within the bladder. Further, in patients with incontinence or fistulae, supravesical urinary diversion is preferable (85).

Some small series reporting on permanent indwelling metal stents (107) have reported high patency rates, whereas other studies have noted primary patency in only 16% (108) to 31% (78). Metal stents made of the thermoexpandable shape memory alloy Memokath 051 may have a better patency rate and fewer problems with epithelial overgrowth (82).

In patients with impassable ureteral strictures, novel approaches have been used to establish drainage. Cornud et al. (109) created a neotract between the ureter and bladder using electrocautery, and Lang (110) and Rosdy (111) used a perforating guidewire to create a ureteroneocystostomy. Fistulas to the alimentary tract were a serious (and fatal) complication in Cornud et al.'s series (109). Mishra et al. (112) reported on inadvertent catheterization of a ureterorectal fistula in a patient with a rectal stump and advanced colon cancer; a double-pigtail stent was placed through and served to keep the obstructed kidney decompressed. Bilbao et al. (113) described a direct translumbar puncture of the ureter with subsequent stent placement in patients in whom ureteral laceration or rigid ureteral kinking prevented stent placement. Extra-anatomic ureteral replacement with a subcutaneous silicone–polytetrafluoroethylene (PTFE) prosthesis has also been reported (114).

Complications

The single most frequent complication of ureteral stenting is occlusion of the stent due to encrustation, which is an unpredictable phenomenon but which appears to correlate with the length of time that a stent has been left in place. About 68% of stents that are indwelling for nine weeks have been found to be obstructed with mucus and microcalculi when they are removed (115,116). In another series, El-Faqih et al. (117) found that in patients in whom stents were placed for treatment of urinary stones, there was minimal morbidity when the indwelling time was six weeks or less. Encrustation was present in 9.2% of stents retrieved before six weeks, but in 47.5% of stents retrieved at 6 to 12 weeks, and in 76.3% of stents retrieved after 12 weeks. In order to minimize the risk of early encrustation, many investigators suggest that all patients should be encouraged to maintain a high fluid intake after stent placement to dilute the urine and that urine infections should be aggressively treated.

Evaluation to confirm stent patency and function can sometimes be difficult. Flank pain may occur with both functioning and nonfunctioning stents and is not a helpful clinical parameter to monitor stent function. Many, though not all, patent stents will reflux on voiding cystourethrography. Diuretic renography is reportedly the most sensitive test in evaluating stent patency (118). Pyelocaliectasis often persists even after relief of obstruction with a ureteral stent, and the upper urinary tract may remain abnormal in appearance. Thus, imaging may be unhelpful in predicting which patients have obstructed stents. Intrarenal Doppler sonography can be used to distinguish between patency and obstruction. Platt et al. (119) reported that obstructed stents were associated with increased mean resistive indices (0.78), whereas patent stents were associated with a resistive index of less than 0.70. Assessment of jets in the urinary bladder with color Doppler ultrasonography has also been used (120) to evaluate stent patency.

Stents should be changed every three to six months, whether cystoscopically by urologists or in a retrograde (per urethral) fashion by radiologists. The physician placing the stent bears the responsibility of making the patient aware of the necessity of follow-up and monitoring. Patients who present with fractured stents (Fig. 6A,B) will often report that they were either unaware of the presence of an indwelling stent or unaware that periodic exchange or removal was necessary.

Severe encrustation on indwelling ureteral stents tends to be at the renal or bladder ends, and this propensity has been attributed to ureteral peristalsis "wiping" clean the ureteral portion of the stent (Fig. 7A,B) (121). A "twinkling" artifact may be seen in encrusted stents on color Doppler sonography (122). Minimally encrusted stents may be removed without event, but more severe encrustation can be complicated to treat and often requires ESWL in combination with endoscopic techniques (Fig. 7A–D) (123–126).

Proximal stent migration can lead to perforation of the renal pelvis or calyces (127), which can result in a urinoma or even catastrophic exsanguination due to erosion of the stent tip into a renal vessel. Stents that have migrated up into the kidney above a lower ureteral stricture or anastomosis can be extracted through a nephrostomy track under fluoroscopic guidance. A second approach is to use ureteroscopy to reposition the caudal end of the stent within the bladder. A stent that is positioned too far cephalad (so that the distal end is no longer within the urinary bladder) is usually related to placement of too short a stent rather than to cephalad migration (128). Distal migration is more common than proximal migration and may be a result of inappropriate positioning.

Stents that are fractured are best approached with a combined percutaneous–endoscopic technique. Although the stent fragments can be removed percutaneously, the fragments tend to be brittle and refracture into smaller pieces when they are grasped with forceps or baskets. Therefore, removal under endoscopic guidance is most likely to result in complete extraction (Fig. 6) (129).

Fistulae between the iliac artery and the ureter have been reported in patients with pelvic surgery, irradiation, and indwelling ureteral stents (130–132). The primary

(A)

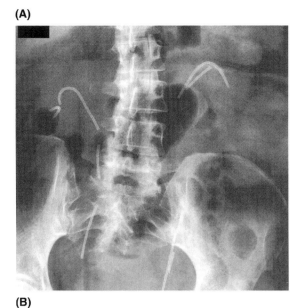

(B)

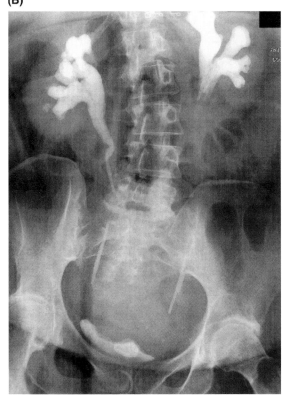

Figure 6 A patient with ureteral stents placed for bilateral ureteral obstruction (same patient as in Fig. 5) presenting two years later with nonspecific urinary complaints. The patient was lost to follow-up after ureteral stent placement. (**A**) Plain film demonstrates fractures of the stents bilaterally. This is not a common complication with modern day stents. (**B**) An IVU showing bilateral moderate hydronephrosis. Note the stent fragment in the urethra. *Abbreviation*: IVU, intravenous urogram.

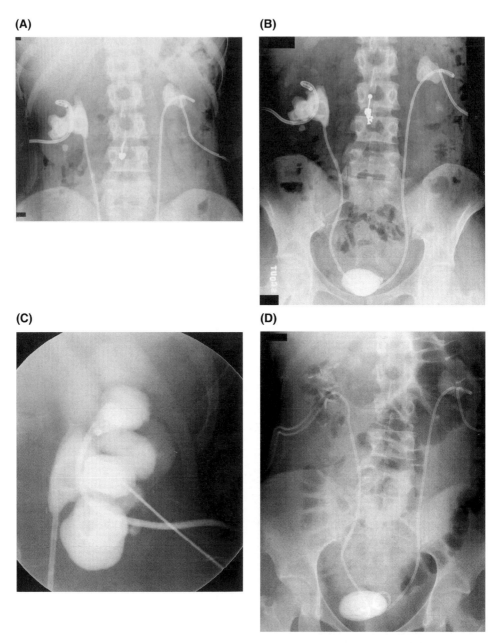

Figure 7 A patient with severely encrusted ureteral stents. (**A,B**) Plain abdominal films demonstrate large calculi that have encrusted on the proximal and distal pigtails of the catheters. The patient has an internalized stent and an externally draining nephrostomy on the right, and a nephroureteral stent on the left. Note the encrustation on the ureteral limb of the right catheter at the L5 level. (**C**) The right kidney was treated first. A new nephrostomy was performed (with patient in prone position) through an interpolar calyx for removal of encrusted stone. The majority of the stone in the right collecting system is obscured by the contrast injected into the right collecting system. (**D**) A follow-up film shows only small residual calculi in the right kidney. The encrustations on the ureteral portion of the stent were treated with SWL and the bladder calculus removed by open surgery. *Abbreviation*: SWL, shock wave lithotripsy.

predisposing factor is compromise of the vascular supply of the ureter, with a fistula occurring where the ureter crosses the iliac artery. Underlying abnormalities of the iliac artery, such as an aneurysm, are additional risk factors. Unsuspected and undiagnosed ureteroarterial fistulas are associated with 52% mortality, whereas a correct preoperative diagnosis allows for 89% of patients to be successfully discharged from the hospital (133). Prompt diagnosis requires an awareness of the condition and referral for selective or subselective arterial injections that may need to be performed in multiple projections. Provocative maneuvers, such as stent removal or manipulation during angiography, may be required during angiography for demonstration of the fistula, particularly if the angiogram is being performed in a quiescent period, when no acute bleeding is occurring.

An indwelling stent can be associated with discomfort in the flank or the pelvis, which can range from severe pain to a mild annoyance. A long intravesical segment can cause significant dysuria and bladder spasms due to irritation of the trigone and may necessitate removal of the stent, but even an appropriately placed stent may cause irritative bladder symptoms. Most patients can be managed with antispasmodics and hydration. Flank pain may be worse during voiding, but some patients complain of flank discomfort even in the nonvoiding state. Intolerance to ureteral stents is neither material-specific nor design-specific. Pryor et al. (134) found no significant differences in patient symptoms in an analysis of stents made of polyurethane, silicone, Silitek, and C-Flex. If there are significant symptoms, an abdominal radiograph is often helpful in assuring that the stent remains well positioned.

Stents are associated with microscopic hematuria in the majority of patients, but gross hematuria and pyuria may also occur (albeit less frequently).

URETERAL STRICTURE DILATION

Iatrogenic causes predominate in the development of ureteral strictures. Gynecologic and general surgical procedures are widely considered to be common causes of ureteral trauma and stricture formation, but endourologic procedures (such as ureteroscopy or ureterolithotomy), which facilitate less invasive management of many conditions, may paradoxically cause ureteral injury (135–137). A 1% to 11% incidence of stricture formation has been reported after upper tract endoscopy (138). Selzman and Spirnak (139) found that urological, gynecological, and general surgical procedures accounted for 42%, 34%, and 24% of ureteral injuries, respectively. Of the urological injuries, 21% occurred during open procedures and 79% during endoscopic procedures, most commonly stone removal (Fig. 4).

Urologic procedures that have been implicated in ureteral stricture formation include transurethral resection of the prostate, radical prostatectomy, ureteral meatotomy, traumatic ureteral catheterization, ureteroneocystostomy, and renal transplantation. Gynecologic procedures that have been associated with strictures include hysterectomy (for benign or malignant disease), cesarean sections, and tubal ligations. Selzman and Spirnak (139) found that radical abdominal hysterectomy accounted for most of the gynecological injuries in their series. Surgical procedures that may cause ureteral trauma and stricture formation are abdominal aortic aneurysm repair, bowel resection, and pelvic exenterations. Selzman and Spirnak (139) found that colorectal surgery and abdominal aortic surgery accounted for most of the ureteral injuries during general surgery and that these injuries were transections (in 62% of cases).

Ureteral strictures can also develop in patients with chronic calculous disease as well as after penetrating abdominal trauma, particularly high-velocity gunshot wounds. Urinary extravasation and ureteral ischemia may contribute to scar formation in these cases and in postoperative strictures (such as ureteroenteral anastomotic strictures associated with urinary diversion). Chronic inflammatory diseases, such as tuberculosis and schistosomiasis, can also cause strictures.

With malignant strictures, the goal of treatment is to provide drainage (percutaneous or internal) so that renal function can be improved. Chronic stenting is often the most reasonable option for these patients. For benign strictures, stenting alone is not the optimal therapy, and attempts are made to relieve the obstruction, with balloon dilation often being the initial mode of therapy. Successful balloon dilation obviates the need for chronic indwelling stents or additional open surgery.

Ureteral dilation can be performed through either an antegrade or retrograde approach or a combination of these two approaches. The antegrade approach is the preferred route, for several reasons. Many strictures that may be impassable by a retrograde approach can be negotiated in an antegrade fashion. More importantly, once dilation and stenting have been completed, the remaining nephrostomy tube can be used to assess the results of the dilation as well as to perform urodynamic tests (such as the Whitaker test) for more physiologic evaluation. The only disadvantage of the antegrade route is the invasiveness of establishing a percutaneous access tract (Fig. 8).

The retrograde approach is the least invasive method of management. Access can be gained by either cystoscopy or ureteroscopy, during which time a retrograde catheter is inserted. This catheter can then be exchanged for guidewires and balloon dilators.

For dilation, reinforced high-pressure balloon catheters are used. A "waist" deformity is seen in the balloon on initial inflation and should disappear with continued or subsequent inflations (Fig. 8D). There is no consensus in the literature regarding the most effective method of dilation, the optimal size of balloon to be used, or the inflation period for the balloon. In experimental studies (140), dilation of the ureter to twice its diameter was well tolerated, but threefold dilation produced changes ranging from hydronephrosis to complete rupture. Inflated balloon diameters in published reports range between 4 and 10 mm, number of inflation cycles from 1 to 10, and the duration of inflation from 30 seconds to 10 minutes (138) to as long as 1 to 16 hours in different series. Similarly, there is no uniformity regarding the number of inflations that should be performed. The various technical approaches have been summarized in reviews by Meretyk et al. (141,142) and Chang et al. (143).

After dilation, there is no consensus regarding the necessity for stenting, with some authors leaving in stents for several days to months and others avoiding stenting altogether. Laboratory studies of ureteral healing demonstrate reepithelialization in 7 to 10 days and muscular healing in six to eight weeks. Thus six weeks of postprocedural stenting appears prudent because the stent serves as a scaffold for organized reepithelialization and smooth muscle growth (144). In published reports, stent sizes have varied between 6 and 16 French, and stenting duration has varied from 2 days to 12 weeks (138). The ultimate outcome may depend more on the nature (and etiology) of the stricture than on the technical nuances of dilation. If a stent is placed after dilation, a 7 to 10 French size is used in native ureters and 6 to 8 French size in transplanted ureters.

As previously mentioned, the stents are left in place for at least six weeks to allow muscular healing while the ureteral caliber is maintained. Nephroureteral

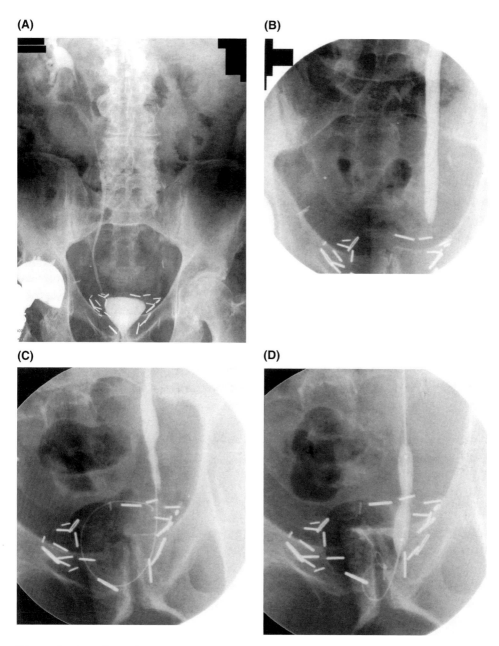

Figure 8 A patient with left distal ureteral stricture following ureteroscopic stone retrieval from left distal ureter (same patient as in Fig. 4). (**A**) There is a high-grade obstruction of the left renal collecting system on IVU with no discernible excretion, one month after uretero-scopic stone removal. (**B**) A PCN was performed, and a catheter advanced into the distal left ureter where contrast injection showed complete occlusion, with no flow into the bladder. (**C**) A guidewire was maneuvered across the stricture. A hydrophilic wire is very useful in this situation. (**D**) Balloon dilation shows a waist in the balloon at the stricture site that was effaced with continuing balloon inflation. A nephroureteral catheter was placed following the procedure (Fig. 5A). The stricture did not respond to balloon dilation, and the patient is being managed with a nephroureteral catheter. *Abbreviations*: IVU, intravenous urogram; PCN, percutaneous nephrostomy.

stents (external–internal stents) are preferred over completely internalized stents (Fig. 5). They are initially left to gravity drainage and can then be capped. The patient is asked to uncap the tube if flank pain, fever, or drainage around the catheter develops. The stent is exchanged for a nephrostomy catheter at the end of six to eight weeks. The efficacy of the dilation can then be assessed by nephrostograms and urodynamic studies before catheter removal. The tube can be safely removed if the opening pressures are low (less than 14 cm of water), the renal pelvic residual volumes are low, and the stricture itself appears to be anatomically improved, with satisfactory flow through the previously strictured segment. If follow-up studies demonstrate a recurrent stricture, a second attempt at dilation is usually made. Subsequent failures are managed with either open surgical repair or chronic stenting, depending on the circumstances.

When balloon dilation is apparently successful, follow-up intravenous urography or renal scans are performed at 1, 6, and 12 months and then periodically, as indicated, to check on the continuing patency of the ureter (145).

Percutaneous ureteroneocystostomy and direct percutaneous ureteral puncture are other techniques that have been used in the management of impassable ureteral strictures (109–111). Electrocautery and rotational atherolytic devices have also been used to recanalize occluded ureters and stenotic UPJs (146–148), but their efficacy remains to be proven.

Ureteroenteral Anastomotic Strictures

Strictures at the anastomosis of the ureter to an ileal conduit urinary diversion or continent urinary pouch or conduit are almost always benign and reportedly occur in 4% to 30% of patients (149–151). One study that compared complications in the different forms of urinary diversion reported the incidence of ureteroenteric strictures in ileal conduits to be 6.5%, compared to 10.0% in the continent reservoir group and 13.6% in patients who underwent ureterosigmoidostomy (150). The predisposing factors are ischemic necrosis and subsequent fibrosis and stricture, due to excessive mobilization and skeletonization of the ureter. Preoperative radiation therapy appears to have a compounding effect. Extravasation at the anastomosis may progress to scarring and subsequently a stricture, and, rarely, recurrent tumor in the ureter may present with obstruction. Stenoses tend to be more prevalent on the left side, probably because of the necessity for high mobilization of the left ureter (to ensure a gradual course to the right), which often requires the middle ureteric artery to be sacrificed (152). Rarely, ureteral obstruction can be due to extrinsic compression by a crossing vessel or to compression at the site where the left ureter is brought through the sigmoid mesocolon into the peritoneal cavity to be anastomosed to the ileal conduit. Strictures can predispose patients to urinary infections, stone formation, and loss of renal function, which can often be clinically silent.

Surgical revision of anastomotic strictures is technically difficult because of fibrotic adhesions from prior surgery and, frequently, prior radiation therapy. Nonoperative interventional therapy has been embraced as an alternative, but results to date have been disappointing and not equivalent to those of surgical repair. However, the lower morbidity of interventional techniques and the ability to perform open repair if the interventional procedures are a failure justify the continuing primary application of interventional and endourologic procedures.

The diagnosis of an anastomotic stricture is made when an intravenous urogram, renal ultrasound, or CT scan demonstrates progressive hydronephrosis and/or a loopogram demonstrates the absence of ureteral reflux in a patient in whom the diagnosis of a stricture is being entertained. Ultrasound examination in this situation, although highly sensitive, demonstrates a specificity of only 50% because of the high prevalence of dilated collecting systems that are not obstructed in patients with ureteroileostomies (153). Both antegrade and retrograde studies are performed in an attempt to define the site, length, degree of narrowing, and possible etiology of the stricture. Brush biopsies are performed if there is a concern that the stricture may be malignant (Fig. 9). There is a consensus that malignant obstruction is best treated by ureteral stenting and drainage.

Ureteroenteral anastomotic strictures are best cannulated through a combined antegrade and retrograde approach (154). Nonrefluxing strictured anastomoses are difficult to catheterize in a transconduit fashion, with success in only 14% to 56% of patients (155,156). Continent diversions, whether cutaneous or orthotopic, are treated by the antegrade route.

The retrograde route is usually successful in catheterizing patent ureteroileal anastomoses in 85% to 100% of patients (Fig. 9) (155–158). The procedure is required in patients with a patent ureteroenteral anastomosis for draining partially obstructing ureteral strictures, for extraction of renal or ureteral calculi in patients who would otherwise require a PCN, and for brush biopsies of filling defects in the collecting systems (Fig. 9). Endoscopy of an ileal conduit is not always successful in identifying or catheterizing the ureteroenteral anastomosis. Retrograde uretero-scopy has been reported to be successful in 10/13 patients with orthotopic ileal neobladder urinary diversion in one series (159).

The radiologic management of a ureteroenteral anastomotic stricture in an ileal conduit consists of performing a PCN, maneuvering a guidewire down the ureter, across the anastomotic stricture, through the ileal conduit, and out the stoma; and then advancing a balloon catheter to the site of the stricture. High-pressure reinforced balloons of 8- to 10-mm diameter and 4- to 10-cm length are preferable. As with bal-loon dilation of other benign ureteral strictures, there is no consensus on the size of the balloon, the ideal period of balloon inflation, the necessity or desirability of repeat inflations, and, lastly, the size of the catheter used to stent the newly dilated anasto-mosis. The ureteral stent placement following the balloon dilation is performed in a retrograde transconduit fashion through the ileal conduit. The stent should have a large lumen with side holes only in the renal pelvis and it should be long enough to extend beyond the stoma into the ileostomy drainage bag. The standard 25 cm–long nephrostomy catheter is not long enough to protrude through the stoma into the drainage bag. Locking loop catheters that are 40 cm to 50 cm long are usually required (Fig. 9). Side holes along the shaft of the catheter should be avoided because intestinal mucus can reflux into the renal pelvis, and predispose to occlusion of drai-nage holes (137,157). The standard double-pigtail ureteral stent, with one pigtail in the renal collecting system and the other end within the conduit, is not appropriate for drainage in patients with urinary diversions to the bowel. The catheter is left in place for roughly six weeks, after which a nephrostogram is performed. If the stricture appears persistent, a second attempt at balloon dilation is made. Because of the high recurrence rate of ureteral strictures after apparently successful balloon dilation, close follow-up is essential to detect stricture recurrence before renal function deteriorates.

Following ureteral dilation in patients with continent diversions, a large-bore self-retaining single-pigtail catheter is placed through the nephrostomy site, with the pigtail end in the pouch, and the catheter is capped externally. This catheter merely stents open the newly dilated segment. An additional nephrostomy catheter is

(A)

(B)

(C)

(D)

(E)

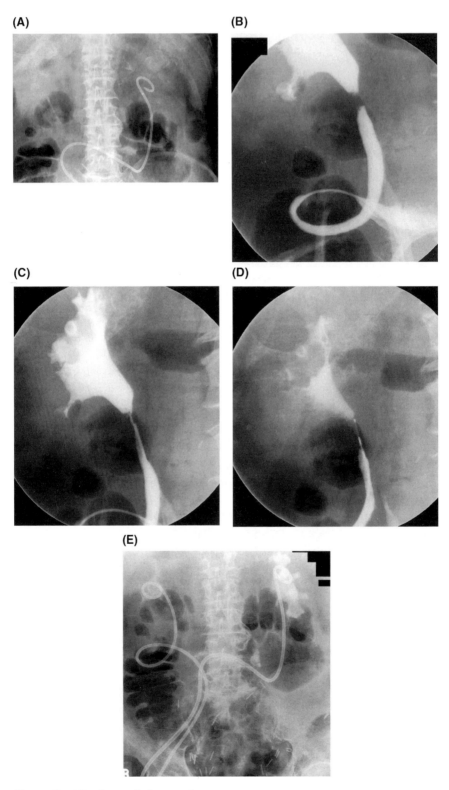

Figure 9 (*Caption on facing page*)

placed to drain the kidney. Placing a stent that can let mucus from the pouch reflux into the renal collecting system is not prudent because the stent can be easily occluded and cause sepsis (137).

Results

The response of strictures to balloon dilation is influenced by such factors as the etiology of the stricture, the length and location of the stricture, the duration of time that the stricture has been present, and the presence of ischemia or dense fibrosis (as in patients who have undergone radical extirpative surgery or have had radiation therapy). The relatively nonischemic strictures associated with endourologic surgery appear to respond better than do ischemic strictures.

Overall, 50% of all benign strictures respond favorably to one attempt at balloon dilation. Lang and Glorioso (160) reported that 91% of strictures less than three months old responded to dilation, compared to 53% of treated strictures that were of more than three months duration. In the presence of ischemia or fibrosis, only 21% of strictures were successfully dilated, whereas 70% of strictures not associated with vascular compromise responded. In a small series, Kim et al. (161) found that balloon dilation and stenting were successful in dilating tuberculous strictures in 75% of cases with good long-term results. Bilharzial strictures also respond to endourologic management, with the longer strictures requiring endoureterotomy (162). Chang et al. (143) reported 100% success in dilating strictures less than 1.5 cm in length, and O'Brien et al. (163) reported no difference in the outcomes whether the interval between ureteral injury and dilation was short or long. They reported a 65% overall success rate in dilating benign ureteral strictures. Kwak et al. (164) found that multiple dilations were of no benefit in prolonging or maintaining ureteral patency.

Strictures related to ureterolithotomy, ureteral endoscopy, and gynecologic surgery responded in 100%, 71%, and 62% of cases respectively, in one series (137). However, strictures associated with radical hysterectomy or retroperitoneal fibrosis responded poorly (33% and 0%, respectively).

Endoscopic incision has been used for treatment of many ureteral strictures that fail balloon dilation. An antegrade, retrograde, or combined approach can be used. Cutting devices in use are a cold knife, electrocautery, lasers, and the Acucise cutting balloon catheter (138). Endoureterotomy success rates range from 55% to 85% for benign ureteral strictures (141,146).

Balloon dilation and stenting have been used to treat UPJ obstruction (both primarily as an alternative to pyeloplasty and in secondary obstruction following

---

Figure 9 (*Figure on facing page*) Eighty-two-year-old man post-cystectomy for bladder cancer and urinary diversion to an ileal conduit. (**A**) A transconduit retrograde nephrostomy catheter was placed on the left side for a stricture at the left ureteroenteral anastomosis. The procedure was performed with a combination of an antegrade–retrograde approach, as described in the text. (**B**) A loopogram demonstrated the right ureteroenteral anastomosis to be patent, but a filling defect is present in the proximal ureter. (**C**) The right ureter was cannulated in a retrograde manner. A patent anastomosis can usually be easily catheterized from the ileal conduit. A high-grade stricture in the proximal ureter was causing hydronephrosis of the right collecting system. (**D**) A brush biopsy of the abnormal area was performed through the retrograde transconduit route and demonstrated transitional cell carcinoma. (**E**) A transconduit retrograde nephrostomy catheter was placed on the right side, as well as on the left side, because the patient was not a surgical candidate.

pyeloplasty). The reported success rate varies from 64% to 86% (165,166). Balloon dilation has been nearly completely superseded by endopyelotomy, which may be more effective in treating UPJ obstruction. Reported success rates with endopyelotomy vary from 32% to 67% (167–169), with higher success rates in treating secondary UPJ obstructions (obstructions occurring after a pyeloplasty) than in treating primary UPJ obstructions (167).

The long-term results of balloon dilation of ureteroenteral anastomotic strictures are poor, indicating that the strictures are resistant to nonoperative therapy. Shapiro et al. (170) reported a patency rate of only 30% at six months and 16% at one year. Similarly, Chang et al. (143) and Kramolowsky et al. (171) reported patency rates of 20% to 38% at one year. Kwak et al. (164) reported a nine-month success rate of 18% for continuing patency of balloon-dilated anastomotic strictures. They found that multiple dilations were of no benefit in maintaining ureteral patency. Overall, the average success rate in many series is 29% at 14 months (138).

The addition of endoscopic electroincision of the stricture to balloon dilation may improve patency rates to 42% to 71% (137,172,173) (average follow-up 16–28 months). Wolf et al. (174) used electrocauteruy and the Acucise cutting balloon and reported success rates of 72%, 51%, and 32% at one, two, and three years respectively; right-sided strictures had a better outcome with 68% of strictures improved at three years versus 17% of left-sided strictures. They also found no correlation between successful treatment and stricture length or stricture diameter but did report a higher success rate with the use of stents that were 12 French or larger, stenting periods of longer than four weeks, and treating strictures less than 24 months after the inciting event. Holmium laser endoureterotomy (175) has a reported success rate of 57% to 83% for right-sided strictures and 38% for left-sided strictures. Injury to the iliac artery has been reported with endoureterotomy (176). Cornud et al. (177) reported that incision of strictures had an actuarial three-year patency rate of 62% and also found that strictures associated with a continent neobladder responded more favorably than did ureteroileal strictures.

Metal stents have also been used to treat anastomotic strictures. To date, the reported series are small. Pollak et al. (108) reported that metallic stents (Wallstent endoprostheses) are ineffective in keeping benign ureteroileal strictures patent. Only one of six stents remained patent at 11 months, with the remainder becoming occluded by hyperplastic tissue growth within the stent. Other series (178) reported 100% patency at 10 and 22 months (178,179). The ultimate role of metal stents in the management of these patients remains in evolution, and judgment has to be deferred till larger cohorts of patients have been studied.

Ureteroenteral Anastomotic Strictures in Continent Diversions

Rates of ureteral obstruction vary depending on the type of pouch and ureteral anastomosis, with a reported 3% incidence for Kock reservoirs (180) and a 10% incidence for the modified Indiana pouch (181). Wilson et al. (181) reported dismal results with combined therapy of balloon dilation and incision of strictures. The failure rate of percutaneous therapy was 83%, whereas subsequent ureteral reimplantation was successful in 91%. They also reported an increased risk for stricture complications in patients who received preoperative radiation therapy, whereas Frazier et al. (150) reported no increase in the risk of long-term complications with radiation therapy. Strictures that develop in patients with orthotopic neobladders appear to respond more favorably than do those in ileal conduits or cutaneous continent diversions (177).

A few technical points need to be emphasized at this juncture. The antegrade route is the safest and most practical approach for stricture dilation because there is no reported experience regarding the feasibility and safety of cannulating nonrefluxing ureterocolonic anastomoses. After dilation, an 8 to 10 French stent is placed across the anastomosis, with its distal end in the colonic pouch and the proximal end obturated to prevent intrarenal reflux of mucus. In addition, a nephrostomy catheter is placed within the renal pelvis to facilitate drainage of the kidney. There are no reports regarding the effect of balloon dilation on the antireflux properties of the anastomosis, but our own experience indicates no significant ureteral reflux when the balloon dilation is successful. After a 6- to 8-week period of stenting, the ureteral stent is removed, and the effects of balloon dilation are assessed by a nephrostogram performed via the remaining nephrostomy catheter. When open surgical repair of the anastomotic stricture becomes necessary, the preoperative placement of a stent across the stricture (through a nephrostomy access) is helpful because it facilitates identification of the ureter (181).

OBSTRUCTED RENAL TRANSPLANTS

Urologic complications occur in 2% to 10% of renal transplant recipients, with ureteral complications accounting for the majority (182–184). The rate of posttransplant ureteral stenosis is 9.7% at five years (182). Ureteral strictures can be related to one or more of the following: postoperative urine leak with periureteral fibrosis, ureteral ischemia with resultant necrosis, selective ureteral rejection, and surgical technique used to harvest the ureter as well as to create the ureteroneocystostomy (UNC) (185–187). Ureteral obstruction due to such intraluminal pathology as a blood clot, fungus ball, or calculus is less common, as is extrinsic compression by the spermatic cord.

The most common site of ureteral obstruction is at the distal ureter, near the UNC site (182,187–189), likely due to the surgical manipulations required to create the anastomosis. Strictures in the proximal and middle ureter are more likely to be ischemic in nature. Urinary obstruction is suspected if the serum creatinine levels increase, urinary output is poor, or if renal ultrasonography or radioisotope renal scan indicate hydronephrosis.

Transplant ureteral leaks are also most frequent at the UNC site and usually present in the second or third postoperative week and almost always within five to six weeks of transplantation (187,188). Leaks are usually the result of ureteral necrosis due to rejection or vascular insufficiency. Extensive dissection during donor nephrectomy can jeopardize the ureteral blood supply because the ureteral vessels traverse the renal hilus and periureteral soft tissues. Urinary leaks are reportedly more common in living donors than with cadaveric kidneys because more dissection is required to harvest a kidney from a living donor (190). Other complications that can affect renal transplants are renal artery stenosis and perirenal fluid collections, which can occur in the early or late postoperative periods.

Technique for Percutaneous Urinary Interventions in Renal Transplants

The standard preprocedural preparations for a PCN are instituted. When planning a percutaneous puncture, it is important to avoid entry into the peritoneum by staying lateral to the lateral border of the transplant and the skin sutures. Transperitoneal punctures are more likely if an upper polar access is used and if the puncture is medial to the skin incision. Real-time ultrasound is useful in directing puncture into an anterolateral calyx with a minimal number of punctures.

Although ultrasound is quite sensitive for detecting hydronephrosis, mild, non-obstructive fullness of the transplant collecting system, which may be merely related to denervation of renal transplants may be difficult to distinguish from fullness of the collecting system due to obstruction. Another cause for mild dilation of the collecting system is reflux through the UNC. Therefore, antegrade pyelography plays a crucial role in confirming the status of the transplant collecting system in patients with suspected obstruction or leak. This procedure confirms the presence of obstruction or leak and helps to localize its site. It may also identify the etiology.

Antegrade pyelography is performed using the previously described standard technique used for nontransplant nephrostomies. If a stricture or occlusion is found, both balloon dilation followed by stenting (188) and stenting alone (184,187) are treatment options. Bhagat et al. (187) used a 4 mm balloon to facilitate placement of a stent in selected patients and used 6 to 10 French double-pigtail ureteral stents (8–10 cm long stents) in all patients. Fontaine et al. (188) balloon dilated all strictures with 5 mm to 8 mm balloons, prior to nephroureteral stent placement. Pappas et al. (184) reported on 13 patients, of whom eight had distal obstruction and four had UPJ or proximal ureteral obstructions. These authors dilated the stricture in only 7 of 12 patients (58%) prior to placement of 24 cm–long double-pigtail ureteral stents in all 12 patients, and the stents were left in place for a mean duration of 15 months. Our own preference (189) is to balloon dilate all ureteral strictures with 6 mm to 10 mm high-pressure balloons (to a pressure of 17 atmospheres) prior to stenting with a nephroureteral catheter. We use commercially available special-order catheters (Cook Inc., Bloomington, Indiana) that are 8 French to 10 French in diameter and have an 8 cm to 10 cm distance between the two pigtails. Only the proximal pigtail is self-retaining (as is the case with nephroureteral catheters used for ureteral stenting in native, nontransplant urinary tracts). Internalized stents reportedly have fewer infection complications because there is no external catheter, but percutaneous access is lost, precluding radiologic evaluation of the strictured segment. Stents were left indwelling without interval change for a mean duration of 15 months in one series (184) and up to two years in another series (187), without evidence of obstruction.

Surgical management of ureteral obstructions is required when the stricture cannot be traversed with a wire, the stricture does not respond to balloon dilation and stenting, or the radiographic findings strongly suggest extrinsic compression by vascular structures or the spermatic cord; however, graft survival appears to be higher in patients treated with ureteral stent placement as opposed to surgery (191).

Balloon dilation of transplant ureteral strictures has been reported to be effective in 40% to 78% of patients (184,187,189–195). Initial technical success in dilating the stricture does not translate into long-term success. Failure of balloon dilation becomes evident usually within weeks of the stent removal. Streem et al. (193) found that all failures presented within 12 months of dilation. Strictures that present early (within three months of surgery) have been reported by some to respond better to balloon dilation and stenting (187–189), but other series have not noted this to be the case (189). Early strictures reportedly respond in 62% to 100% of cases and late strictures (greater than three months) respond in 16% to 66% of cases (194). Endoureterotomy, which involves incision of the stricture, has also been used for UNC strictures (195,196). The results and indications for endoureterotomy are still in evolution, with the reported series all consisting of only a few patients each.

Prolonged ureteral stenting alone may be effective in treating transplant ureteral strictures (184,187). Bhagat et al. (187) reported that 69% (18 of 26) of early obstructions and 33% (5 of 15) of late obstructions (overall success rate of 57%—25 of 44 patients) responded to a stenting period of an average of 75 days, and the failures were treated with either surgery or chronic stent placement. Pappas et al. (184) reported that 75% of their cases responded successfully.

Strictures that develop at the UNC site appear to respond better to balloon dilation than do strictures at other sites in the ureter (188). This may be related to the ischemic nature of strictures in the proximal and middle ureter, whereas strictures at the ureteral anastomotic site are related to either errors in surgical technique or periureteral fibrosis.

Ureteral leaks also occur most frequently at the UNC; Bhagat et al. (187) reported that 80% of leaks were at the UNC and 50% of leaks were associated with stenoses. Ureteral stenting is effective in promoting healing and resolution of the leak in 59% to 80% of cases (187,188). If ureteral leak persists, surgical repair is usually required.

The only complication that is unique to a transplant nephrostomy is intraperitoneal leak of contrast due to inadvertent puncture of the peritoneum (187). This problem usually resolves spontaneously, without any adverse event. Because the patients are immunocompromised, special vigilance is required to avoid precipitating septicemia when percutaneous interventions are performed. Still, minor urinary tract infections can reportedly occur in as many as 38% of patients after the procedure (188).

PCN FOR STONE DISEASE

Percutaneous management of stone disease (PCNL), shock wave lithotripsy (SWL), and ureteroscopy have all had a significant impact on the management of upper urinary tract stone disease. Percutaneous management of urinary tract calculi is currently limited to patients who are not candidates for SWL or ureteroscopy. Percutaneous techniques are also used to salvage SWL or ureteroscopic failures. Open surgical procedures for stone disease are currently performed in only 1% to 2% of cases (197).

The widespread worldwide availability of SWL, its efficacy, and its relative noninvasiveness compared to PCNL make it the treatment of choice for most renal and ureteral calculi. However, with the introduction of second- and third-generation SWL machines, which appear to be less effective in stone fragmentation than the original unmodified Dornier HM-3 SWL machine (197), the role of ureteroscopy in stone treatment is being reassessed.

Indications for PCNL

SWL relies on stone fragmentation and propulsion of the fragments into the urinary bladder by urine flow and peristalsis. PCNL is therefore indicated when calculus fragmentation and passage would be suboptimal, so that the patient would not be rendered stone-free. The indications for PCNL are listed in Table 1.

Stone Size

As the size of stones increases to greater than 2 cm to 3 cm, the fragmentation efficiency with SWL decreases, necessitating multiple SWL attempts for complete breakup and, often, ancillary procedures to aid the passage of calculus particles (198–200).

Table 1 Indications for PCNL for Upper Tract Urinary Calculi

Stone size: large stones (greater than 2–2.5 cm), staghorn calculi
Stone composition: cystine calculi, failure of fragmentation with SWL
Urinary obstruction + stones: UPJ obstruction, ureteral strictures
Compromised urine drainage + stones: stones in dependent dilated calyces, stones in calyceal
   diverticula
Abnormal body habitus
Symptomatic stones during pregnancy
Certain removal of all calculous material important; e.g., for airline pilots
Stones for which other treatment modalities have failed
Stones in renal transplants
Stones following urinary diversion

Abbreviations: PCNL, percutaneous nephrostolithotomy; SWL, shock wave lithotripsy; UPJ, ureteropelvic junction.

Therefore, for most large stones, including staghorn calculi, SWL is not the treatment of choice (Fig. 2). Only 30% to 35% of stones larger than 2.5 cm to 3.0 cm may be rendered stone-free with SWL, compared to 70% to 90% of those treated with PCNL (201). Furthermore, 60% to 75% of patients with stones greater than 2.5 cm in size treated with SWL require additional procedures such as repeat SWL, PCNL, ureteroscopy, PCN, or stone manipulation, compared to 30% of patients treated primarily with PCNL (198). There is also a direct correlation between the size of the stone being treated with SWL and the subsequent accumulation of stone fragments (steinstrassen) in the distal ureter. Fedullo et al. (202) reported that the prevalence of steinstrassen was 17% when the calculi being treated were smaller than 10 mm, 26% when stones were 10 mm to 19 mm, 61% when stones were 20 mm to 29 mm, and 57% when stones were 30 mm or larger. It should be noted that a single stone larger than 25 mm to 30 mm has a different significance than several stones that are each 5 mm. The former is initially better managed with percutaneous techniques, whereas SWL is better for multiple smaller stones that are scattered throughout the collecting system and therefore less accessible to percutaneous techniques. Although each stone may be targeted easily for SWL, the presence of multiple stones does decrease the efficiency of SWL and the stone-free rate when compared to that of a single small stone.

Staghorn Calculi

Staghorn calculi are most commonly composed of struvite and are associated with recurrent urinary tract infections. Complete stone removal is essential in these patients because failure to do so allows persistence of infection and the eventual regrowth of the stone (Fig. 2). Other stones that may occasionally have a staghorn configuration are cystine stones, uric acid stones, and, rarely, calcium oxalate monohydrate stones. Staghorn calculi can range in size from a surface area that is less than 250 mm^2 to greater than 5000 mm^2 (200).

The primary approach to staghorn calculi should be by PCNL. Branched staghorn stones that fill the majority of the collecting system pose special problems in removal because stones located deep in infundibulae and calyces may be difficult to reach from the initial percutaneous tract or tracts. The most efficacious method of treating such staghorn calculi is by the so-called sandwich technique (203–205). PCNL is initially used to rapidly remove large volumes of easily accessible stone with ultrasonic or electrohydraulic lithotripsy ("debulking"). If infundibulocalyceal fragments are inaccessible from the nephrostomy tract by the usual endourological techniques, SWL is used to break up the small volumes of remaining stones, followed by PCNL to remove the residual fragments. Some advocate a second percutaneous procedure to remove the stone gravel because stone fragments have a tendency to remain in dilated collecting systems for prolonged periods. Others allow the stone fragments to pass spontaneously after adjunctive SWL (206,207).

PCNL followed by SWL and second-look nephroscopy, if necessary, has been shown to be the most cost-effective method of treating staghorn calculi (208). Martin et al. (209) reported that in their 97 patients with complete staghorn stones, 46% were treated with one session of PCNL alone, 40% in two stages (PCNL + SWL), 10% in three stages, and 4% in four stages. Patients treated in one or two stages were more likely to be stone-free than those treated in three or four stages.

In patients with partial staghorn calculi, monotherapy with SWL is an option. Lingeman (200) reported that patients with staghorn calculi that were less than $500 \, mm^2$ in size and with no dilatation of the collecting system could be made stone-free in more than 90% of cases with SWL alone. They cautioned, however, that such small-volume staghorn calculi are uncommon, making up only 3% of the staghorn stones treated in their series.

If staghorn calculi are considered as a group, reported stone-free rates for PCNL alone vary from 71% to 86% (210,211), compared to 84.2% for PCNL with or without SWL (200). Even though the addition of SWL at first glance appears to confer little advantage over PCNL alone as far as the stone-free success rate is concerned, the combination of the two procedures minimizes or eliminates the need for multiple renal accesses as well as for secondary endourologic procedures.

Still, only a minority of staghorn calculi require the addition of SWL to PCNL. During initial PCNL, efforts should be made to remove as much stone material as possible. If residual stone material is unavoidable, efforts should be directed toward removing enough stone material so that the residual stone burden is less than 2.0 to 2.5 cm in diameter (and thus more effectively treated with SWL).

To summarize, the effectiveness of SWL monotherapy in treating staghorn stones is directly proportional to the stone burden (212), with stone-free rates of 91.7% for staghorn stones smaller than $500 \, mm^2$ and 51.2% for larger stones (213). In contrast, the efficacy of PCNL is excellent irrespective of stone size, except when extremely large staghorn calculi (greater than $2500 \, mm^2$) are treated, with stone-free rates of approximately 85%.

Urinary Obstruction/Compromised Urinary Drainage

Urinary stasis can predispose to calculus formation. Examples of stones forming in association with obstruction are those in patients with UPJ obstruction (Fig. 10), calculi in calyceal diverticula, and stones in dilated lower pole calyces, malrotated kidneys, ectopic kidneys, horseshoe kidneys, and in patients with obstruction due to renal cysts or other renal masses. Changes in ureteral caliber or course due to congenital anomalies (retrocaval ureter, crossed ectopia), previous surgery (uretero-lithotomy, ureteral reimplantation), and chronic obstruction with resultant tortuos-ity or retroperitoneal processes (retroperitoneal fibrosis, tumors) can also impede ureteral drainage, leading to stone formation in these patients as well.

Although SWL can successfully break up the calculi in these situations, the frag-ments are unlikely to pass even when the stones are extensively fragmented (214).

(A)

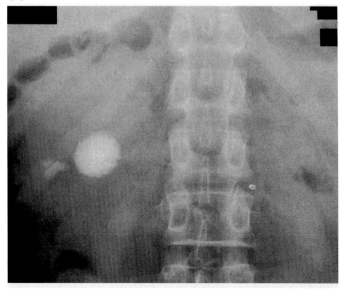

(B)

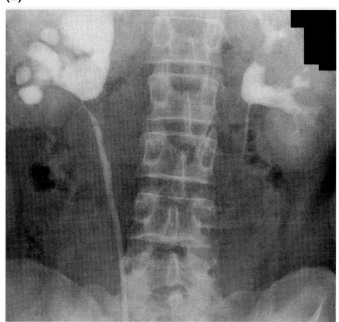

Figure 10 Large calculus in a patient with a UPJ obstruction. (**A**) A 2.5 cm spiculated calculus is seen in the right renal pelvis. There is also a smaller interpolar stone. (**B**) An IVU demonstrates marked right UPJ narrowing. Both the large size of the stone and the UPJ narrowing are contraindications for SWL and make PCNL the treatment of choice. *Abbreviations*: IVU, intravenous urogram; PCNL, percutaneous nephrostolithotomy; SWL, shock wave lithotripsy; UPJ, ureteropelvic junction.

A study that compared SWL for stones in abnormal and normal urinary tracts found that although fragmentation rates were similar for the two groups, clearance rates of fragments were significantly different (78% vs 56%) (215). PCNL is often preferred to SWL in these situations because percutaneous removal of the calculi circumvents the anatomic abnormalities that prevent stone passage. For example, absolute stone-free rates with SWL in patients with such renal anomalies as horse-shoe kidneys and pelvic kidneys average 62% (216), with many patients requiring multiple SWL treatments as well as additional procedures such as PCNL and ureteroscopy to render them stone-free. A recent multicenter study reported that primary PCNL in patients with horseshoe kidneys had an 87.5% success rate in making patients stone-free, but major complications were reported in 9% of patients (217). The availability of small-caliber, flexible, actively deflectable ureteroscopes and holmium laser lithotripsy (which is an effective lithotrite to vaporize and fragment stones) has positioned ureteroscopy as an effective alternative to PCNL and SWL in treating stones in anomalous kidneys, with a reported posttreatment stone-free rate of 75% in one small series (216).

Transplanted Kidneys

Calculi that occur in transplanted kidneys can be effectively treated with PCNL (218,219). Percutaneous dilation of the tract may be difficult due to perirenal fibrosis that may occur in some patients, but the approach is otherwise similar to that used in native kidneys.

UPJ Obstructions (Specific Considerations)

In patients with UPJ obstruction, PCNL is often combined with endopyelotomy. Endopyelotomy incisions are made along the posterior and lateral margins of the UPJ, with the incisions extending through the ureteral wall into the periureteric fat. Such an approach avoids the vascular structures that are usually located anteriorly and medially. After the procedure, the ureter is stented for six to eight weeks with a large-bore stent. The reported success for relief of obstruction varies from 64% to 86% (165,167). When an endopyelotomy is planned, PCNL access through a posterior interpolar calyx or upper polar calyx provides the most direct and straight access to the UPJ.

Calyceal Diverticula

Calculi occur in about 40% of calyceal diverticula and are usually asymptomatic and of little clinical significance. However, they may be associated with flank pain and/or chronic urinary tract infections (220). Open surgery with either marsupialization or excision of the diverticulum and fulguration or closure of the narrow neck is highly successful. Occasional patients may also be treated with partial or, rarely, total nephrectomy.

SWL of stones within calyceal diverticula has poor results, and stone-free rates of only 20% to 25% have been reported (221–223). Curiously, relief of symptoms can occur even if the patient is not rendered stone-free, although residual fragments do eventually grow and become symptomatic again. Percutaneous procedures are therefore advocated (224–226) as the safe and effective alternative for the management of symptomatic calyceal diverticular calculi. Retrograde ureteroscopic techniques (227), as well as a combined technique using both retrograde flexible ureteroscopy and simultaneous calyceal puncture, have also been used. The percutaneous technique consists of direct puncture of the symptomatic diverticulum (224–226) followed by tract dilation to 24 French to 34 French and nephroscopic stone extraction. Subsequently, either the neck of the diverticulum is dilated to 18 French to 34 French to enlarge its connection to the collecting system or the diverticular cavity is obliterated by electrocoagulation. The treatment of stones within anteriorly positioned diverticula can be technically challenging. Percutaneous techniques result in a stone-free rate of 95% to 100% (224–226), with obliteration of the diverticulum in 80% of patients and a marked decrease in size in the remaining 20% (224). These results are far superior to those obtainable by SWL and justify the use of PCNL as a preferred treatment, despite its greater invasiveness.

Stones in Dependent Calyces

The clearance of stones and stone fragments from the dependent calyces, i.e., the lower pole of the kidneys, is variable, unpredictable, and problematic after SWL, and especially so if stones occur in association with lower pole hydronephrosis. When the stone burden is small and located in a nondilated collecting system, stone fragments are more likely to be propelled and expelled out of the lower dependent calyces by the coaptation of the nondilated calyces and infundibula during normal peristalsis (228). Coaptation of the calyces and infundibula is less likely in hydronephrotic collecting systems where peristalsis is often diminished or absent. There is a tendency for the fragments of lower pole calculi to remain within the dependent calyces after SWL, and these retained stone particles in the lower pole can serve as a nidus for stone growth. Lingeman et al. (228) reported stone-free rates of 90% for PCNL versus 59% for SWL and also noted that results of SWL correlated inversely with the stone burden treated, whereas the results of PCNL were independent of the stone burden. With stones that were 1 cm to 2 cm in size or larger than 2 cm, stone-free rates with SWL were 56% and 33%, compared to 89% and 94%, respectively, for PCNL. Albala et al. (229) reported that with stones greater than 1 cm in the lower poles, retreatment or auxiliary procedures were needed in 36% (15/42) after SWL compared with 11% (4/38) undergoing PCNL. Stone recurrence rates in the lower pole following SWL range from 22% to 58% (230,231).

Gerber (232) reported that despite the poor published results for treating lower pole stones greater than 2 cm with SWL, 21% of urologists in their survey still preferred and recommended SWL over PCNL, whereas 65% of urologists treated 1 cm to 2 cm lower pole stones with SWL despite stone-free rates of just 41% to 56% (228,233,234). Thus, although SWL continues to be the preferred initial therapy for lower pole stones, as well as upper pole stones, by many urologists, the proven success and efficacy of PCNL in treating these calculi would argue for PCNL being the therapeutic modality of choice.

It remains unclear whether calyceal and infundibular anatomy can be predictive of lower pole stone clearance. Some factors that may be influential are the lower infundibular length-to-diameter ratio, overall infundibular diameter, and the number of minor calyces (233,234).

Need for PCNL in Stones of Different Composition

The composition of a given calculus is critical when one is deciding on the best method of management. Certain calculi are readily fragmented by ultrasonic lithotripsy but are refractory to SWL, making PCNL the treatment of choice.

Calculi composed of cystine fragment unreliably with SWL, requiring a greater number of treatments and total number of shocks compared to other calculi (235). Because many patients with these calculi are plagued with multiple stone events, which have required multiple previous interventions and can be anticipated to do so again, a trial of SWL for cystine stones less than 2 cm in size is reasonable. Rough, spiculated cystine stones that have recently formed respond better to SWL than do homogeneous, smooth, long-standing stones (236). High-power machines, such as the HM-3, also appear to be more effective. For stones larger than 2 cm, proceeding directly to PCNL is the best option. All stone material must be removed at the time of the percutaneous procedure to ensure that the patient will remain stone-free. Medical treatment (with acetylcysteine) has been unreliable in removing residual fragments (237), but its efficacy may be improved by infusing the drugs through percutaneously placed catheters.

Stones composed of calcium oxalate dihydrate and struvite break up well with SWL or any other form of power lithotripsy, whereas stones composed either partially or completely of calcium oxalate monohydrate do not respond well to SWL. With these stones, the volume of the stone is the main determinant of the most desirable mode of therapy.

Uric acid calculi respond well to SWL but not to ultrasonic lithotripsy.

Anatomic Abnormalities and Abnormal Body Habitus

A misshapen body habitus, such as that caused by scoliosis or, more commonly, morbid obesity, may make SWL unfeasible because the patients cannot be positioned so that the stone is in the focal point of the machine. PCNL may also be technically demanding in these patients but carries fewer risks than open surgery does. A preprocedural CT scan is helpful in such patients to evaluate the anatomy and plan an access route that avoids bowel and other viscera (238). PCNL has also been successfully applied in the treatment of calculus disease in anomalous kidneys, such as crossed-fused renal ectopia, horseshoe kidneys, and pelvic kidneys. These complicated cases also call for extensive preprocedural planning.

Need for Complete Stone Fragment Removal

If the presence of residual fragments is unacceptable to the patient for psychological or occupational reasons (airline pilots being the classic example), PCNL is an optimal option because of its superior stone-free rate of 95% to 98%.

Symptomatic Stones During Pregnancy

Renal colic affects 1 in 1500 pregnancies, usually during the second and third trimesters. Conservative treatment consisting of analgesia and hydration is effective in most patients, and the renal calculi pass spontaneously in 75% of patients (239). More aggressive therapy is required in patients with refractory pain, sepsis, renal insufficiency (particularly if there is a solitary kidney), and colic-induced preterm labor. Therapeutic interventions during pregnancy are restricted to drainage of the affected collecting system by either a ureteral stent placed in a retrograde fashion or a PCN. Ureteral stents can be placed with local anesthesia and are usually well tolerated during pregnancy (240,241). Endoluminal ultrasound has been used to place a ureteral stent (242), thus avoiding the potential risks of radiation exposure. If stent placement fails, PCN is performed.

SWL as well as ultrasonic and laser lithotripsy are contraindicated during pregnancy. Therefore, definitive therapy for the calculus is best postponed until six weeks postpartum. PCNL, ureteroscopic stone extraction, and open surgery (pyelolithotomy or ureterolithotomy) have all been performed during pregnancy (240), and general anesthesia can safely be administered during pregnancy (243). Because radiologic monitoring during ureteroscopy is not essential and can be eliminated, it is preferred over PCNL if stone extraction is deemed necessary (244).

Technique

Two primary components in the percutaneous therapy of upper urinary tract calculi are the establishment of an access tract and the actual stone removal itself.

Accurate access is the essential underpinning of a successful PCNL. A well-placed access tract can simplify a complex procedure, and, conversely, a poorly placed track may make it impossible to remove even the most accessible of calculi. Fluoroscopic control is usually preferred for the procedure, especially if the calculi are radio-opaque. CT is useful in preprocedural planning in patients with aberrant anatomy, in that the liver, spleen, colon, and pleural space can be avoided by the proposed tract (238,245).

If the calculus is located in a calyx or diverticulum, access should be obtained through that particular calyx or diverticulum. For large-volume calculi, a lower pole or interpolar calyceal puncture through a subcostal approach offers the advantages of avoiding the pleura while being certain of clearing the dependent lower pole calyces of calculi (Figs. 2 and 3). A stone-free rate of greater than 95% can be achieved using a subcostal approach (246). An intercostal puncture may be performed to access an upper pole calyx, usually to extract upper pole staghorn calculi, for concurrent endopyelotomy, and in patients with a large stone burden (247–252).

Narasimhan et al. (247) used an intercostal approach in 24% of their cases. In two of the three patients in whom access was above the 11th rib, thoracic complications requiring treatment (hydrothorax, pneumothorax) occurred. The authors recorded no clinically significant complications in cases where the puncture was below the 11th rib and into a middle or lower calyx. Fuchs and Forsyth (248) used an intercostal approach in 30% of their patients, of whom 5% had a major thoracic complication. The authors of both series (247,248) recommend that access above the 11th rib be avoided. Hopper and Yakes (57) performed CT on prone patients to estimate the risks associated with a puncture between the 10th and 11th ribs and found that an 11th–12th rib intercostal approach would puncture the right lung in 14% of patients and the left lung in 29% of patients in expiration. The risk of puncturing the liver and spleen was minimal in full expiration. However, the risk to the lungs was considered to be prohibitive with a 10th–11th intercostal approach, regardless of the degree of respiration. Munver et al. (252) used a supracostal approach in 33% of their cases (27% of tracks above the 11th rib and 73% above the 12th rib) and reported complications in 34% of supra–11th rib procedures and 9.7% incidence in supra–12th rib procedures. Intrathoracic complications were 16 times greater with supra–11th rib access, when compared with supra–12th rib, and 46 times greater than with subcostal access (intrathoracic complications in 23.1% of supra–11th rib access vs 1.4% of supra–12th rib and 0.5% of subcostal access). Thoracic complications in these patients include intraoperative hydrothorax/hemothorax, nephropleural fistula, and pneumothorax. Seven of eight intrathoracic complications occurred in supracostal cases in Munver et al.'s series (252). Kekre et al. reported a 10% thoracic complication rate (251).

PCNL is customarily performed with the patient in the prone position but has also been performed with the patient in a lateral decubitus position (253) and with the patient in the supine position when he or she is unable to lie prone (254,255). After the puncture is made, a 0.038-inch guidewire is placed into the collecting system and maneuvered into the ureter. Depending on the circumstances unique to the institution, tract dilation may be performed at the same sitting, in the radiology suite, or in the operating room immediately after the nephrostomy (246,256), with the urologists then extracting the calculus under nephroscopic guidance. Experience has proven that tracts can be dilated acutely to 24 French to 30 French with no adverse effects; this approach considerably shortens hospitalization and physician time (256). In most cases, bleeding associated with the tract dilation does not hamper visibility enough to require postponing the procedure.

Tract dilation is a painful procedure and requires that the patient be under either general anesthesia (preferably) or regional anesthesia. The dilation can be performed with tapered-tip fascial dilators of 10 French to 30 French size or high-pressure tract balloons measuring 10 cm in length and 10 mm in width when inflated. Tract dilation should be performed with fluoroscopic monitoring, with care being taken to avoid perforating the medial aspect of the renal pelvis when the stiff dilators are advanced.

Depending on the size and complexity of a stone, multiple access tracts may be necessary to remove it in entirety (257,258). The addition of SWL to PCNL can reduce the number of tracts required, with SWL being used to fragment the residual stone and the fragments then being extracted through the existing nephrostomy tract.

Simultaneous bilateral PCNL has been described for bilateral staghorn calculi (259), with no significant difference in the results or complication rate when compared with unilateral PCNL (Fig. 11).

Small calculi can be directly extracted through the sheath using forceps or a basket. For larger calculi, some form of lithotripsy is used to break the stone into smaller fragments. Ultrasonic lithotripsy is frequently used. The vibrating probe breaks up the calculus, and the fragments are aspirated through the hollow probe. For particularly hard stones, electrohydraulic lithotripsy or laser is used. Flexible nephroscopy is valuable in identifying and breaking up calyceal and ureteral fragments.

After the procedure, the collecting system is inspected to ensure a stone-free state. It is standard practice to leave in a ureteral catheter and a large-bore nephrostomy tube (20 French to 24 French Malecot catheters or Foley catheters) after the procedure to provide reliable drainage of urine, tamponade the tract, and allow the renal puncture to heal, and to permit access to the collecting system if additional procedures are required. The nephrostomy catheter is then removed in 48 hours to one week after a nephrostogram demonstrates no leaks from the collecting system and no residual stones. However, the routine placement of nephrostomy tubes after an uncomplicated PCNL with complete calculus clearance is increasingly being questioned due to the discomfort associated with the presence of a large-bore nephrostomy tube (260,261). In one series (262), 30 patients were randomized to receive a standard (20 French) nephrostomy drainage catheter, small-bore (9 French) nephrostomy drainage catheter, or no nephrostomy drainage. All patients with no postprocedural nephrostomy drainage catheters had antegrade placement of a 6 French double-J stent for four weeks. All three groups had a similar duration of hematuria and decrease in hematocrit postprocedure, but analgesic requirements were the highest in the large catheter group and the lowest in the no-catheter group. The tubeless group also had the shortest hospital stay and the smallest amount of

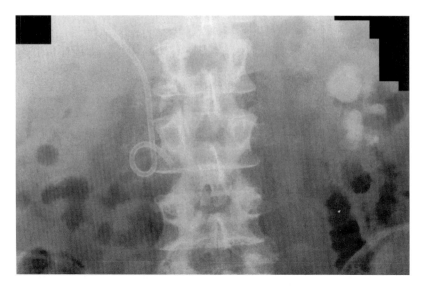

Figure 11 Patient with bilateral renal calculi (same patient as Fig. 2). After successful percutaneous removal of right renal calculi, left renal stones were removed percutaneously. Although bilateral simultaneous stone removal has been described, we prefer to treat one kidney at a time in patients with bilateral stones.

postoperative percutaneous site urine leak. Totally tubeless PCNL has also been reported elsewhere as a safe and effective procedure (263). Exclusion criteria for a tubeless approach are more than two percutaneous accesses, significant perforation of the collecting system, a large residual stone burden, significant postoperative bleeding, ureteral obstruction, and renal anomaly.

Contraindications

An uncorrected bleeding diathesis is the only absolute contraindication for PCNL. Also, the procedure should not be performed if a stone-bearing kidney is uninfected and nonfunctioning. A relative contraindication is the inability to establish a safe access tract.

Complications

Bleeding

Substantial arterial bleeding occurs in 0.5% to 1.5% of patients (264). Stoller et al. (265) reported an average blood loss of 2.8 g/dL hemoglobin for an uncomplicated one-stage, single-puncture PCNL. A twofold increase in blood loss occurred in patients treated for complicated staghorn calculi, who required multiple punctures, and in patients with renal pelvic perforation. Davidoff and Bellman (266) reported that in their experience, balloon dilation of the tract was associated with less renal hemorrhage and lower transfusion rates than tract dilation performed with sequential Amplatz dilators.

Vascular injury during the placement of the access tract or tract dilation can occasionally lead to pseudoaneurysms, arteriovenous fistulas, perinephric hematomas, and loss of functional parenchyma. Initial puncture into a calyx rather than an infundibulum or the renal pelvis is preferable and the approach is the least likely to cause major vascular injury (Fig. 4A–C).

Injury to Adjacent Organs

The colon can be punctured if it is positioned posterior to the kidney. In one series, CT scanning showed that the ascending colon was more posterior than the lower pole of the right kidney in 39.4%, and the descending colon was more posterior than the lower pole of the left kidney in 30.6% of patients (267). Furthermore, in 75% of patients, the colon moved more posteriorly when patients were placed in the prone position (compared to in the supine position).

When colonic injury occurs, it may not be obvious until the postprocedure nephrostogram demonstrates colonic filling with contrast. If the colonic puncture is small, the injury can be managed conservatively by draining the kidneys with a double-pigtail ureteral stent placed from below and then pulling the nephrostomy tube into the colon, leaving the nephrostomy tube to drainage and thus act as a colostomy tube. The tract usually seals in a few days (55,56). If a more serious injury occurs, open repair may be required (268).

Injury to the duodenum is uncommon and occurs if the large-bore dilators perforate the medial aspect of the right renal pelvis and then enter the duodenum during track dilation.

Injury to the liver and spleen is uncommon, especially if a puncture is performed with the patient in full expiration.

Pleural and lung injuries have been previously discussed. These injuries are usually recognized when the nephrostogram is done. A chest tube may be required if a large amount of pleural fluid accumulates.

Sepsis

The need for prophylactic antibiotics is unclear in patients with sterile urine undergoing PCNL even though a short course of antibiotics is often administered. A rise in temperature is common after stone removal. Postoperative bacteremia and pyrexia have been reported in up to 34% and 74% of patients respectively (269,270), but a 2% rate of bacteremia after percutaneous surgery with antibiotic prophylaxis is probably most reflective of current procedures (270).

Perforation

During the process of stone removal, the renal pelvis can be perforated by a sharp fragment of stone or by one of the instruments (such as the ultrasound probe) in as many as 10% of cases (271). Most such perforations heal within 12 to 24 hours provided adequate urine drainage is maintained. Serial nephrostograms show that even sizable renal pelvic and ureteral lacerations heal in a few days without stricture formation. A calculus can extrude through a urothelial tear. If it is not recognized at endoscopy, it will usually become obvious on postprocedural radiographs, although antegrade or retrograde contrast injections may sometimes be necessary for confirmation (272). Extruded calculi will be closely related to the collecting system and ureter, yet be outside these structures on different projections. Renal pelvic extrusions should be treated with nephrostomy drainage, whereas ureteral tears should be treated with stenting for a few weeks. In the absence of infection, extrusion of calculus material into the perinephric and periureteral tissues appears to be of no clinical consequence (272). Extraureteral infected stones are also initially managed by placement of a ureteral stent and a course of intravenous antibiotics (271), with close follow-up to monitor for complications such as a retroperitoneal abscess.

Entrapped Nephrostomy Tube

Malecot tubes are often placed after PCNL to allow residual fragments to drain. If the renal pelvis is small and intrarenal, tissue bridges can grow through the wings of the Malecot tube, making it resistant to removal (65,273,274). Therefore, it is unwise to place a Malecot type of nephrostomy catheter for more than two to three weeks in patients with small, intrarenal pelves.

REFERENCES

1. Goodwin WE, Casey WC, Woolf W. Percutaneous trocar (needle) nephrostomy in hydronephrosis. JAMA 1955; 157:891–894.
2. Levin DC, Flanders SJ, Spettell CM, Bonn J, Steiner RM. Participation by radiologists and other specialists in percutaneous vascular and nonvascular interventions: findings from a seven-state database. Radiology 1995; 196:51–54.
3. Smith Ad. Editorial: Percutaneous punctures—is this the endourologist's turf? J Urol 1994; 152:1982–1983.
4. Pearle MS. Editorial comment. J Endourol 2002; 16:96.
5. Bird VG, Fallon B, Winfield HN. Practice patterns in the treatment of large renal stones. J Endourol 2003; 17:355–363.
6. Farrell TA, Hicks MS. A review of radiologically guided percutaneous nephrostomies in 303 patients. J Vasc Interv Radiol 1997; 8:769–774.
7. Shokeir AA, El-Diasty T, Eassa W, et al. Diagnosis of ureteral obstruction in patients with compromised renal function: the role of noninvasive imaging modalities. J Urol 2004; 171:2303–2306.
8. Shokeir AA, El-Diasty T, Eassa W, et al. Diagnosis of noncalcareous hydronephrosis: role of magnetic resonance urography and noncontrast computed tomography. Urology 2004; 63:225–229.
9. Abo El-Ghar ME, Shokheir AA, El-Diasty TA, et al. Contrast enhanced spiral computerized tomography in patients with chronic obstructive uropathy and normal serum creatinine: a single session for anatomical and functional assessment. J Urol 2004; 172:985–988.
10. Zielonko J, Studniarek M, Markuszewski M. MR urography of obstructive uropathy: diagnostic value of the method in selected clinical groups. Eur Radiol 2003; 13:802–809.
11. Banner MP, Ramchandani P, Pollack HM. Interventional procedures in the upper urinary tract. Cardiovasc Intervent Radiol 1991; 14:267–284.
12. Silverman SG, Mueller PR, Pfister RC. Hemostatic evaluation before abdominal interventions: an overview and proposal. AJR 1990; 154:233–238.
13. Payne CS. A primer on patient management problems in interventional radiology. AJR 1998; 170:1169–1176.
14. Rohrer MJ, Michelotti MC, Nahrwold DL. A prospective evaluation of the efficacy of preoperative coagulation testing. Ann Surg 1988; 208:554–557.
15. Millward SF. Percutaneous nephrostomy: a practical approach. J Vasc Interv Radiol 2000; 11:955–964.
16. Gray RR, So CB, McLoughlin RF, et al. Outpatient percutaneous nephrostomy. Radiology 1996; 198:85–88.
17. Lee WJ, Mond DJ, Patel M, Pillari GP. Emergency percutaneous nephrostomy: technical success based on level of operator experience. J Vasc Interv Radiol 1994; 5:327–330.
18. McDermott VG, Schuster MG, Smith TP. Antibiotic prophylaxis in vascular and interventional radiology. AJR 1997; 169:31–38.
19. Larsen E, Gasser T, Madsen P. Antibiotic prophylaxis in urologic surgery. Urol Clin North Am 1986; 13:591–604.
20. Ryan MJ, Ryan BM, Smith TP. Antibiotic prophylaxis in interventional radiology. J Vasc Interv Radiol 2004; 15:547–556.

21. Classen DC, Evans RS, Pestonik SL. The timing of prophylactic administration of anti-biotics and the risk of surgical wound infection. New Engl J Med 1992; 326:281–286.

22. Cochran ST, Barbaric ZL, Lee JJ, Kashfian P. Percutaneous nephrostomy tube placement: an outpatient procedure. Radiology 1991; 179:843–847.

23. Spies JB, Rosen RJ, Lebowitz AS. Antibiotic prophylaxis in vascular and interventional radiology: a rational approach. Radiology 1988; 166:381–387.

24. Barbaric ZL, Hall T, Cochran ST, et al. Percutaneous nephrostomy: placement under CT and fluoroscopy guidance. AJR 1997; 169:151–155.

25. Ozden E, Yaman O, Soygur T, et al. Sonography guided percutaneous nephrostomy: success rates according to the grade of hydronephrosis. J Ankara Med Sch 2002; 24:69–72.

26. von der Recke P, Nielsen MB, Pedersen JF. Complications of ultrasound guided nephrostomy: a 5-year experience. Acta Radiol 1994; 35:452–454.

27. Dyer RB, Regan JD, Kavanagh PV, et al. Percutaneous nephrostomy with extensions of the technique: step by step. Radiographics 2002; 22:503–525.

28. Chien GW, Bellman GC. Blind percutaneous renal access. J Endourol 2002; 16:93–95.

29. LeMaitre L, Mestdagh P, Marecaux-Delomez J, et al. Percutaneous nephrostomy: placement under laser guidance and real-time CT fluoroscopy. Eur Radiol 2000; 10:892–895.

30. Stables DP. Percutaneous nephrostomy: techniques, indications and results. Urol Clin North Am 1982; 9:15–29.

31. Sampaio FJB, Zanier JFC, Aragao AHM, Favorita LA. Intrarenal access: 3-dimensional anatomical study. J Urol 1992; 148:1769–1773.

32. Lee WJ, Patel U, Patel S, GP Pillari. Emergency percutaneous nephrostomy: results and complications. J Vasc Interv Radiol 1994; 5:135–139.

33. Gupta S, Gulati M, Uday Shankar K, Rungta U, Suri S. Percutaneous nephrostomy with real time sonographic guidance. Acta Radiol 1997; 38:454–457.

34. Reznek RH, Talner LB. Percutaneous nephrostomy. Radiol Clin North Am 1984; 22:393–406.

35. Gupta S, Gulati M, Suri S. Ultrasound-guided percutaneous nephrostomy in non-dilated pelvicaliceal systems. J Clin Ultrasound 1998; 26:177–179.

36. Lewis S, Patel U. Major complications after percutaneous nephrostomy—lessons from a department audit. Clin Radiol 2001; 59:171–179.

37. Riddell AM, Charig MJ. A survey of current practice in out of hours percutaneous nephrostomy insertion in the United Kingdom. Clin Radiol 2002; 57:1067–1069.

38. Camunez F, Echenagusia A, Prieto ML, et al. Percutaneous nephrostomy in pyonephrosis. Urol Radiol 1989; 11:77–81.

39. Pearle MS, Pierce HL, Miller GL, et al. Optimal method of urgent decompression of the collecting system for obstruction and infection due to ureteral calculi. J Urol 1996; 160:1260–1264.

40. Bell AD, Rose SC, Starr NK, Jaffe RB, Miller FJ Jr. Percutaneous nephrostomy for nonoperative management of fungal urinary tract infections. J Vasc Interv Radiol 1993; 4:311–315.

41. Pappas P, Stravodimos KG, Mitropoulos D, et al. Role of percutaneous urinary diversion in malignant and benign obstructive uropathy. J Endourol 2000; 14:401–405.

42. Feng MI, Bellman GC, Shapiro CE. Management of ureteral obstruction secondary to pelvic malignancies. J Endourol 1999; 13:521–524.

43. Docimo SG, Dewolf WC. High failure rate of indwelling ureteral stents in patients with extrinsic obstruction: experience at two institutions. J Urol 1989; 142:277–279.

44. Hoe JWM, Tung KH, Tan EC. Reevaluation of indications for percutaneous nephrostomy and interventional uroradiological procedures in pelvic malignancy. Br J Radiol 1993; 71:469–472.

45. Markowitz DM, Wong KT, Laffey KJ, et al. Maintaining quality of life after palliative diversion for malignant ureteral obstruction. Urol Radiol 1989; 11:129–132.

46. Ekici S, Sahin A, Ozen H. Percutaneous nephrostomy in the management of malignant ureteral obstruction secondary to bladder cancer. J Endourol 2001; 15:827–829.

47. Ramchandani P, Cardella JF, Grassi CJ, et al. Quality improvement guidelines for percutaneous nephrostomy. J Vasc Interv Radiol 2001; 12:1247–1251.

48. Ramchandani P, Lewis CA, Bakal C, et al. (Committee of the Interventional and Cardiovascular radiology Commission). ACR practice guideline for the performance of percutaneous nephrostomy. Effective 1/1/02, pp. 335–343.

49. Cope C, Zeit RM. Pseudoaneurysms after nephrostomy. AJR 1982; 139:255–261.

50. Clark TW, Abraham RJ, Flemming BK. Is routine micropuncture access necessary for percutaneous nephrostomy? A randomized trial. Can Assoc Radiol J 2002; 53:87–91.

51. Zagoria RJ, Dyer RB. Do's and don't's of percutaneous nephrostomy. Acad Radiol 1999; 6:370–377.

52. Cronan JJ, Dorfman GS, Amis ES, Denny DF Jr. Retroperitoneal hemorrhage after percutaneous nephrostomy. AJR 1985; 144:801–803.

53. Nosher JL, Ericksen AS, Trooskin SZ, et al. Antibiotic bonded nephrostomy catheters for percutaneous nephrostomies. Cardiovasc Intervent Radiol 1990; 13:102–106.

54. Varkarakis J, Su Li-Ming, Hsu THS. Air embolism from pneumopyelography. J Urol 2003; 169:267.

55. Leroy AJ, Williams HJ Jr, Bender CE, et al. Colon perforation following percutaneous nephrostomy and renal calculus removal. Radiology 1985; 155:83–85.

56. Miller G, Summa J. Transcolonic placement of a percutaneous nephrostomy tube: recognition and treatment. J Vasc Interv Radiol 1997; 8:401–403.

57. Hopper KD, Yakes WF. The posterior intercostal approach for percutaneous renal procedures: risk of puncturing the lung, spleen and liver as determined by CT. AJR 1990; 154:115–117.

58. Neto ACL, Tobias-Machado M, Juliana RV, et al. Duodenal damage complicating percutaneous access to kidney. Sao Paulo Med J 2000; 118:116–117.

59. Reinberg Y, Moore LS, Lange PH. Splenic abscess as a complication of percutaneous nephrostomy. Urology 1989; 34:274–276.

60. Picus D, Weyman PJ, Clayman RV, McClennan BL. Intercostal space nephrostomy for percutaneous stone removal. AJR 1986; 147:393–397.

61. Marx MV. The radiation dose in interventional radiology study: knowledge brings responsibility. J Vasc Interv Radiol 2003; 14:947–951.

62. Miller DL, Balter S, Cole PE, et al. Radiation doses in interventional radiology procedures: the RAD-IR study. I. Overall measurement of dose. J Vasc Interv Radiol 2003; 14:711–727.

63. Miller DL, Balter S, Cole PE, et al. Radiation doses in interventional radiology procedures: the RAD-IR study. II. Skin dose. J Vasc Interv Radiol 2003; 14:977–990.

64. Pollack HM, Banner MP. Replacing blocked or dislodged percutaneous nephrostomy and ureteral stent catheters. Radiology 1982; 145:203–205.

65. Stewart LH, Kernohan RM, Loughridge WG. Nephrostomy tubes resistant to removal. Br J Urol 1992; 70:213–214.

66. Cronan JJ, Marcello A, Horn DL, et al. Antibiotics and nephrostomy tube care: preliminary observations: Part I. Bacteriuria. Radiology 1989; 172:1041–1042.

67. Cronan JJ, Horn DL, Marcello A, et al. Antibiotics and nephrostomy tube care: preliminary observations: Part II. Bacteremia. Radiology 1989; 172:1043–1045.

68. Zagoria RJ, Hodge RG, Dyer RB, et al. Percutaneous nephrostomy for treatment of intractable hemorrhagic cystitis. J Urol 1993; 149:1449–1451.

69. Beiko DT, Knudsen BE, Denstedt JD. Advances in ureteral stent design. J Endourol 2003; 17:195–199.

70. Chew BH, Knudsen BE, Denstedt JD. Advances in ureteral stent design and construction. Contemp Urol 2004; 10:16–20.

71. Holmes SAV, Kirby RS, Whitfield HN. Urinary tract prostheses and their biocompatibility. Br J Urol 1993; 71:378–383.

72. Mardis HK, Kroeger RM, Morton JJ, et al. Comparative evaluation of materials used for internal ureteral stents. J Endourol 1993; 7:105–115.

73. Mardis HK, Kroeger RM. Ureteral stents: materials. Urol Clin North Am 1988; 15:471.

74. Rackson ME, Mitty HA, Lossef SV, et al. Biocompatible copolymer ureteral stent: maintenance of patency beyond 6 months. AJR 1989; 153:783–784.

75. Cardella JF, Castaneda-Zuniga WR, Hunter DW, et al. Urine-compatible polymer for long term ureteral stenting. Radiology 1986; 161:313–318.

76. Pauer W, Lugmayr H. Metallic Wallstents: a new therapy for extrinsic ureteral obstruction. J Urol 1992; 148:281–284.

77. Lugmayr H, Pauer W. Self expanding metal stents for palliative treatment of malignant ureteral obstruction. AJR 1992; 159:1091–1094.

78. Lugmayr H, Pauer W. Wallstents for the treatment of extrinsic malignant ureteric obstruction: midterm results. Radiology 1996; 198:105–108.

79. Flueckiger F, Lammer J, Klein GE, et al. Malignant ureteral obstruction: preliminary results of treatment with metallic self expandable stents. Radiology 1993; 186:169–173.

80. van Sonnenberg E, D'Agostino HB, O'Laoide R, et al. Malignant ureteral obstruction: treatment with metal stents—technique, results and observations with percutaneous intraluminal US. Radiology 1994; 191:765–768.

81. Cussenot O, Bassi S, Desgrandchamps F, et al. Outcomes of non-self-expandable metal prostheses in strictured human ureter: suggestions for future developments. J Endourol 1993; 7:205–209.

82. Kulkarni R, Bellamy E. Nickel–titanium shape memory alloy Memokath 051 ureteral stent for managing long-term ureteral obstruction: 4-year experience. J Urol 2001; 166:1750–1754.

83. Lingeman JE, Preminger GM, Berger Y, et al. Use of a temporary ureteral drainage stent after uncomplicated ureteroscopy: results from a phase II clinical trial. J Urol 2003; 169:1682–1688.

84. Schlick RW, Plantz K. In vitro results with special plastics for biodegradable endourethral stents. J Endourol 1998; 12:451–455.

85. Dyer RB, Chen MY, Zagoria RJ, et al. Complications of ureteral stent placement. Radiographics 2002; 22:1005–1022.

86. Mitty HA, Dan SJ, Train JS. Antegrade ureteral stents: technical and catheter related problems with polyethylene and polyurethane. Radiology 1987; 165:439–443.

87. Mitty HA. Ureteral stenting facilitated by antegrade transurethral passage of guide wire. AJR 1984; 142:831–832.

88. D'Souza R, Tait P, Thomson RW, et al. Case report: an alternative approach to stenting the ureter. Br J Radiol 1993; 66:460–461.

89. Watson GMT, Patel U. Primary antegrade ureteric stenting: prospective experience and cost-effectiveness analysis in 50 ureters. Clin Radiol 2001; 56:568–574.

90. Patel U, Abubacker MZ. Ureteral stent placement without postprocedural nephrostomy tube: experience in 41 patients. Radiology 2004; 230:435–442.

91. Greenstein A, Shoval Y, Chen J, et al. Incidental extraction of double pigtail catheter during nephrostomy removal. Urol Radiol 1989; 11:121–122.

92. Seymour H, Patel U. Ureteral stenting: current status. Semin Intervent Radiol 2000; 17:351–366.

93. Amendola MA, Banner MP, Pollack HM, Gordon RL. Fluoroscopically guided pyeloureteral interventions by using a perurethral transvesical approach. AJR 1989; 152:97–102.

94. Babel SG, Winterkorn KG. Retrograde catheterization of the ureter without cystoscopic assistance: preliminary experience. Radiology 1993; 187:547–549.

95. Huang T-Y, Perkins T, Mader G. Retrograde placement of internal double-J ureteral stents by using cystographic guidance. AJR 1994; 163:371–372.

96. Babel SG, Winterkorn KG. Primary retrograde placement of ureteral stents by radiologists. AJR 1995; 164:1555.

97. deBaere T, Denys A, Pappas P, et al. Ureteral stents: exchange under fluoroscopic control as an effective alternative to cystoscopy. Radiology 1994; 190:887–889.
98. Yedlicka JW, Aizpuru R, Hunter DW, et al. Retrograde replacement of internal double-J ureteral stents. AJR 1991; 156:1007–1009.
99. Pilcher JM, Patel U. Choosing the correct length of ureteric stent: a formula based on the patient's height compared with direct ureteric measurement. Clin Radiol 2002; 57:59–62.
100. Eiley DM, McDougall EM, Smith AD. Techniques for stenting the normal and obstructed ureter. J Endourol 1997; 11:419–429.
101. Herrera M, Brawerman S. The endocatheter ruler: a useful new device. AJR 1982; 139:828–829.
102. Wills MI, Gilbert HW, Chadwick DJ, et al. Which ureteric stent length? Br J Urol 1991; 68:440.
103. Yossepowitch O, Lifshitz DA, Dekel Y, et al. Predicting the success of retrograde stenting for managing ureteral obstruction. J Urol 2001; 166:1746–1749.
104. Chung SY, Stein RJ, Landsittel D, et al. 15-year experience with the management of extrinsic ureteral obstruction with indwelling ureteral stents. J Urol 2004; 172:592–595.
105. Fine H, Gordon RL, Lebensart PD. Extracorporeal shock wave lithotripsy and stents: fluoroscopic observations and a hypothesis on the mechanisms of stent function. Urol Radiol 1989; 11:37.
106. Rotaru P, Yohannes P, Alexianu M, et al. Management of malignant extrinsic compression of the ureter by simultaneous placement of two ipsilateral ureteral stents. J Endourol 2001; 15:979–983.
107. Slavis SA, Wilson RW, Jones RJ, et al. Long-term results of permanent indwelling Wallstents for benign mid-ureteral strictures. J Endourol 2000; 14:577–581.
108. Pollak JS, Rosenblatt MM, Egglin TK, et al. Treatment of ureteral obstructions with the Wallstent endoprosthesis: preliminary results. J Vasc Interv Radiol 1995; 6:417–425.
109. Cornud FE, Casanova JP, Bonnel DH, et al. Impassable ureteral strictures: management with percutaneous ureteroneocystostomy. Radiology 1991; 180:451–454.
110. Lang EK. Percutaneous ureterocystostomy and ureteroneocystostomy. AJR 1988; 150:1065–1068.
111. Rosdy E. Percutaneous transrenal ureteroneocystostomy. J Endourol 1999; 13:369–372.
112. Mishra VC, Rao AR, Desai AR, et al. A unique extra-anatomic urinary diversion. J Endourol 2004; 18:57–58.
113. Bilbao JI, Longo JM, Martin-Palance A, et al. Direct percutaneous ureteral approach for the treatment of ureteral stenosis or obstruction. J Vasc Interv Radiol 1992; 3:553–555.
114. Jabbour ME, Desgrandchamps F, Angelescu E, et al. Percutaneous implantation of subcutaneous prosthetic ureters: long-term outcome. J Endourol 2001; 15:611–614.
115. Thomas R. Indwelling ureteral stents: impact of material and shape on patient comfort. J Endourol 1993; 7:137–140.
116. Ramsay JWA, Crocker RP, Ball AJ, et al. Urothelial reaction to ureteric intubation: a clinical study. Br J Urol 1987; 60:504.
117. El-Faqih SR, Shamsuddin AB, Chakrabarti A, et al. Polyurethane internal ureteral stents in treatment of stone patients: morbidity related to indwelling times. J Urol 1991; 146:1487–1491.
118. Fox CW Jr, Vaccaro JA, Kiesling FJ Jr, et al. Determination of indwelling ureteral stent patency: comparison of standard contrast and nuclear cystography and Lasix renography. Urology 1994; 43:442–445.
119. Platt JR, Ellis JH, Rubin JM. Assessment of internal ureteral stent patency in patients with pyelocaliectases: value of renal duplex sonography. AJR 1993; 161:87–90.
120. Haferkamp A, Brkovic D, Wiesel M, et al. Role of color-coded Doppler sonography in the assessment of internal ureteral stent patency. J Endourol 1999; 13:199–203.
121. Singh I, Gupta MP, Hemal AK, et al. Severely encrusted polyurethane ureteral stents: management and analysis of potential risk factors. Urology 2001; 58:526–531.

122. Trillaud H, Pariente J-L, Rabie A, et al. Detection of encrusted indwelling ureteral stents using a twinkling artifact revealed on color Doppler sonography. AJR 2001; 176: 1446–1448.

123. Bukkapatnam R, Seigne J, Helal M. 1-step removal of encrusted retained ureteral stents. J Urol 2003; 170:1111–1114.

124. Lam JS, Gupta M. Tips and tricks for the management of retained ureteral stents. J Endourol 2002; 16:733–741.

125. Monga M, Klein E, Castaneda-Zuniga WR, et al. The forgotten indwelling ureteral stent: a urological dilemma. J Urol 1995; 153:1817–1819.

126. Somers WJ. Management of forgotten or retained indwelling ureteral stents. Urology 1996; 47:431–435.

127. Salazar JE, Johnson JB, Scott RL. Perforation of renal pelvis by internal ureteral stents. AJR 1984; 143:816–818.

128. Slaton JW, Kropp KA. Proximal ureteral stent migration: an avoidable complication. J Urol 1996; 155:58–61.

129. Leroy AJ, Williams HJ, Segura JW, et al. Indwelling ureteral stents: percutaneous management of complications. Radiology 1986; 158:219–222.

130. Quillin SP, Darey MD, Picus D. Angiographic evaluation and therapy of ureteroarterial fistulas. AJR 1994; 162:873–878.

131. Vandersteen DR, Saxon RR, Fuchs E, et al. Diagnosis and management of ureteroiliac artery fistula: value of provocative arteriography followed by common iliac artery embolization and extraanatomic arterial bypass grafting. J Urol 1997; 158:754–758.

132. Batter SJ, McGovern FJ, Cambria RP. Ureteroarterial fistula: case report and review of the literature. Urology 1996; 48:481–489.

133. Keller FS, Barton RE, Routh WD, et al. Gross hematuria in two patients with ureteral ileal conduits and double-J stents. J Vasc Interv Radiol 1990; 1:69–79.

134. Pryor JL, Langley MJ, Jenkins AD. Comparison of symptom characteristics of indwelling ureteral catheters. J Urol 1991; 145:719.

135. Netto NR, Ferreira U, Lemos GC, et al. Endourological management of ureteral strictures. J Urol 1990; 144:631.

136. Kramolowsky EV, Tucker RD, Nelson CMK. Management of benign ureteral strictures: open surgical repair or endoscopic dilation. J Urol 1989; 141:285.

137. Van Arsdalen KN, Banner MP. The management of ureteral and anastomotic strictures. Probl Urol 1992; 6:420–432.

138. Hafez KS, Wolf JS. Update on minimally invasive management of ureteral strictures. J Endourol 2003; 17:453–464.

139. Selzman AA, Spirnak JP. Iatrogenic ureteral injuries: a 20-year experience in treating 165 injuries. J Urol 1996; 155:878–881.

140. Selmy G, Hassovna M, Begin LR, et al. Effect of balloon dilation of ureter on upper tract dynamics and ureteral wall morphology. J Endourol 1993; 7:211–219.

141. Meretyk S, Albala DM, Clayman RV, et al. Endoureterotomy for treatment of ureteral strictures. J Urol 1992; 147:1502.

142. Meretyk S, Albala DM, Kavoussi LR, et al. Endosurgery: noncalculus applications in the upper urinary tract. In: Clayman RU, ed. Monographs in Urology. Florida: Medical Directions, 1991:68–89.

143. Chang R, Marshall FF, Mitchell S. Percutaneous management of benign ureteral strictures and fistulas. J Urol 1987; 137:1126.

144. Lee CK, Smith AD. Role of stents in open ureteral surgery. J Endourol 1993; 7: 141–144.

145. Beckmann CF, Roth RA, Bihrle W. Dilatation of benign ureteral strictures. Radiology 1989; 172:437–441.

146. Chandhoke PS, Clayman RV, Stome AM, et al. Endopyelotomy and endoureterotomy with the Acucise ureteral cutting balloon device: preliminary experience. J Endourol 1993; 7:45–51.

147. Cardella JF, Hunter DW, Castaneda-Zuniga WR, et al. Electrolysis for recanalization of urinary collecting system obstructions: a percutaneous approach. Radiology 1985; 155:87–90.

148. Uflacker R, Wholey MH. A new low-speed rotational atherolytic device for ureteral recanalization. AJR 1988; 151:1157–1158.

149. Schmidt JD, Hawtrey CE, Flocks RH, et al. Complications, results and problems of ileal conduit diversions. J Urol 1973; 109:210–216.

150. Frazier HA, Robertson JE, Paulson DF. Complications of radical cystectomy and urinary diversion: a retrospective review of 675 cases in 2 decades. J Urol 1992; 148: 1401–1405.

151. Gburek BM, Lieber MM, Blute ML. Comparison of Studer ileal neobladder and ileal conduit urinary diversion with respect to perioperative outcome and late complications. J Urol 1998; 160:721–723.

152. Vandenbroucke F, Van Poppel H, Vandeursen H, et al. Surgical versus endoscopic treatment of nonmalignant uretero-ileal anastomotic strictures. Br J Urol 1993; 71:408–412.

153. Cronan JJ, Amis ES, Scola FH, et al. Renal obstruction in patients with ileal loops: US evaluation. Radiology 1986; 158:647–648.

154. Delvecchio FC, Kuo RL, Iselin CE, et al. Combined antegrade and retrograde endoscopic approach for the management of urinary-diversion associated pathology. J Endourol 2000; 14:251–256.

155. Zaleski GX, Funaki B, Newmark G. Placement of retrograde nephroureteral stents through ileal conduits. AJR 1998; 170:1275–1278.

156. Drake MJ, Cowan NC. Fluoroscopy guided retrograde ureteral stent insertion in patients with a ureteroileal urinary conduit: method and results. J Urol 2002; 167:2049–2051.

157. Tal R, Bachar GN, Belenky A. External-internal nephro-uretero-ileal stents in patients with an ileal conduit: long-term results. Urology 2004; 63:438–441.

158. Banner MP, Amendola MA, Pollack HM. Anastomosed ureters: fluoroscopically guided transconduit retrograde catheterization. Radiology 1989; 170:45–49.

159. Nelson CP, Wolf JS, Montie JE, et al. Retrograde ureteroscopy in patients with ortho-topic ileal neobladder urinary diversion. J Urol 2003; 170:107–110.

160. Lang EK, Glorioso LW III. Antegrade transluminal dilatation of benign ureteral stric-tures: long-term results. AJR 1988; 150:131–134.

161. Kim SH, Yoon HK, Park JH, et al. Tuberculous stricture of the urinary tract: antegrade balloon dilation and ureteral stenting. Abdom Imaging 1993; 18:186–190.

162. El-Abd SA, El-Sharaby MD, El-Shaer AF, et al. Long-term results of endourological and percutaneous management of ureteral strictures in Bilharzial patients. J Endourol 1996; 10:35–43.

163. O'Brien WM, Maxted WC, Pahira JJ. Ureteral stricture: experience with 31 cases. J Urol 1988; 140:737.

164. Kwak S, Leef JA, Rosenblum JD. Percutaneous balloon catheter dilation of benign ureteral strictures: effect of multiple dilation procedures on long-term patency. AJR 1995; 165:97–100.

165. Gerber GS, Lyon ES. Endopyelotomy: patient selection, results and complications. Urology 1994; 43:2–10.

166. McClinton S, Steyn JH, Hussey JK. Retrograde balloon dilatation for pelviureteric junction obstruction. Br J Urol 1993; 71:152–155.

167. Knudsen BE, Cook AJ, Watterson JD, et al. Percutaneous antegrade endopyelotomy: long term results from one institution. Urology 2004; 63:230–234.

168. Albani JM, Yost AJ, Streem SB. Ureteropelvic junction obstruction: determining dur-ability of endourological interventions. J Urol 2004; 171:579–582.

169. Sofras F, Livadas K, Alivizatos G, et al. Retrograde acucise endopyelotomy: is it worth the cost? J Endourol 2004; 18:466–468.

170. Shapiro MJ, Banner MP, Amendola MA, et al. Balloon catheter dilation of ureteroenteric strictures: long-term results. Radiology 1988; 168:385–387.

171. Kramolowsky EV, Clayman RV, Weyman PJ. Endourological management of ureteroileal anastomotic strictures: is it effective?. J Urol 1987; 137:390–394.

172. Kramolowsky EV, Clayman RV, Weyman PJ. Management of ureterointestinal anastomotic strictures: comparison of open surgical and endourological repair. J Urol 1988; 139:1195–1198.

173. Cornud F, Mendelsberg M, Chretien Y, et al. Fluoroscopically guided percutaneous transrenal incision of ureterointestinal anastomotic strictures. J Urol 1992; 147:578–581.

174. Wolf JS Jr, Elashry OM, Clayman RV. Long-term results of endoureterotomy for benign ureteral and ureteroenteric strictures. J Urol 1997; 158:759–764.

175. Laven BA, O'Connor RC, Steinberg GD, et al. Long-term results of Antegrade endoureterotomy using the holmium laser in patients with ureterointestinal strictures. Urology 2001; 58:924–929.

176. Roth S, Schmidt C, Weyand M, et al. Nearly fatal injury of iliac artery after inaccurate incision of ureterointestinal stricture in orthotopic neobladder. J Urol 1996; 155: 640–641.

177. Cornud F, Chretien Y, Helenon O, et al. Percutaneous incision of stenotic ureteroenteric anastomosis with a cutting balloon catheter: long-term results. Radiology 2000; 214:358–362.

178. Rapp DE, Laven BA, Steinberg GD, et al. Percutaneous placement of permanent metal stents for treatment of ureteroanastomotic strictures. J Endourol 2004; 18:677–681.

179. Palascak P, Bouchareb M, Zachoval R, et al. Treatment of benign ureterointestinal anastomotic strictures with permanent ureteral Wallstent after Camey and Wallace urinary diversion: long term follow up. J Endourol 2001; 15:575–580.

180. Freeman JA, Skinner DG. Orthotopic urinary diversion. Contemp Urol 1995; 6:29–41.

181. Wilson TG, Moreno JG, Weinberg A, et al. Late complications of the modified Indiana pouch. J Urol 1994; 151:331–334.

182. Kinnaert P, Hall M, Janssen F, et al. Ureteral stenosis after kidney transplantation: true incidence and long term follow up after surgical correction. J Urol 1985; 133:17.

183. Makisalo H, Eklund B, Salmela K, et al. Urological complications after 2084 consecutive kidney transplantations. Transplant Proc 1997; 29:152–153.

184. Pappas P, Giannopoulos A, Stravodimos KG, et al. Obstructive uropathy in the transplanted kidney: definitive management with percutaneous nephrostomy and prolonged ureteral stenting. J Endourol 2001; 15:719–723.

185. Thrasher JB, Temple DR, Spees EK. Extravesical versus Leadbetter-Politano ureteroneocystostomy: a comparison of urological complications in 320 renal transplants. J Urol 1990; 144:1105–1109.

186. Swierzewski SJ III, Konnak JW, Ellis JH. Treatment of renal transplant ureteral complications by percutaneous techniques. J Urol 1993; 149:986–987.

187. Bhagat VJ, Gordon RL, Osorio RW, et al. Ureteral obstructions and leaks after renal transplantation: outcome of percutaneous antegrade ureteral stent placement in 44 patients. Radiology 1998; 209:159–167.

188. Fontaine AB, Nijjar A, Rangaraj R. Update on the use of percutaneous nephrostomy/balloon dilation for the treatment of renal transplant leak/obstruction. J Vasc Interv Radiol 1997; 8:649–653.

189. Kim JC, Banner MP, Ramchandani P, et al. Balloon dilation of ureteral strictures after renal transplantation. Radiology 1993; 186:717–722.

190. Waltzer WC, Frischer Z, Shabtal M, et al. Early aggressive management for the prevention of renal allograft loss and patient mortality following major urologic complications. Clin Transplant 1992; 6:318–322.

191. Kashi SH, Lodge JPA, Giles GR, et al. Ureteric complications of renal transplantation. Br J Radiol 1992; 70:139–143.

192. Voegeli ER, Crummy AB, McDermott JC, et al. Percutaneous dilation of ureteral strictures in renal transplant patients. Radiology 1988; 169:185–188.

193. Streem SB, Novick AC, Steinmuller DR, et al. Long-term efficacy of ureteral dilation for transplant ureteral stenosis. J Urol 1988; 140:32–35.

194. Yong AA, Ball ST, Pelling MX, et al. Management of ureteral strictures in renal transplants by antegrade balloon dilatation and temporary internal stenting. Cardiovasc Intervent Radiol 1999; 22:385–388.

195. Erturk E, Burzon DT, Waldman D. Treatment of transplant ureteral stenosis with endoureterotomy. J Urol 1999; 161:412–414.

196. Bhayani SB, Landman J, Slotoroff C, et al. Transplant ureter stricture: Acucise endoureterotomy and balloon dilation are effective. J Endourol 2003; 17:19–22.

197. Kerbl K, Rehman J, Landman J, et al. Current management of urolithiasis: progress or regress? J Endourol 2002; 16:281–288.

198. Segura JW. Percutaneous nephrolithotomy: technique, indications and complications. AUA Update Ser 1993; 12:154–159.

199. Lingeman JE, Zafar FS. Lithotripsy systems. In: Smith AD, ed. Smith's Textbook of Endourology. St. Louis: Quality Medical Publishing, 1996:553–589.

200. Lingeman JE. Staghorn stones: the continued challenge. AUA Update Ser 1993; 12:146–151.

201. Al-Kohlany KM, Shokeir AA, Mosbah A, et al. Treatment of complete staghorn stones: a prospective randomized comparison of open surgery versus percutaneous nephrolithotomy. J Urol 2005; 173:469–473.

202. Fedullo LM, Pollack HM, Banner MP, et al. The development of steinstrassen after ESWL: frequency, natural history and radiologic management. AJR 1988; 151: 1145–1147.

203. Streem SB, Lammert G. Long term efficacy of combination therapy for struvite staghorn calculi. J Urol 1992; 147:563.

204. Schulze H, Hertle L, Kutlar A, et al. Critical evaluation of treatment of staghorn calculi by percutaneous nephrolithotomy and ESWL. J Urol 1989; 141:822–825.

205. Streem SB, Yost A, Dolmatch B, et al. Combination "sándwich" therapy for extensive renal calculi in 100 consecutive patients: immediate, long term and stratified results from a 10-year experience. J Urol 1997; 158:342–345.

206. Miller K, Bachor R, Sauter T, et al. Percutaneous nephrolithotomy/ESWL vs stent/ ESWL for large stones and staghorn calculi: what have we learned? J Endourol 1989; 3:287.

207. Chaussy CG, Fuchs GJ. Current state and future developments of noninvasive treatment of human urinary stones with extracorporeal shock wave lithotripsy. J Urol 1989; 141:782.

208. Chandhoke PS. Cost-effectiveness of different treatment options for staghorn calculi. J Urol 1996; 156:1567–1571.

209. Martin X, Tajra LC, Gelet A, et al. Complete staghorn stones: percutaneous approach using one or more multiple accesses. J Endourol 1999; 13:367–368.

210. Chibber PJ. Percutaneous nephrolithotomy for large and staghorn calculi. J Endourol 1993; 7:293–295.

211. Patterson DE, Segura JW, LeRoy AJ. Long term follow up of patients treated by percutaneous ultrasonic lithotripsy for struvite staghorn calculi. J Endourol 1987; 1:777.

212. Van Deursen H, Baert L. Extracorporeal shock wave lithotripsy monotherapy for staghorn stones with the second generation lithotripters. J Urol 1990; 143:252.

213. Lingeman JE, Coury TA, Newman DM, et al. Comparison of results and morbidity of percutaneous nephrostolithotomy and extracorporeal shock wave lithotripsy. J Urol 1987; 138:485.

214. Kirkali Z, Esen AA, Mungan MU. Effectiveness of extracorporeal shock wave lithotripsy in the management of stone bearing horseshoe kidneys. J Endourol 1996; 10:13–15.

215. Demirkesen O, Yaycioglu O, Onal B, et al. Extracorporeal shockwave lithotripsy for stones in abnormal urinary tracts: analysis of results and comparison with normal urinary tracts. J Endourol 2001; 15:681–685.
216. Weizer AZ, Springhart WP, Ekeruo WO, et al. Ureteroscopic management of renal calculi in anomalous kidneys. Urology 2005; 65:265–269.
217. Raj GV, Auge BK, Weizer AZ, et al. Percutaneous management of calculi within horseshoe kidneys. J Urol 2003; 170:48–51.
218. Francesca F, Felipetto R, Mosca F, et al. Percutaneous nephrolithotomy of transplanted kidneys. J Endourol 2002; 16:225–227.
219. Lu H-F, Shekarriz B, Stoller M. Donor-gifted allograft urolithiasis; early percutaneous management. Urology 2002; 59:25–27.
220. Grasso M, Lang G, Loisides P, et al. Endoscopic management of the symptomatic caliceal diverticular calculus. J Urol 1995; 153:1878–1881.
221. Psihramis KE, Dretler SP. Extracorporeal shock wave lithotripsy of caliceal diverticula calculi. J Urol 1987; 138:707–711.
222. Ritchie AWS, Parr NJ, Moussa SA, et al. Lithotripsy for calculi in caliceal diverticula? Br J Urol 1990; 66:6–8.
223. Hendrikx AJM, Bierkens AF, Bos R, et al. Treatment of stones in caliceal diverticula: extracorporeal shock wave lithotripsy versus percutaneous nephrolitholapaxy. Br J Urol 1992; 70:478–482.
224. Bellman GC, Silverstein JI, Blickensderfer S, et al. Technique and follow up of percutaneous management of caliceal diverticula. Urology 1993; 42:21–25.
225. Donnellan SM, Harewood LS, Wenn DR. Percutaneous management of caliceal diverticular calculi: technique and outcome. J Endourol 1999; 13:83–88.
226. Auge BK, Munver R, Kourambas J, et al. Endoscopic management of symptomatic caliceal diverticula: a retrospective comparison of percutaneous nephrolithotripsy and ureteroscopy. J Endourol 2002; 16:557–563.
227. Fuchs AM, David RD, Fuchs GJ. Treatment of stones in caliceal diverticuli using retrograde endoscopic approach. J Endourol 1990; 4:109.
228. Lingeman JE, Siegel YI, Steele B, et al. Management of lower pole nephrolithiasis: a critical analysis. J Urol 1994; 151:663–667.
229. Albala DM, Assimos DG, Clayman RV, et al. Lower pole 1: a prospective randomized trial of extracorporeal shock wave lithotripsy and percutaneous nephrostolithotomy for lower pole nephrolithiasis: initial results. J Urol 2001; 166:2072–2080.
230. Graff J, Diederichs W, Schulze H. Long-term follow up in 1003 extracorporeal shock wave lithotripsy patients. J Urol 1988; 140:479.
231. McCullough DL. Extracorporeal shock wave lithotripsy and residual stone fragments in lower calices: letter to the editor. J Urol 1989; 141:140.
232. Gerber GS. Management of lower-pole caliceal stones. J Endourol 2003; 17:501–503.
233. Sumino Y, Mimata H, Tasaki Y, et al. Predictors of lower pole stone clearance after extracorporeal shock wave lithotripsy. J Urol 2002; 168:1344–1347.
234. Sorensen CM, Chandhoke PS. Is lower pole calyceal anatomy predictive of extracorporeal shock wave lithotripsy success for primary lower pole kidney stones?. J Urol 2002; 168:2377–2382.
235. Hockley NM, Lingeman JE, Hutchinson CL. Relative efficacy of extracorporeal shock wave lithotripsy and percutaneous nephrostolithotomy in the management of cystine calculi. J Endourol 1989; 3:273.
236. Motola JA, Smith AD. Therapeutic options for the management of upper tract calculi. Urol Clin North Am 1990; 17:191.
237. Knoll LD, Segura JW, Patterson DE. Long term follow up in patients with cystine urinary calculi treated by percutaneous ultrasonic lithotripsy. J Urol 1988; 140:246.
238. Matlaga BR, Shah OD, Zagoria RJ, et al. Computerized tomography guided access for percutaneous nephrolithotomy. J Urol 2003; 170:45–47.

239. Cass AS, Smith CS, Gleich P. Management of urinary calculi in pregnancy. Urology 1986; 28:370–372.

240. Drago JR, Rohner TJ, Chez RA. Management of urinary calculi in pregnancy. Urology 1982; 20:578–581.

241. Loughlin KR, Bailey RB Jr. Internal ureteral stents for conservative management of ureteral calculi during pregnancy. New Engl J Med 1986; 315:1647–1649.

242. Wolf MC, Hallander JB, Salisz JA, et al. A new technique for ureteral stent placement during pregnancy using endoluminal ultrasound. Surg Obstet Gynecol 1992; 175: 575–576.

243. Shnider SM, Webster GM. Maternal and fetal hazards of surgery during pregnancy. Am J Obstet Gynecol 1965; 92:891–900.

244. Watterson JD, Girvan AR, Beiko DT, et al. Ureteroscopy and holmium:YAG laser lithotripsy: an emerging definitive management strategy for symptomatic ureteral calculi in pregnancy. Urology 2002; 60:383–387.

245. Ng CS, Herts BR, Streem SB. Percutaneous access to upper pole renal stones: role of prone 3-dimensional computerized tomography in inspiratory and expiratory phases. J Urol 2005; 173:124–126.

246. Bush WH, Brannen GE, Burnett LL, et al. Ultrasonic renal lithotripsy: single stage percutaneous technique and adjuvant radiological procedures. Radiology 1984; 152:387–390.

247. Narasimhan DL, Jacobsson B, Vijayan P, et al. Percutaneous nephrolithotomy through an intercostal approach. Acta Radiol 1991; 32:162–165.

248. Fuchs EF, Forsyth MJ. Supracostal approach for percutaneous ultrasonic lithotripsy. Urol Clin North Am 1990; 17:99–102.

249. Wong C, Leveillee RJ. Single upper pole percutaneous access for treatment of ≥5-cm complex branched staghorn calculi: is shockwave lithotripsy necessary. J Endourol 2002; 16:477–481.

250. Golijanin D, Katz R, Verstandig A, et al. The supracostal percutaneous nephrostomy for treatment of staghorn and complex kidney stones. J Endourol 1998; 12:403–405.

251. Kekre NS, Gopalakrishnan GG, Gupta GG, et al. Supracostal approach in percutaneous nephrolithotomy: experience with 102 cases. J Endourol 2001; 15:789–791.

252. Munver R, Delvecchio FC, Newman GE, et al. Critical analysis of supracostal access for percutaneous renal surgery. J Urol 2001; 166:1242–1246.

253. Gofrit ON, Shapiro A, Donchin Y, et al. Lateral decubitus position for percutaneous nephrolithotripsy in the morbidly obese or kyphotic patient. J Endourol 2002; 16:383–386.

254. Shoma AM, Eraky I, El-Kenawy MR, et al. Percutaneous nephrolithotomy in the supine position: technical aspects and functional outcome compared with the prone position. Urology 2002; 60:388–392.

255. Ng M-T, Sun W-H, Cheng C-W, et al. Supine position is safe and effective for percutaneous nephrolithotomy. J Endourol 2004; 18:469–474.

256. LeRoy AJ, May GR, Segura JW, et al. Rapid dilatation of percutaneous nephrostomy tracks. AJR 1984; 142:355–357.

257. Lang EK, Glorioso LW. Multiple percutaneous access routes to multiple calculi, calculi in caliceal diverticula and staghorn calculi. Radiology 1986; 158:211–214.

258. Mercado S, Hunter DW, Castaneda-Zuniga WR. The double puncture: an effective percutaneous technique for removing complex, multiple renal calculi. Radiology 1986; 158:207–209.

259. Holman E, Salah MA, Coth C. Comparison of 150 simultaneous bilateral and 300 unilateral percutaneous nephrolithotomies. J Endourol 2002; 16:33–36.

260. Limb J, Bellman GC. Tubeless percutaneous renal surgery: review of first 112 patients. Urology 2002; 59:527.

261. Pietrow PK, Auge BK, Lallas CD, et al. Pain after percutaneous nephrolithotomy: impact of nephrostomy tube size. J Endourol 2003; 17:411–414.

262. Desai MR, Kukreja RA, Desai MM, et al. A prospective randomized comparison of type of nephrostomy drainage following percutaneous nephrostolithotomy: large bore versus small bore versus tubeless. J Urol 2004; 172:565–567.

263. Aghamir SMK, Hosseini SR, Gooran S. Totally tubeless percutaneous nephrolithotomy. J Endourol 2004; 18:647–648.

264. Patterson DE, Segura JW, LeRoy AJ, et al. The etiology and treatment of delayed bleeding following percutaneous lithotripsy. J Urol 1985; 133:447.

265. Stoller ML, Wolf JS, St Lezin MA. Estimated blood loss and transfusion rates associated with percutaneous nephrolithotomy. J Urol 1994; 152:1977–1981.

266. Davidoff R, Bellman GC. Influence of technique of percutaneous tract creation on incidence of renal hemorrhage. J Urol 1997; 157:1229–1231.

267. Hopper KD, Sherman JL, Williams MD, et al. The variable anteroposterior position of the retroperitoneal colon to the kidneys. Invest Radiol 1987; 22:298–302.

268. Vallancien G, Capdeville R, Veillon B, et al. Colonic perforation during percutaneous nephrolithotomy: case report. J Urol 1985; 134:1185.

269. Rao PN, Dube AD, Weightman NC, et al. Prediction of septicemia following endourological manipulation for stones in the upper urinary tract. J Urol 1991; 146:955–960.

270. Dogan HS, Sahin AS, Cetinkaya Y, et al. Antibiotic prophylaxis in percutaneous nephrolithotomy: prospective study in 81 patients. J Endourol 2002; 16:649–653.

271. Evans CP, Stoller ML. The fate of the iatrogenic retroperitoneal stone. J Urol 1993; 150:827–829.

272. Verstandig AG, Banner MP, Van Arsdalen KN, et al. Upper urinary tract calculi: extrusion into perinephric and periureteric tissues during percutaneous management. Radiology 1986; 158:215–218.

273. Koolpe HA, Lord B. Eccentric nephroscopy for the incarcerated nephrostomy. Urol Radiol 1990; 12:96.

274. Sardina JI, Bolton DM, Stoller ML. Entrapped Malecot nephrostomy tube: etiology and management. J Urol 1995; 153:1882–1883.

14

Image-Guided Ablation of Renal Tumors

J. Louis Hinshaw and Fred T. Lee Jr.
Department of Radiology, University of Wisconsin, Madison, Wisconsin, U.S.A.

INTRODUCTION

Renal cell carcinoma (RCC) is an increasingly common clinical problem with 36,160 new cases and 12,660 deaths predicted for 2005 (1). These numbers represent a doubling of the incidence during the last 50 years. This increase is secondary to a combination of (i) an overall increase in the incidence of RCC (2), which is of uncertain etiology, and (ii) a tremendous increase in serendipitous identification of small RCC on cross-sectional imaging performed for other indications (3). As a result, there has been a fivefold increase in the diagnosis of small, less than 3 cm RCC during the last 20 years (4). These tumors tend to grow slowly with a linear growth rate of 0 to 1.1 cm/yr (5), and are frequently diagnosed in older patients. The early diagnosis of these tumors is changing the prognosis and management of the disease. Historically, RCC was frequently diagnosed only after mass effect symptoms or gross hematuria became evident. As a result, the tumor was often very large and metastatic at the time of diagnosis. Thus, RCC had a very poor prognosis and management focused on chemotherapeutic interventions and surgical debulking. If the patient was a surgical candidate, radical nephrectomy was considered the standard of care (6).

Surgical techniques designed to remove the tumor, yet spare renal tissue and function, have been aggressively developed in recent years for the treatment of small, asymptomatic tumors. Partial nephrectomy has proven to have local recurrence and survival rates similar to that for radical nephrectomy for small RCC (7). The associated improvement in postoperative renal function can be particularly important in older patients who often have multiple comorbidities. Unfortunately, radical and partial nephrectomies have significant associated morbidity and mortality, and usually require a prolonged period of recuperation. Laparoscopic techniques have decreased postoperative recovery time, but are technically difficult and still require extensive peritoneal or retroperitoneal dissections. Despite these limitations, open or laparoscopic partial nephrectomy is now considered the standard of care for the treatment of small RCC at most institutions (7,8).

Because of the success of local tumor resection for the treatment of RCC, there has been increasing interest in the development of even less invasive techniques.

Tumor ablation has been in use since the early 1900s for the treatment of bladder tumors. Being familiar with these methodologies, urologists began utilizing intraoperative ultrasound (US)-guided cryoablation for the treatment of RCC during the 1990s (9–12). Early clinical results have been promising, and indicate that the efficacy of this technique for the treatment of small tumors is comparable to both radical and partial nephrectomy. Percutaneous image-guided ablation has enjoyed tremendous success in the treatment of liver and prostate cancer recently (13,14), and has potential as a less invasive alternative therapy for small RCC (15–18). In many instances, small renal tumors are ideally suited to treatment with percutaneous ablation techniques. The retroperitoneal location decreases the likelihood of significant postablation bleeding, the perirenal fat insulates surrounding structures from inadvertent damage, and the exophytic location of most renal tumors makes targeting straightforward. In this chapter, the indications for ablative treatment of renal tumors, ablation modalities, and currently utilized techniques will be reviewed.

INDICATIONS

Appropriate patient selection is the first step to managing a successful tumor ablation program, and requires a thorough knowledge of the indications and limitations of the ablation technologies, as well as the more traditional therapies. A cooperative multidisciplinary approach is important, and for the treatment of RCC, involvement of urologists and oncologists can help assure that the appropriate treatment option is pursued.

Percutaneous tumor ablation is quickly becoming a viable option for many patients. In particular, patients with significant comorbidities and contraindications to surgical intervention should be considered for ablation because of its excellent safety profile (15–18). Patients who have compromised renal function, a solitary kidney, or a syndrome that places them at risk for multiple RCC (i.e., von Hippel-Lindau), or who refuse surgery, should also be considered for possible ablation. The role of ablation for the treatment of RCC that can reasonably be treated with either ablation or resection is evolving, and is currently up to the discretion of the individual patient and his or her physician.

The size of a renal tumor, its location within the kidney, and the proximity of adjacent structures should be considered when evaluating a tumor for possible ablation. The size of the tumor is directly correlated with the likelihood of metastatic disease. Once a tumor reaches 5 cm in diameter, it is much more likely to have metastasized (19,20), thus limiting the role of any local therapy. The size of the tumor is also directly linked to the technical difficulty of performing an ablation. With the currently available technologies, successfully ablating a tumor larger than 3.0 cm can be challenging (15). The difficulty is primarily related to the need for multiple overlapping ablations when larger tumors are involved. Multiple ablations can be difficult to monitor and control (21). Increasing the size of the ablation zone also increases the likelihood of inadvertently damaging adjacent structures. The location of the tumor within the kidney is also important. In particular, centrally and/or anteriorly positioned tumors can be problematic. Centrally located tumors are resistant to ablation due to the "heat sink effect" of the large vessels within the renal hilum (22). These vessels disperse the heat, resulting in sparing of the tumor directly adjacent to the vessels. This has been confirmed in clinical trials, where centrally located tumors have been associated with a higher rate of incomplete ablation, as compared with parenchymal or exophytic tumors (15). Centrally located tumors are also associated with a higher rate of injury to the collecting system (15). Ablation of lower pole tumors is associated with a higher risk of ureteral injury and subsequent stricturing. These injuries can require prolonged stenting or ureteral resection. Anteriorly located tumors are often located in close proximity to the colon. Inadvertent thermal injury of the colon has been associated with poor patient outcome and even death in patients who have undergone hepatic radiofrequency (RF) ablation (23). In an effort to avoid this complication, anteriorly located tumors are often surgically resected, or ablated as part of an intraoperative procedure. Retraction of the colon during the ablation protects the colon from injury.

Research into techniques to increase the size of the ablation zone and make central/anterior tumors more approachable for percutaneous ablation is ongoing (24). However, taking the limitations of current technology and techniques into account, ablation is presently best suited to the treatment of exophytic/parenchymal RCC less than 5 cm in diameter. Centrally located tumors should be considered if they are less than 3 cm in diameter, and anteriorly located tumors should be approached with intraoperative techniques if the colon or other viscera is in close proximity, and is not able to be displaced. After determining that a patient is a suitable candidate for tumor ablation, the appropriate patient management, image guidance, ablation modality, and methodology must be established.

PATIENT PREPARATION/ANESTHESIA

The use of a mild bowel prep prior to the ablation procedure results in improved tumor visualization under US due to less bowel gas, and a decrease in the incidence of postprocedure ileus. Nothing per oral after midnight before the procedure allows either conscious sedation or general anesthesia to be administered safely. The use of antibiotics prior to ablation is controversial. Some institutions routinely use prophylactic antibiotics to provide coverage for skin organisms; however, there is currently no compelling data to indicate that this is necessary. Despite this, at the present time, at our institution, we administer 1 mg Kefzol IV just prior to the procedure.

There is also no consensus as to the most appropriate procedural anesthesia. In general, renal ablation is less painful than liver ablation due to the retroperitoneal location of the kidneys, but there still may be substantial pain resulting from the procedure. General anesthesia, conscious sedation, or a combination of the two has been utilized with success at different institutions. General anesthesia has significant procedural advantages over conscious sedation, including decreased patient movement during the ablation, decreased patient discomfort, and improved patient monitoring. However, general anesthesia is resource and personnel intensive, and can have risks and complications that are magnified in a medically unfit population. Thus, there is no preferred type of procedural anesthesia and practitioners have had success with both methods. One special circumstance that must be considered is when the tumor is adjacent to the adrenal gland. Heating of the adrenal gland during RF ablation can result in a hypertensive crisis (25). Therefore, in cases where the target tumor is close to the adrenal, it is important to have anesthesia support on hand to manage any lability in blood pressure. Placing an arterial line prior to the procedure for blood pressure monitoring is also very helpful in the management of these patients.

IMAGE GUIDANCE

Image guidance consists of five basic parts—planning, targeting, monitoring, controlling, and assessment of response (26). Computed tomography (CT) is the primary modality for planning prior to ablation of a renal tumor. The high spatial resolution and ability of CT to visualize adjacent structures, as well as to evaluate patients concurrently for evidence of metastatic disease, makes it superior to US for preprocedural evaluation. Magnetic resonance imaging (MRI) can perform a comparable role, particularly in patients with renal insufficiency.

US continues to play an important role for evaluating the malignant potential of indeterminate renal masses (27,28), and is the preferred imaging modality for tumor targeting during the ablation procedure in many institutions, including at the University of Wisconsin Clinical Science Center (UW CSC). This is not only because of the real-time feedback available with US, which allows rapid applicator positioning, but also because of its portability, excellent soft tissue resolution, and relatively low cost. The limitations of CT for targeting RCC as compared to US include the frequent difficulty of visualizing RCC on noncontrast CT, the comparatively limited approach path allowed by CT, the relatively thick imaging plane, which makes applicator positioning less precise, and the greater time (compared with US) required to position the applicator under CT guidance (29). CT fluoroscopy can speed the ablation procedure, but increases the radiation dose to the patient and physician (30). MRI has many advantages for use as a targeting modality, including multiplanar imaging capabilities, exceptional soft tissue differentiation, real-time fluoroscopic capabilities, and the ability to directly measure tissue temperature with MR thermometry based on gradient echo imaging (31,32). Despite these theoretical advantages over both US and CT (33,34), access to interventional magnets continues to be very limited, even in tertiary care facilities, and as a result, MRI-guided tumor ablation is not currently a viable option for most radiologists.

Monitoring an ongoing ablation can be difficult regardless of whether CT or US is being utilized. This is particularly true for RF and the other heat-based ablation techniques. The high temperatures produced by these modalities result in the release of water vapor. The water vapor distorts the US beam, producing "dirty shadowing," often obscuring the tumor being targeted, as well as surrounding normal parenchyma (35,36) (Fig. 1). On CT, the water vapor is visualized as small gas bubbles, allowing for improved definition of the involved area, but unfortunately, the gas bubbles do not closely correlate with the area of tissue necrosis (36). Cryoablation is more easily monitored than the heat-based methods of ablation, because the iceball produced during the ablation is readily seen by US, CT, and MRI (Fig. 2A and B). The iceball is identified as a regular, well-defined, hyperechoic line with dense posterior acoustic shadowing by US and as a region of low attenuation [0 Houston units (HU)] on CT and low signal on T1-weighted MRI images (37–40). If there is an appropriate acoustic window with US, the iceball can be evaluated from multiple angles, allowing superb definition of the involved area. Unlike the heat-based methods, the imaging changes are closely correlated with the area of tissue necrosis. In fact, the iceball identified on US corresponds to the portion of the ablated tissue that reaches a temperature of $0°C$. At a depth of 1 mm to this region is the transition point at which the ablated tissue reaches a temperature of $-20°C$ or less. Complete cell death generally results at a temperature of $-20°C$ (41). Controlling the ablation is intimately linked to monitoring the ablation and thus can be difficult, particularly with the heat-based mechanisms. Appropriate planning and knowledge of

(A)

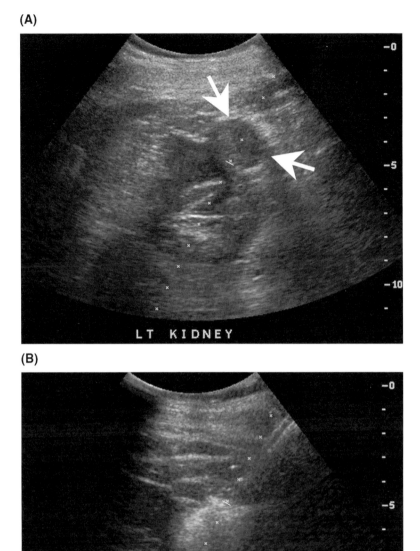

(B)

Figure 1 RF ablation monitored with US. (**A**) An exophytic renal tumor (*arrows*) was targeted under US guidance. The dotted line is the biopsy guide, indicating the predicted path for the RF probe. (**B**) When monitored by US, gas bubbles form around the probe, obscuring the area with "dirty shadowing." The bubbles do resolve over time, but complicate subsequent targeting, making the sequence of probe positioning very important. *Abbreviations*: RF, radiofrequency; US, ultrasound.

(A)   **(B)**

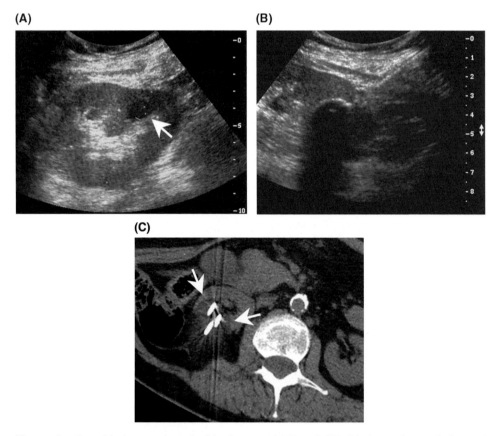

(C)

Figure 2 Cryoablation monitored with ultrasound US and CT. (**A**) A new hypoechoic renal tumor (*arrow*) was identified in a transplant kidney. (**B**) The tumor was targeted and ablated under US guidance. The leading edge of the ice ball is identified as a hyperechoic interface with dense posterior acoustic shadowing. (**C**) In a different patient, the ice ball is identified on CT as a zone of low attenuation (0 Hounsfield units). It is easy to distinguish the line of demarcation between the ice ball and unaffected tissues (*arrows*). *Abbreviations*: CT, computed tomography; US, ultrasound.

the ablation size associated with a particular applicator is important to ensuring complete ablation and avoiding inadvertent damage to surrounding structures.

Assessing response to ablation should be performed soon after the procedure itself. At Wisconsin, most tumor ablations are performed with the patient on the CT scanner. Targeting is usually performed with US guidance, and the ablation is monitored with a combination of US and CT fluoroscopy as necessary. Performing the ablation on the CT scanner allows a diagnostic contrast-enhanced CT to be performed while the patient is still under general anesthesia. US contrast agents have been used in hepatic tumor ablations to evaluate response to treatment, but the role of these materials in the treatment of RCC has not yet been evaluated (42). If the tumor is not completely ablated, additional ablations are performed in the same setting to ensure adequate treatment of the entire tumor. Note that a "tumor ghost" is usually identified on immediate postablation imaging regardless of the ablation modality utilized (Fig. 3). In the case of cryoablation, the tumor becomes revascularized, and appears hypervascular immediately after the final thaw due to preservation

(A)

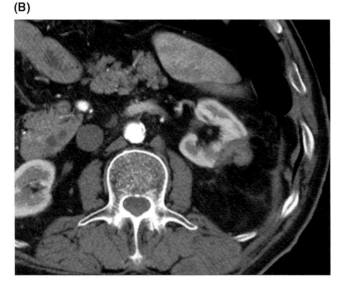

(B)

Figure 3 "Tumor ghost" after RF ablation of a RCC. (**A**) An exophytic RCC (*arrow*) was identified incidentally on a CT scan performed for other reasons. The tumor was subsequently targeted and ablated with RF, using a combination of US and CT guidance. (**B**) A diagnostic contrast enhanced CT performed immediately after the ablation shows the "tumor ghost." The tumor often does decrease in size, likely secondary to dessication, but will not resolve. More importantly, there is no residual enhancement of the tumor itself, and the lack of adjacent renal enhancement shows there is an adequate margin. *Abbreviations*: CT, computed tomography; RCC, renal cell carcinoma; RF, radiofrequency; US, ultrasound.

of the blood vessel walls. Tumor vessels thrombose approximately 48 to 72 hours postablation and the tumor then slowly resorbs over the course of 12 to 18 months (Fig. 4). The heat-based ablations cause immediate vascular thrombosis within the tumor, and these vessels never revascularize. Therefore, any residual tumor enhancement should be considered evidence of incomplete ablation (43). Because vessels

(A)

(B)

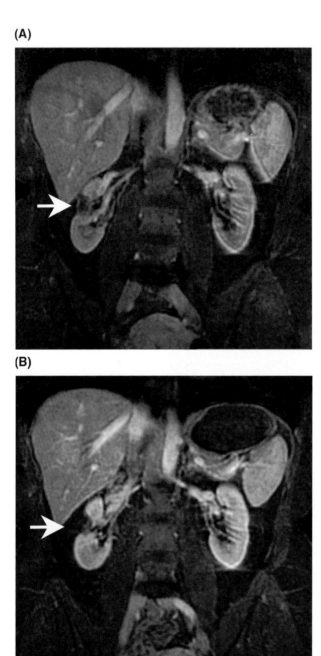

Figure 4 Tumor regression after ablation. (**A**) A contrast-enhanced T1-weighted image obtained one month after ablation of an RCC identifies the tumor and shows some subtle smooth peripheral enhancement (*arrow*). This kind of enhancement is often seen in the immediate postablation period and is not necessarily concerning. (**B**) Follow-up imaging six months later shows that the peripheral enhancement has resolved and the tumor mass has almost entirely resorbed (*arrow*), indicating complete ablation. *Abbreviation*: RCC, renal cell carcinoma.

do not have access to the tumor after treatment, tumors treated with heat-based modalities are slow to resorb, sometimes taking more than 24 months to completely resorb. Thus, the first several CT scans obtained after ablation with heat-based modalities should be primarily focused on evaluating for residual tumor enhancement.

IMAGE-GUIDED TUMOR ABLATION MODALITIES

There are a variety of different tumor ablation modalities available (44). These can be divided into the heat-based technologies [i.e. RF, microwave (MW), high-intensity focused US, and laser] and cryoablation. RF ablation and cryoablation are the most mature technologies and are the most extensively studied and clinically applied techniques. The other technologies are in development and have attributes that may prove beneficial as the technology continues to evolve. This section details the various technologies and their relative strengths and weaknesses. At present, clinical experience is too limited to establish one technology as clearly superior to any other. Therefore, the choice of which ablation modality to use in a particular case should be based upon the individual's comfort level with an ablation technology and the requirements of a given case.

RF Ablation

Mechanism

RF ablation is the most widely applied and thoroughly studied of the ablation technologies. The potential for local tumor destruction by RF was first appreciated when McGahan et al. published a paper detailing their work with in vivo porcine liver ablation using a rudimentary RF applicator based on the Bovie electrocautery system (45). Subsequently, there have been rapid improvements in the technology and it is now in widespread clinical use for the ablation of hepatic malignancies. In 1997, the first use of RF ablation was reported in the kidney (46), followed by the first percutaneous renal tumor ablation in 1998 (47), and during the last several years, multiple clinical series have been reported. These studies have established the safety and short-term efficacy of RF ablation for the treatment of renal tumors (15–18).

In RF ablation, a high-frequency alternating current (approximately 450 kHz) is applied to an electrode. Grounding pads are used to establish an electrical circuit through the body from the electrodes to the pads. The current agitates the tissue ions surrounding the electrode, thus creating molecular friction and heat. Because the surface area of the electrode is relatively small in comparison to the grounding pads, the current density around the electrode is quite high. This results in significant energy deposition and tissue heating around the electrode, but ideally not at the grounding pads. When the temperature reaches 50°C, the tissue coagulates (48). It is very important to apply the grounding pads correctly, because severe skin burns can result from incorrect pad placement. Four fundamental considerations for ground pad placement are as follows:

1. Pads should be placed equidistant from the ablation zone to avoid preferential heating of the nearest pad.
2. The long axis of the pad should be placed to receive the current.

3. Pads should never be placed superficial to a metal prosthesis or other metal object to avoid arcing.
4. The current path should not cross the heart if possible, especially if the patient has a pacemaker.

There are two primary factors that limit the size of the ablation zone when using RF. RF only creates ionic agitation, and thus only actively heats the tissues that are within a few millimeters of the electrode (49). This significantly limits the size of the ablation zone because the remainder of the tissue heating is due to thermal conduction. Utilizing a needle-shaped electrode, this dependence on thermal conduction limits the ablation zone to approximately 1.6 cm, even under ideal circumstances (45). The energy dispersion related to flowing blood at tissue vessel interfaces ("heat sink effect") (50) further limits the size of the ablation zone and results in thermal protection of perivascular tissue and tumor (51). As a result, vessels larger than 2 mm can be spared along with the surrounding tissues. This effect at least partially explains the difficulty in obtaining complete ablation of centrally located renal tumors located adjacent to large vessels in the renal hilum (15). Also, because the active heating only occurs in the tissues directly adjacent to the electrode, these tissues can reach very high temperatures. This is problematic because when tissue temperature reaches 100°C, tissue boiling, dessication, and charring occurs. As a result, eschar forms around the active portions of the electrode. This eschar acts as an effective insulator, limiting further current deposition (52). Many modifications have been made to the electrodes and the generators to overcome these limitations, and ablation zones up to 7 cm in diameter can now be achieved in some circumstances, by using multiple-prong electrodes and saline infusion (52).

Current Ablation Technology

There are currently three companies with Food and Drug Administration (FDA)-approved devices available in the United States. The companies have modified the electrodes in different ways in an attempt to optimize the ablation zone size. The multiple-prong, expandable array is utilized by two devices (Fig. 5) (Starburst/Starburst XL, Rita Medical Systems, Mountain View, California; LeV-een needle electrode, Radiotherapeutics, Natick, Massachusetts) and involves placement of a needle cannula from which multiple electrode tines are deployed in an umbrella-shaped array. Each prong produces a discrete ablation zone and the conglomerate ablation can be quite large. An internally cooled electrode (Fig. 6) (Cool-tip single and cluster electrodes, Valleylab, Boulder, Colorado) has a cooled perfusate that flows within an internal lumen during the ablation. Active cooling of the electrode and adjacent tissues decreases the high temperatures encountered in close proximity to the RF probe, and thus decreases tissue charring. The decreased eschar formation results in decreased impedance, allowing more current deposition. The multiple-prong and triple internally cooled (cluster) electrodes have increased surface area as compared to a single electrode, which also decreases impedance and allows more current to be deposited in tissue when compared to a single electrode.

A developing technique is the use of perfused or "wet" electrodes (52). These electrodes have an opening in the active tip through which fluids are infused, usually before or during an ablation. Normal or hypertonic saline is usually used. This technique increases the size of the thermal ablation zone by multiple mechanisms. The saline acts to conduct the electricity and heat more efficiently than soft tissue. There is also direct osmotic damage to the tissues from hypertonic saline. If the infusion is

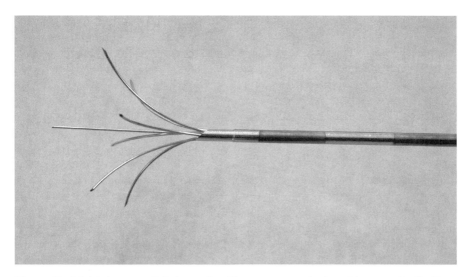

Figure 5 Multiple-prong RF electrodes. The prongs are deployed in an umbrella-like config-uration after image-guided placement of the needle cannula into the target. The increased surface area and span of the multiple prongs result in an increase in the size of the ablation zone. *Abbreviation*: RF, radiofrequency.

performed during the ablation, heated fluid is forced into the tissues (53). All of these factors lead to a larger zone of ablation. However, there is also a relative loss of control over the ablation zone because the infusate diffuses along tissue planes and can flow to unexpected locations, sometimes quite distant from the electrode itself (53,54). This lack of control has been a significant issue for hepatic ablations, but will probably not be as important for the kidney. Gerota's fascia should help contain the infusate, thus limiting collateral damage.

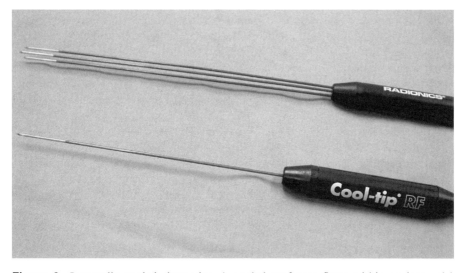

Figure 6 Internally cooled electrodes. A cooled perfusate flows within an internal lumen, decreasing charring and eschar formation on the electrode. This decreases impedance and thus increases the size of the ablation zone. The cluster electrode gives a larger zone of ablation than the single electrode (Radionics, Medford, Massachusetts).

During the last several years, RF generators and their current-control algo-rithms have improved. RF generators are capable of generating higher currents (up to 2.0 amp), leading to larger zones of ablation. The control of current deposition is based upon a feedback loop that modulates the current based upon impedance, cur-rent, or temperature. Fine-tuning the rate of current deposition allows maximum energy deposition while minimizing the amount of tissue charring that occurs. In addition, a multiple electrode system has now become clinically available. This system (Switching Controller Valleylab, Boulder, Colorado) can power up to three electrodes by switching at each impedance spike. As our understanding of the electrical and thermal properties of specific tissues increases, it is likely that different ablation algorithms will become available for different tissues and tumors (55).

Methods of Application

RF ablation can be performed during conventional open surgery, at laparoscopy, or as an image-guided percutaneous technique. Small-gauge RF probes and the inherent cautery associated with heat-based ablation decreases the likelihood of significant postprocedure hemorrhage. Applying the knowledge acquired during the development of hepatic ablation technology should speed the growth of renal RF ablation and ablation in general as an image-guided, percutaneous technique. Surgical or laparoscopic techniques should be reserved for cases with confounding variables that would make a percutaneous approach difficult or risky.

Results

The treatment of RCC with ablative techniques is a rapidly evolving, relatively young field, and as a result, only short-term outcome data are available. The data to this point are extremely promising with excellent primary and secondary local control and an exceptional safety profile (Table 1). However, because of the indolent course of many small RCCs, several more years of follow-up will be required to provide data that can be meaningfully compared with the results of radical and partial nephrectomy. Interpretation of the data, particularly when it comes to eval-uating the limitations of ablation, is also confounded by the rapid improvements in the technology and techniques of ablation. Because of these improvements, the indi-cations have been rapidly expanding and will continue to do so. Tumors that were considered unapproachable by ablation several years ago are now routinely treated in clinical practice. Also, as with many developing therapies, many of the patients included in clinical trials are poor candidates for traditional treatments and often have significant comorbidities. This may bias survival data to some extent.

Overall, the treatment of small (<3 cm) parenchymal tumors and frankly exo-phytic tumors has been very successful with minimal side effects and excellent local control. The ablation of larger (particularly >5 cm) or central tumors has been more difficult with a higher local recurrence and incomplete treatment rate (15–18). This led to at least one additional ablation session for approximately 25% of the central tumors (15). Results should continue to improve during the next several years as patient selection, RF technology, and the experience of practitioners progresses.

Cryoablation

Mechanism

Cryoablation is the antithesis of the heat-based ablation modalities. It is the applica-tion of cold temperatures to tissue, resulting in irreversible cell damage and death.

Table 1 Results of RF Ablation Trials

Author	Year	Number of tumors treated	Mean F/u (mo)	Device	Local control
Pavlovich et al. (56)	2002	24	2	Rita Model 500 (22) Rita Model 30 (2)	19/24 No retreatments were performed
Roy-Choudhury et al. (18)	2003	11	17.1	Radionics	11/11
Gervais et al. (15)	2003	42	13.2	Radionics (38) Starburst XL (4)	36/42 5/13 for central tumors
Farrell et al. (16,24)	2003	35	9	Radionics (23) Starburst and Starburst XL (12)	35/35
Mayo-Smith et al. (17)	2003	38	9	Radionics	37/38
Zagoria et al. (57)	2004	27	7	Radionics	20/22 2 refused retreatment
Veltri et al. (63)	2004	18	14	RITA	17/18
Lewin et al. (64)	2004	10	22.7	Radionics	10/10
Hwang et al. (65)	2004	24	12.7	Radionics	23/24
Boss et al. (58)	2005	12	10.3	Valleylab (MRI guided)	12/12
Varkarakis et al. (59)	2005	56	27.5	RITA (31) Boston Scientific (25)	53/56
Gervais et al. (60)	2005	100	27.6	Valleylab (92) RITA Starburst XL (8)	90/100
Mahnken et al. (61)	2005	15	13.9	LeVeen	15/15
Matsumoto et al. (62)	2005	109	19.4	RITA Starburst XL	109

Abbreviation: RF, radiofrequency.

Cryoablation has been used for more than a century to ablate tumors in superficial structures such as the skin, cervix, and breast. More recently, its uses have been expanded to include the ablation of tumors involving deeper structures including the prostate, liver, and kidney. Initially, cryoablation was applied exclusively at open conventional surgery (40), but as the probe size has decreased, there has been more interest in utilizing cryoablation percutaneously.

The mechanism by which cryoablation produces cell death is a combination of extracellular and intracellular ice crystal formation (66,67). Extracellular ice crystal formation damages the cell by direct physical damage to the cellular membrane by the ice crystals and by creating an osmotic gradient between the extracellular and intracellular compartments (67). This osmotic gradient creates a fluid shift out of the cell, resulting in dehydration and cell death. Intracellular ice crystal formation directly damages the cell membrane and intracellular proteins, leading to cell death

(58). Similar to RF ablation, cryoablation causes small blood vessels to thrombose, resulting in additional cytotoxic effects related to ischemia (41,68). However, the "heat sink effect" seen in RF is manifested as a "cold sink" in cryoablation and results in relative tissue sparing around large blood vessels (41). Vessels up to 3 mm can be completely frozen during cryoablation. Except for the small capillaries, these vessels often recanalize after thawing. Because the recanalized vessel is often perfusing necrotic tissue, there is a higher risk of postprocedure hemorrhage associated with cryoablation. Vessels larger than 3 mm tend to be spared, along with their perivascular tissues (69).

The critical temperature required to accomplish complete necrosis of a given tissue is dependent upon the tissue type, but is typically between -20 and $-50°C$. This temperature is usually achieved within a millimeter or two of the edge of the iceball created during cryoablation (41,70). As a result, estimating the expected zone of cell death based upon the imaging findings is relatively precise. Techniques that can increase the efficiency of cryoablation include multiple freeze–thaw cycles, an increased rate of freezing, and colder temperatures (71,72). Two freeze–thaw cycles are standard at most institutions.

Current Technology

The development of argon gas–based cryoablation systems has expanded the use of cryoablation from a primarily intraoperative technique to its consideration as a viable option for percutaneous use. Early cryoablation technology utilized liquid nitrogen (LN_2) as the cryogen. These systems were cumbersome, difficult to maintain, and required large probes (3.0–8.0 mm OD). The large probe size limited percutaneous use because of the difficulty and danger in placing such a large applicator percutaneously, but also because of the perceived risk of significant postprocedure hemorrhage related to the large access portal. Endocare Inc. (Irvine, California) (Fig. 7) and Galil Medical (Wallingford, Connecticut) are the only two companies that currently manufacture an argon-based system in the United States. Argon-based systems function by circulating argon gas under high pressure through the probe tip. The argon gas expands rapidly in the probe and creates very low temperatures on the order of $-150°C$ (Joule–Thompson phenomenon). The argon gas tanks are smaller and can be stored for longer periods of time than LN_2 tanks. The response times of the system are much quicker because the argon gas is relatively less viscous and therefore, more rapidly circulated. These systems use helium gas to speed the thawing process, which can significantly decrease the time necessary to perform an ablation. And perhaps most importantly, argon-based systems utilize smaller cryoprobes (currently as small as 17 gauge), which has expanded their use in image-guided percutaneous applications.

Methods of Application

The use of cryoablation has been primarily intraoperative in the past (73). In this setting, the probes are placed under direct visual guidance, usually in combination with intraoperative US. As image-guided percutaneous cryoablation becomes more prevalent, several advantages over the heat-based ablation modalities have become apparent. For one, multiple cryoablation probes can be placed simultaneously at the beginning of the procedure. They can then be activated simultaneously, creating a large conglomerate zone of freezing. This allows zones of ablation up to 12 cm in diameter, much larger than can be created with current heat-based ablation methods.

(A)

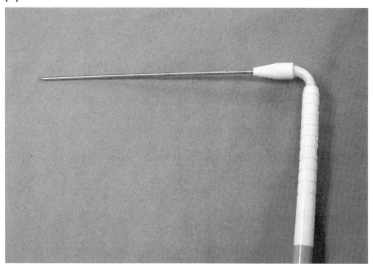

(B)

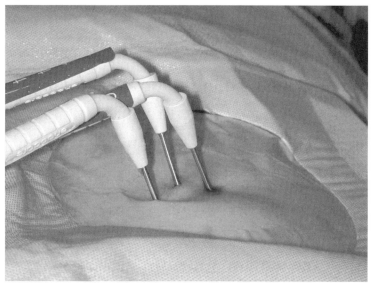

Figure 7 Cryoprobes. (**A**) Argon gas cryoablation systems utilize probes with much smaller diameters. These systems have made percutaneous cryoablation feasible. (**B**) Because multiple probes can be placed simultaneously, large zones of ablation can be achieved. The low profile of these angled probes allow the patient to be placed in the CT gantry both during and after positioning. *Abbreviation*: CT, computed tomography.

Positioning all of the probes prior to the ablation also allows more precise placement, because the targeted area is not obscured by the sequelae of previous ablations. Also, because the probes can be individually controlled, and the ice ball is easily identified with both US and CT, the shape and size of the ablation can be closely monitored and controlled. Overall, this can result in a very significant reduction in procedure time and improved control over the ablation zone, particularly when larger tumors are being ablated. A multiprobe RF system is now currently available and has shown promising results in animal studies (74). An effective multiprobe RF ablation system would obviate some of the advantages of multiprobe cryoablation.

Results

Cryoablation has been in use as an intraoperative technique for the treatment of RCC since the late 1990s. Early results show comparable local control and survival rates when compared with nephron-sparing surgical techniques (9–12). The safety profile may even be slightly more advantageous. The experience with percutaneous cryoablation of renal tumors is currently very limited, with no large clinical trials. However, early case series and case study results are promising. The largest series to date involved 19 patients, of whom 17 were successfully ablated at the first treatment. No complications were encountered (Table 2) (75). As with all the ablation modalities, repeat ablations can be performed as needed if the initial treatment is incomplete.

High-Intensity Focused US

High-intensity focused ultrasound (HIFU) is the use of highly focused powerful US beams that converge on the target tissue (82). The US beams vibrate the tissues and create heat. Physical therapists and athletic trainers have used similar, but less powerful US units for years (83). These units are used for heating deep muscle groups to encourage healing. When the transducer is focused in an appropriate manner, the heating can be marked and target temperatures in excess of 50°C are possible. Although the energy is primarily focused into the target tissues, skin burns secondary to nontarget energy deposition have been a problem experimentally.

HIFU is theoretically a near-ideal ablation modality. It is completely noninvasive because it does not require placement of an applicator, allows concurrent imaging during an ablation, and can ablate a precise tissue volume. However, the

Table 2   Result of Image-Guided Cryoablation Trials

Author	Year	Number of tumors treated	Mean F/u (mo)	Approach	Local success rate
Gill et al. (10)	2000	34	16.2	Laparoscopic	34/34
Rukstalis et al. (11)	2001	29	16	Open	29/29
Lee et al. (12)	2003	20	14.2	Laparoscopic	19/20
Shingleton and Sewell (37)	2003	12	17	Percutaneous	10/12
Harb et al. (75)	2003	19	18	Percutaneous	17/19 2 recurrences in pts with VHL
Cestari et al. (80)	2004	37	NR	Laparoscopic	36/37
Moon et al. (81)	2004	16	9.6	Laparoscopic	16/16
Desai et al. (77)	2005	89	24.6	Laparoscopic	87/89
Silverman et al. (78)	2005	26	14	Percutaneous	24/26
Gill et al. (79)	2005	60	36	Laparoscopic	58/60
Hruby et al. (76)	2006	11	11.3	Laparoscopic	11/11

Abbreviation: VHL, von Hippel-Lindau.

theoretical advantages of HIFU have yet to be translated into clinical results due to a large number of technological and logistic problems that, to date, have not been solved. The time required to reach ablative temperatures can be up to 20 minutes, even under ideal circumstances. Because the patient and the transducer are not coupled together, any movement over that time period can result in the dispersal of the energy into nontarget tissues. This can result in incomplete ablations or the ablation of nontarget tissues. Respiratory motion alone can be enough to interfere with accurate ablation. Another limitation is that the tissues do not change their imaging appearance during treatment, making monitoring of the ablation and assessment of response to treatment essentially impossible (84). Despite these limitations, Kohrmann et al. used HIFU to successfully ablate two of three renal tumors without significant complications (85). There is active research into solving these and other problems, using respiratory gating and computer-guided targeting systems. If significant improvements are made, HIFU will become an appealing abla- tion modality because of its noninvasive nature. However, a reliable commercial product is not yet available.

MW Ablation

MW ablation is a promising ablation technology that is used extensively in Asia, but has not yet been widely applied in the United States. To date, only a single company (Vivant Medical, Mountain View, California) has FDA approval for MW ablation. The MW ablation mechanism of cell death is identical to that of RF, because heat is again utilized to denature and destroy cells. However, the transfer of energy is dif- ferent and there are several theoretical advantages of MW over RF, which have not been optimized or fully explored to this point. MW ablation probes make use of electromagnetic waves (30–3000 MHz) that are identical to those used in a MW oven. These electromagnetic waves produce an electromagnetic field around the MW antenna and similar to RF, they produce ion agitation and heat. However, the electromagnetic field does not require an electrical circuit and is not dependent on direct physical contact for energy transfer. As a result, no grounding pads are required and theoretically, a much larger zone of active heating can be achieved (49,86). This also means that the transfer of energy is not affected nearly as much by the charring that occurs in the surrounding tissues. As a result, temperatures approaching 150°C can be achieved (87). Similar to cryoablation, multiple MW antennae can be placed simultaneously at the beginning of the procedure with the associated benefits discussed above. Overall, MW should theoretically achieve a more uniform and predictable zone of necrosis than RF; however, there are still significant technological and procedural limitations to be overcome.

Unfortunately, with current technology, the probe sizes remain quite large and the ablation sizes are relatively small. The most widely utilized system (Microtaze, Azwell, Osaka, Japan) uses a 14-gauge antenna, which is introduced through a 13-gauge cannula. Despite the large size of the probe, this system is only capable of producing a 1.6 cm diameter zone of ablation (88). Obviously technical improve- ments need to be made, and with this goal in mind, several other MW systems are currently in development (Vivant Medical, Mountain View, California; Microsulis, Ltd., Bath, England). As a result of these limitations, percutaneous image-guided MW ablation has only been applied on a limited basis for the treatment of RCC. MW has been used as an intraoperative nephron-sparing surgical technique for renal tumor enucleation in Asia (89). The results thus far have been comparable to other nephron-sparing surgical techniques. Although MW holds much promise as an ablation modality and rapid improvements in the technology are expected, it is not yet ready for widespread clinical application in the treatment of RCC.

Laser Ablation

Lasers work under the same theory as the other heat-based ablation techniques. After placement of a laser fiber in the tumor to be ablated, the laser is activated and the tissue is heated to temperatures in excess of 50°C. The transfer of thermal energy is by photon energy transfer, with conduction of heat away from the laser source. Lasers have been used extensively in the treatment of superficial tumors, most notably of the skin, cervix, and esophagus. In fact, in the esophagus, lasers have been used in conjunction with photosensitizers (i.e., photodynamic therapy) to ablate tumors. In this technique, a photosensitizer, mainly a porphyrin or a porphyrin derivative, is administered to the patient. These agents accumulate preferentially in the neoplastic cells, and then a light source (laser or filament) is placed in the esophagus. The light excites the porphyrin molecule and ultimately results in the production of a highly cytotoxic oxygen "singlet." The resulting necrosis and inflammation effectively ablates the tumor, while decreasing some of the side effects seen with thermally mediated laser ablation of the esophagus.

Lasers have been used quite extensively for the ablation of hepatic tumors and, in fact, have the largest published clinical trial of any of the ablation modalities. The results in that trial were exceptional, with a 98% local control rate and only a 3.5% complication rate (90). However, there has been relatively little experience with the use of lasers for renal tumor ablation. In fact, there is only one clinical trial in the literature, and the results of that trial were not very promising. Nine patients were treated in the trial using MRI-guided laser ablation. The results were given in percent decrease in viable tumor, because no complete ablations were achieved. The viable tumor decrease ranged from 29.5% to 73.7% (91). The laser fibers are also more expensive and more fragile than RF probes, making them less appealing unless other significant advantages become evident clinically. More work needs to be done, possibly on the use of photosensitizers, before laser ablation can be recommended for treatment of RCC.

TECHNIQUE

The placement of an ablation applicator is technically identical to performing an image-guided percutaneous biopsy, with a few caveats. The techniques for percutaneous placement of the probe under US, CT, and MRI guidance are well described and will not be reviewed here. However, there are some techniques specific to performing ablations, which will be discussed. The most important part of performing a successful ablation is appropriate planning prior to beginning the ablation. The tumor size, location, and proximity to blood vessels, the renal pelvis, and bowel must be taken into account.

Positioning of the applicator(s) correctly is critical to obtaining complete tumor ablation in all three dimensions. This requires a full understanding of both the geometry of the tumor itself, and the ablation zones possible with the chosen ablation modality. It is also important to place the applicator as precisely as possible on the first pass, because it is possible to seed the tract when repositioning an ablation applicator after puncturing the tumor. If it is necessary to reposition the applicator, the tract should be ablated (92). The tract is ablated by heating the applicator to ablative temperatures with the heat-based modalities, or by creating a small ice ball around the cryoprobe. This technique should also be used when removing the applicator at the end of an ablation, both to prevent tumor seeding of the ablation tract and, in the case of the heat-based modalities, to reduce the risk of postablation hemorrhage.

Because multiple ablations are usually required to ablate tumors larger than 2 cm in diameter, particularly if they are centrally located, the sequelae of previous ablations and their effect on tumor visualization can be problematic. Evaluating the response of the tumor to treatment also becomes more complicated when multiple ablations have been performed. This is particularly true with heat-based ablation technologies, where gas bubbles produced during the ablation can obscure the tumor (35). Thus, overlapping ablations performed in a sequential manner, beginning along the deep margin of the tumor and moving progressively more superficially, allow for complete ablation of larger tumors and prevent obscuration of residual tumor (21). With cryoablation, a commonly utilized technique involves placement of cryoprobes into the periphery of the tumor, approximately 1.0 to 2.0 cm from the outer border, equidistant from each other. The probes are simultaneously activated, creating a large conglomerate ice ball. The geometry and size of the ice ball can be manipulated by varying the input to the probes.

Optimal tumor ablation requires strategic applicator placement, with attention to subsequent ablations, adjacent structures, and the attributes of the ablation technology being utilized. With careful technique, inadvertent damage to adjacent structures is relatively unlikely for ablations involving the kidney because of its retroperitoneal location, but when it occurs it can be associated with significant complications.

SIDE EFFECTS AND COMPLICATIONS

Untoward effects encountered after a procedure are divided into side effects and complications. Side effects are defined as common undesired consequences of the procedure, which rarely result in substantial morbidity (26). Complications are further subdivided into major and minor complications. Major complications are those that might threaten the patient's life if left untreated, lead to significant morbidity or mortality, or result in a significant change in the course of hospitalization. All other complications are considered minor (26).

Postablation pain is the most commonly encountered side effect. Simply placing the applicator can result in significant soft tissue trauma, particularly because multiple passes are frequently performed through essentially the same tract. With the heat-based ablation modalities, the thermal damage to the renal capsule, abdominal wall, and diaphragm can result in tremendous postablation pain. In the immediate postablation period, patient-controlled analgesia or oral narcotic analgesics may be necessary. Cryoablation is relatively well tolerated with less significant discomfort after the ablation. Infusion of 5% dextrose in water into the peritoneal cavity between the liver and diaphragm is being used at the UW CSC to insulate the diaphragm during RF ablation of hepatic tumors located adjacent to the diaphragm. The technique has resulted in a significant decrease in postablation pain for these patients. The role for this and similar techniques in renal ablations has yet to be evaluated.

Postablation syndrome is a frequently encountered side effect, described as fever, malaise, and body aches encountered in the immediate postablation period (93). This syndrome has been well documented for liver ablation, but it is unclear how severe this problem is after renal tumor ablation. However, it is anticipated that renal ablation will provoke a similar response based on the volume of ablation. For the liver, the severity of the syndrome appears related to the volume of tissue ablated. The symptoms respond well to anti-inflammatory therapy, implying that the syndrome is related to the inflammation that develops around the necrotic tissues (93). At UW CSC, anti-inflammatory medications are given prior to ablation and 48 hours postablation to decrease the severity of both the postablation pain and the post-ablation syndrome.

Complications are relatively infrequent after percutaneous renal tumor ablation (15–18). Hemorrhage is usually reported as a minor complication, but could also be considered a side effect because it is almost always self-limited and rarely results in significant morbidity. The coagulation associated with heat-based ablation limits postprocedure bleeding. Cryoablation does not have this effect and theoretically, should have a higher rate of hemorrhage. However, significant hemorrhage has been very infrequent with either ablation modality in the clinical setting (75). Skin burns at ground pad sites are another relatively common minor complication seen most frequently early in the experience with RF ablation. However, the rate of skin burns has been substantially reduced as the proper number and appropriate positioning of ground pads have been established for the various generators and devices.

Major complications occur in less than 2% of reported image-guided renal tumor RF ablations, and there have been no reported deaths (15–18). Nephron-sparing surgery on the other hand is associated with a major complication 14% of the time, and has a 1% to 2% mortality rate (7).

One of the more common complications encountered with RF ablation thus far is injury to the lumbar plexus, which is associated with a postprocedure syndrome consisting of pain, paresthesia, and numbness in the flank and groin (16,56). The lumbar plexus is located along the anterior aspect of the psoas muscle and is most susceptible to injury when a posteriorly positioned tumor is being ablated. Thus far, these symptoms have been self-limited and usually resolve within one to two months (16,56).

Another significant complication that has been reported after RF ablation of centrally and inferiorly located tumors is thermal injury to the ureter (15). Ureteral injuries are concerning because they can lead to stricturing and resulting urinary tract obstruction that threatens the function of the kidney. The placement of a ureteral stent prior to the ablation is being evaluated experimentally and theoretically may decrease the likelihood of ureteral stricturing for two reasons. When left in place, the stent may mechanically prevent stricturing, even if the urothelium is injured. Also, the stent provides the opportunity to lavage the renal collecting system with cold fluid during heat-based ablations and with warm fluid during cryoablations. This lavage fluid might protect the ureter from achieving temperatures necessary for significant damage to the urothelium. Water, dextrose, or saline can be used as lavage fluid for many types of ablations; however, saline should not be used for lavage during RF ablation. As previously mentioned, saline is an electrical conductor and in this instance its use might actually promote/exacerbate ureteral injury. To date, no definitive data are available to indicate whether the use of ureteral stents and lavage is clinically efficacious.

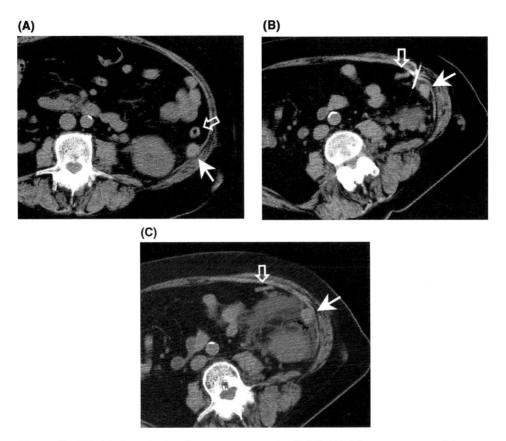

Figure 8 RF ablation of a locally recurrent anterior RCC. (**A**) After an unsuccessful percutaneous ablation, this patient underwent partial nephrectomy. A follow-up CT scan identified a local recurrence (*arrow*) in the renal bed, closely adjacent to the descending colon (*open arrow*). Because inadvertent damage to the colon can result in significant morbidity, this tumor would usually be approached laparoscopically. Infusion of sterile water or D5W into the perirenal space can be used to insulate and displace the colon. (**B**) In this case, a needle was placed between the mass (*arrow*) and the descending colon (*open arrow*) under CT guidance. (**C**) D5W was infused through the needle, displacing the colon anteriorly (*open arrow*). This allowed the recurrent mass (*arrow*) to be safely ablated percutaneously. *Abbreviations*: RF, radiofrequency; RCC, renal cell carcinoma; CT, computed tomography; D5W, 5% dextrose in water.

Most anterior renal tumors have been ablated intraoperatively due to the risk of injuring the adjacent colon. A developing technique for RF or DSW is the infusion of sterile water into the perirenal space between the kidney and the colon (Fig. 8). Theoretically, the fluid protects the colon from injury both by separating the colon from the kidney spatially, but also by acting as an insulating agent, because it is nonconductive. Early results using this technique are very promising (24). Infusing fluid to protect adjacent structures may also be helpful for preventing ureteral and lumbar plexus injuries. Because water might not provide similar protection for cryoablation, esophageal dilator balloons are placed in the anterior perirenal space to act as a spacer prior to cryoablation of anterior renal tumors (75). The full potential of these techniques has not yet been realized, but as they become better studied, and are refined, their use may allow the indications for percutaneous tumor ablation to expand further.

IMAGING FOLLOW-UP

There is no consensus as to the frequency and timing of imaging after ablation. At UW CSC, the follow-up protocol is an immediate postprocedure CT, followed by a CT at 1, 3, 6, and 12 months. If there is no evidence of recurrence at 12 months, follow-up is decreased to every six months. Contrast-enhanced CT or MRI is generally utilized for follow-up imaging. The tissues surrounding the ablated tumor often show concentric, symmetric enhancement in the first six months after an ablation (26). This is likely related to inflammation associated with the tissue necrosis. Irregular, nodular enhancement around the periphery of the ablated area, or any enhancement within the ablated tumor itself are concerning, as is any increase in the size of the ablated tumor (Fig. 9). With most tumors, local recurrence usually occurs within one year. However, because of the slow growth rate of small RCC (5), recurrences may take longer to manifest. The length of time necessary for the follow-up of a RCC ablation is yet to be determined.

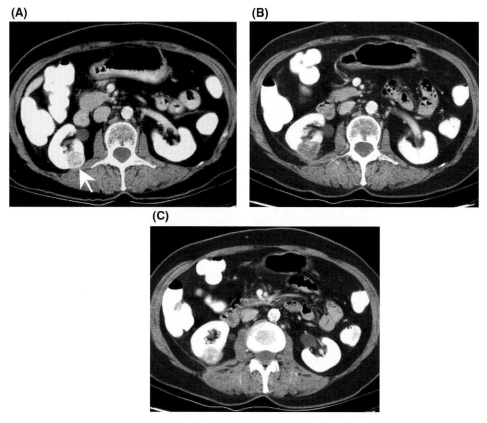

Figure 9 Identification of local recurrence on follow-up imaging. (**A**) A posteriorly located right RCC (*arrow*) underwent percutaneous cryoablation. Immediate post-ablation imaging (not shown) identified no residual enhancement, but was complicated by adjacent hemorrhage. (**B**) Follow-up CT three months later showed a large portion of the tumor was necrotic and had no residual enhancement. (**C**) However, along the inferior aspect of the tumor, there was brisk nodular enhancement, indicating local recurrence. A second ablation was performed and there has been no further evidence of recurrence. *Abbreviations*: RCC, renal cell carcinoma; CT, computed tomography.

Tumors that have imaging findings consistent with RCC are not usually biopsied prior to definitive treatment because there is evidence to suggest that imaging is as good as, or better than percutaneous biopsy for diagnosing RCC (94,95), and there is also a small risk of tumor seeding during the biopsy. However, with smaller renal tumors, the imaging findings are often not as clear cut and because there is no tissue sample available after an ablation procedure, some investigators biopsy renal tumors prior to an ablation. The results of this biopsy are often used to guide the intensity of follow-up imaging, but rarely have an impact on the decision to perform an ablation.

CONCLUSION

Ablation of renal tumors using image-guided ablation techniques is an exciting and promising field. Ablation techniques may eventually replace the more traditional surgical alternatives for the treatment of certain renal tumors and are already gaining clinical acceptance in nonoperative patients. Long-term clinical outcome studies comparing ablation techniques with partial/radical nephrectomy will be difficult to perform because the ablation systems and techniques are developing rapidly and preliminary results are likely to become outdated very quickly. However, these studies are still needed, and will contribute to determining the true role of image-guided ablation in the treatment of RCC. It is likely that, over the next few years, routine use of percutaneous ablation for treating some renal tumors will become much more widely established.

REFERENCES

1. Ahmedin J, Murray T, Ward E, et al. Cancer statistics 2005. Cancer J Clin 2005; 55: 10–30.
2. Chow WH, Devesa SS, Warren JL, Fraumeni JF. Rising incidence of renal cell cancer in the United States. JAMA 1999; 281:1628–1631.
3. Jayson M, Sanders H. Increased incidence of serendipitously discovered renal cell carcinoma. Urology 1998; 51:203–205.
4. Jemal A, Thomas A, Murray T, Thun M. Cancer statistics, 2002. Cancer J Clin 2002; 52:23–47.
5. Bosniak MA, Birnbaum BA, Krinsky GA, Waisman J. Small renal parenchymal neoplasms: further observations on growth. Radiology 1995; 197:589–597.
6. Robson CJ, Churchill BM, Anderson W. The results of radical nephrectomy for renal cell carcinoma. J Urol 1969; 101:297–301.
7. Uzzo RC, Novick AC. Nephron sparing surgery for renal tumors: indications, techniques and outcomes. J Urol 2001; 166:6–18.
8. Fergany AF, Hafez KS, Novick AC. Long-term results of nephron sparing surgery for localized renal cell carcinoma: 10-year followup. J Urol 2000; 163:442–445.
9. Rodriguez R, Chan D, Bishoff J, et al. Renal ablative cryosurgery in selected patients with peripheral renal masses. Urology 2000; 55:25–30.
10. Gill I, Novick A, Meraney A, et al. Laparoscopic renal cryoablation in 32 patients. Urology 2000; 25:748–753.
11. Rukstalis D, Khorsandi M, Garcia F, Hoenig D, Cohen J. Clinical experience with open renal cryoablation. Urology 2001; 57:34–39.
12. Lee D, McGinnis D, Feld R, Strup S. Retroperitoneal laparoscopic cryoablation of small renal tumors: intermediate results. Urology 2003; 61:83–88.

13. Livraghi T, Goldberg SN, Lazzaroni S, Solbiati L, Gazelle GS. Hepatocellular carcinoma: radiofrequency ablation of medium and large lesions. Radiology 2000; 214:761–768.
14. Curley SA, Izzo F, Delaria P, et al. Radiofrequency ablation of unresectable primary and metastatic hepatic malignancies: results in 123 patients. Ann Surg 1999; 230:1–8.
15. Gervais D, McGovern F, Arellano R, McDougal WS, Mueller P. Renal cell carcinoma: clinical experience and technical success with radiofrequency ablation of 42 tumors. Radiology 2003; 226:417–424.
16. Farrell MA, Charboneau WJ, DiMarco DS, et al. Imaging-guided radiofrequency ablation of solid renal tumors. AJR 2003; 180:1509–1513.
17. Mayo-Smith W, Dupuy D, Parikh P, Pezzullo J, Cronan J. Imaging-guided percutaneous radiofrequency ablation of solid renal masses: techniques and outcomes of 38 treatment sessions in 32 consecutive patients. AJR 2003; 180:1503–1508.
18. Roy-Choudhury S, Cast J, Cooksey G, Puri S, Breen D. Early experience with percutaneous radiofrequency ablation of small solid renal masses. AJR 2003; 180:1055–1061.
19. Hafez KS, Fergany AF, Novick AC. Long-term results of nephron sparing surgery for localized renal cell carcinoma: impact of tumor size on patient survival, tumor recurrence and TNM staging. J Urol 1999; 162:1930–1933.
20. Butler BP, Novick AC, Miller DP, et al. Management of small unilateral renal cell carcinomas: radical versus nephron-sparing surgery. Urology 1995; 45:34–40.
21. Dodd GD 3rd, Frank MS, Aribandi M, Chopra S, Chintapalli KN. Radiofrequency thermal ablation: computer analysis of the size of the thermal injury created by overlapping ablations. AJR 2001; 177:777–782.
22. Goldberg SN, Hahn PF, Tanabe KK, et al. Percutaneous radiofrequency ablation: does perfusion-mediated tissue cooling limit coagulation necrosis? J Vasc Interv Radiol 1998; 9:101–111.
23. Livaraghi T, Solbiati L, Meloni MF, Gazelle GS, Halpern EF, Goldberg SN. Treatment of focal liver tumors with percutaneous radiofrequency ablation: complications encountered in a multi-center study. Radiology 2003; 226:441–451.
24. Farrell MA, Charboneau JW, Callstrom MR, Reading CC, Engen D, Blute M. Paranephric water instillation: a technique to prevent bowel injury during percutaneous renal radiofrequency ablation. AJR 2003; 181:1315–1317.
25. Onik G, Onik C, Medary I, et al. Life threatening hypertensive crisis in two patients undergoing hepatic radiofrequency ablation. AJR 3002; 181:295–297.
26. Goldberg SN, Charboneau JW, Dodd G III, Deputy L. Image-guided tumor ablation: proposal for standardization of terms and reporting criteria. Radiology 2003; 228:335–345.
27. Zagoria R, Dyer R. The small renal mass: detection, characterization, and management. Abdom Imaging 1998; 23:256–265.
28. Fowler C, Reznek R. The indeterminate renal mass. Imaging 2001; 13:27–43.
29. Dodd GD 3rd, Soulen MC, Kane RA, et al. Minimally invasive treatment of malignant hepatic tumors: at the threshold of a major breakthrough. Radiographics 2000; 20:9–27.
30. Nawfel RD, Judy PF, Silverman SG, et al. Patient and personnel exposure during CT fluoroscopy-guided interventional procedures. Radiology 2000; 216:180–184.
31. Silverman S, Tunicali K, Adams D, et al. MR imaging-guided percutaneous cryotherapy of liver tumors: initial experience. Radiology 2000; 217:657–664.
32. Harada J, Dohi M, Mogami T, Fukuda K, Miki K, Furuta N. Initial experience of percutaneous renal cryosurgery under the guidance of a horizontal open MRI system. Radiat Med 2001; 19:291–296.
33. Vogl TJ, Straub R, Eichler K, Woitaschek D, Mack MG. Malignant liver tumors treated with MR imaging-guided laser-induced thermotherapy: experience with complications in 899 patients. Radiology 2002; 225:367–377.
34. Boaz TL, Lewin JS, Chung YC, et al. MR monitoring of MR-guided radiofrequency thermal ablation of normal liver in an animal model. J Magn Reson Imaging 1998; 8:64–69.
35. Varghese T, Zagzebske JA, Chen Q, et al. Ultrasound monitoring of temperature change during radiofrequency ablation: preliminary in-vivo results. Ultras Med Biol 2002; 28:321–329.

36. Cha C, Lee FT Jr, Gurney J, et al. CT versus sonography for monitoring radiofrequency ablation in a porcine liver. AJR 2000; 175:705–711.

37. Shingleon WB, Sewell PE Jr. Percutaneous renal tumor cryoablation with magnetic resonance imaging guidance. J Urol 2001; 167:1587–1592.

38. Lee FT Jr, Chosy SG, Littrup P, Warner T, Kuhlman J, Mahvi D. CT-monitored percutaneous cryoablation in a pig liver model: pilot study. Radiology 1999; 211: 687–692.

39. Tacke J, Speetzen R, Heschel I, Hunter DW, Rau G, Gunther RW. Imaging of interstitial cryotherapy—an in vitro comparison of ultrasound, computed tomography, and magnetic resonance imaging. Cryobiology 1999; 38:250–259.

40. Onik G, Cooper C, Goldberg HI, Moss AA, Rubinsky B, Christianson M. Ultrasonic characteristics of frozen liver. Cryobiology 1984; 21:321–328.

41. Weber SM, Lee FT Jr, Warner TF, Chosy SG, Mahvi DM. Hepatic cryoablation: US monitoring of extent of necrosis in normal pig liver. Radiology 1998; 207:73–77.

42. Meloni MF, Goldberg SN, Livraghi T, et al. Hepatocellular carcinoma treated with radiofrequency ablation: comparison of pulse inversion contrast-enhanced harmonic sonography, contrast-enhanced power Doppler sonography, and helical CT. AJR 2001; 177:375–380.

43. Goldberg SN, Gazelle GS, Compton CC, Mueller PR, Tanabe KK. Treatment of intrahepatic malignancy with radiofrequency ablation: radiologic-pathologic correlation. Cancer 2000; 88:2452–2463.

44. Murphy D, Gill I. Energy-based renal tumor ablation: a review. Sem Urol Oncol 2001; 19:133–140.

45. McGahan JP, Brock JN, Tessluk H, Gu WZ, Schneider P, Browning PD. Hepatic ablation with the use of radio-frequency electrocautery in the animal model. J Vasc Interv Radiol 1992; 3:291–297.

46. Zlotta AR, Wildschutz T, Raviv G, et al. Radiofrequency interstitial tumor ablation is a possible new modality for treatment of renal cancer: ex vivo and in vivo experience. J Endourol 1997; 11:251–258.

47. McGovern FJ, Wood BJ, Goldberg SN, Mueller PR. Radiofrequency ablation of renal cell carcinoma via image-guided needle electrodes. J Urol 1999; 161:599–600.

48. Goldberg SN, Gazelle GS, Mueller PR. Thermal ablation therapy for focal malignancy: a unified approach to underlying principles, techniques, and diagnostic imaging guidance. AJR 2000; 174:323–331.

49. Organ LW. Electrophysiologic principles of radiofrequency lesion making. Appl Neurophysiol 1976; 39:69–76.

50. Lu DS, Raman SS, Vodopich DJ, Wang M, Sayre J, Lassman C. Effect of vessel size on creation of hepatic radiofrequency lesions in pigs: assessment of the "heat sink" effect. AJR 2002; 178:47–51.

51. Tungjitkusolmun S, Staelin ST, Haemmerich D, et al. Three-dimensional finite element analyses for radio-frequency hepatic tumor ablation. IEEE Trans Biomed Eng 2002; 49:3–9.

52. Goldberg SN, Gazelle GS, Solbiati L, Rittman WJ, Mueller PR. Radiofrequency tissue ablation: increased lesion diameter with a perfusion electrode. Acad Radiol 1996; 3: 636–644.

53. Kettenbach J, Wolfgang K, Rucklinger E, Gustorff B, Hupfl M, Wolf F. Percutaneous saline-enhanced radiofrequency ablation of hepatic tumors: initial experience in 26 patients. AJR 2003; 180:1537–1545.

54. Boehm T, Malich A, Goldberg SN, et al. Radiofrequency tumor ablation: internally cooled electrode versus saline-enhanced technique in an aggressive rabbit tumor model. Radiology 2002; 222:805–813.

55. Ahmed M, Liu Z, Afzal KS, et al. Radiofrequency ablation: effect of surrounding tissue composition on coagulation necrosis in a canine tumor model. Radiology 2004; 230: 761–767.

56. Pavlovich CP, Walther MM, Choyke PL, et al. Percutaneous radiofrequency ablation of small renal tumors: initial results. J Urol 2002; 167:10–15.

57. Zagoria RJ, Hawkins AD, Clark PE, et al. Percutaneous CT-guided radiofrequency ablation of renal neoplasms: factors influencing success. AJR 2004;183:201–207.

58. Boss A, Clasen S, Kuczyk M, et al. Magnetic resonance-guided percutaneous radiofrequency ablation of renal cell carcinomas: a pilot clinical study. Invest Radiol 2005; 40(9):583–590.

59. Varkarakis IM, Allaf ME, Inagaki T, et al. Percutaneous radio frequency ablation of renal masses: results at a 2-year mean followup. J Urol 2005; 174(2):456–460.

60. Gervais DA, McGovern FJ, Arellano RS, McDougal WS, Mueller PR. Radiofrequency ablation of renal cell carcinoma: part 1, Indications, results, and role in patient management over a 6-year period and ablation of 100 tumors. Am J Roentgenol 2005; 185(1): 64–71.

61. Mahnken AH, Rohde D, Brkovic D, Gunther RW, Tacke JA. Percutaneous radiofrequency ablation of renal cell carcinoma: preliminary results. Acta Radiol 2005; 46(2):208–214.

62. Matsumoto ED, Johnson DB, Ogan K, et al. Short-term efficacy of temperature-based radiofrequency ablation of small renal tumors. Urology 2005; 65(5):877–881.

63. Veltri A, De Fazio G, Malfitana V, et al. Percutaneous US-guided RF thermal ablation for malignant renal tumors: preliminary results in 13 patients. Eur Radiol 2004; 14(12):2303–2310.

64. Lewin JS, Nour SG, Connell CF, et al. Phase II clinical trial of interactive MR imaging-guided interstitial radiofrequency thermal ablation of primary kidney tumors: initial experience. Radiology 2004; 232(3):835–845.

65. Hwang JJ, Walther MM, Pautler SE, et al. Radio frequency ablation of small renal tumors: intermediate results. J Urol 2004; 171(5):1814–1818.

66. Mazur P. The role of intracellular freezing in the death of cells cooled at supraoptimal rates. Cryobiology 1977; 14:251–271.

67. Gill W, Fraser J. Repeated freeze-thaw cycles in cryosurgery. Nature 1968; 219:410–413.

68. Kahlenber MS, Volpe C, Klippenstein DL, Penetrante RB, Petrelli NJ, Rodriquez-Bigas MA. Clinicopathologic effects of cryotherapy on hepatic vessels and bile ducts in a porcine model. Ann Surg Onc 1998; 5:713–718.

69. Weber SM, Lee FT Jr, Chinn DO, Warner TF, Chosy SG, Mahvi DM. Perivascular and intralesional tissue necrosis after hepatic cryoablation: results in a porcine model. Surgery 1997; 122:742–747.

70. Chosy SG, Nakada SY, Lee FT Jr, Warner TF. Monitoring renal cryosurgery: predictors of tissue necrosis in swine. J Urol 1998; 159:1370–1374.

71. Ravikumar TS, Steele G Jr, Kame R, King V. Experimental and clinical observations on hepatic cryosurgery for colorectal metastases. Cancer Res 1991; 5:6323–6327.

72. Tatsutani K, Rubinsky B, Onik G, Dahiya R. Effect of thermal variables on frozen human primary prostatic adenocarcinoma cells. Urology 1996; 48:441–447.

73. Lee FT Jr, Mahvi DM, Chosy SG, et al. Hepatic cryosurgery with intraoperative US guidance. Radiology 1997; 203:465–470.

74. Lee FT Jr, Haemmerich K, Wright AS, Mahvi DM, Sampson L, Webster J. Multiple probe radiofrequency ablation: pilot study in an animal model. J Vasc Interv Radiol 2003; 14:1437–1442.

75. Harb T, Littrup PJ, Silva J, Harvill M, Gaisinsky I. Cryotherapy of Primary Renal Cell Carcinoma and Local Recurrences After Nephrectomy: Techniques and Early Outcomes. RSNA Scientific Assembly and Annual Meeting Program, 2003:495.

76. Hruby G, Reisiger K, Venkatesh R, Yan Y, Landman J. Comparison of laparoscopic partial nephrectomy and laparoscopic cryoablation for renal hilar tumors. Urology 2006; 67(1):50–54.

77. Desai MM, Aron M, Gill IS. Laparoscopic partial nephretomy versus laparoscopic cryoablation for the small renal tumor. Urology 2005; 66(5 suppl):23–28.

78. Silverman SG, Tuncali K, vanSonnenberg E, Morrison PR, Shankar S, Ramaiya N, Richie JP, et al. Renal tumors: MR imaging–guided percutaneous cryotherapy-initial experience in 23 patients. Radiology 2005; 236(2):716–724.

79. Gill IS, Remer EM, Hasan WA, Strezmpkowski B, Spaliviero M, Steinberg AP, Kaouk H, Desai MM, Novic AC, et al. Renal cryoablation: outcome at 3 years. J Urol 2005; 173(6):1903–1907.

80. Cestari A, Guazzoni G, dell'Acqua V, Nava L, Cardone G, Balconi G, Naspro R, Montorsi F, Rigatti P, et al. Laparoscopic cryoablation of solid renal masses: intermediate term followup. J Urol 2004; 172(4 Pt 1):1267–1270.

81. Moon TD, Lee FT Jr, Hedican SP, Lowry P, Nakada SY. Laparoscopic cryoablation under sonographic guidance for the treatment of small renal tumors. J Endourol 2004; 18(5):436–440.

82. Kennedy JE, Ter Jaar GR, Cranston D. High intensity focused ultrasound: surgery of the future? Br J Radiol 2003; 76:590–599.

83. Tiidus PM. Massage and ultrasound as therapeutic modalities in exercise-induced muscle damage. Can J Appl Physiol 1999; 24:267–278.

84. Watkin NA, Morris SB, Rivens IH, et al. High-intensity focused ultrasound ablation of the kidney in a large animal model. J Endourol 1997; 11:191–196.

85. Kohrmann K, Michel M, Gaa J, Marlinghaus E, Alhen P. HIFU as non-invasive therapy for multilocal RCC: case study and review of the literature. J Urol 2002; 167:2397–2403.

86. Skinner MG, Iizuka MN, Kolios MC, Sherar MD. A theoretical comparison of energy sources—microwave, ultrasound, and laser—for interstitial thermal therapy. Phys Med Biol 1998; 43:3535–3547.

87. Wright AS, Lee FT Jr, Mahvi DM. Hepatic microwave ablation with multiple antennae results in synergistically larger zones of coagulation necrosis. Ann Surg Onc 2003; 10: 275–283.

88. Seki T, Wakabayashi M, Nakagawa T, et al. Ultrasonically guided percutaneous microwave coagulation therapy for small hepatocellular carcinoma. Cancer 1994; 74:817–825.

89. Matsui Y, Fujikawa K, Iwamura J, Oka H, Fukuzawa S, Takeuchi H. Application of the MTC: is it beneficial to partial nephrectomy? Urologia Internationalis 2002; 69:27–32.

90. Vogl T, Straub R, Eichler K, Woitaschek D, Mack M. Modern alternatives to resection of metastases-MR-guided laser-induced thermotherapy and other local ablative techniques. Therap Umschau 2001; 58:718–725.

91. Dick EA, Joarder R, De Jode M, Wragg P, Vale J, Gedroyc W. Magnetic resonance imaging-guided laser thermal ablation of renal tumors. BJU Int 2002; 90:814–822.

92. Llovet JM, Vilana R, Bianchi L, et al. Increased risk of tumor seeding after percutaneous radiofrequency ablation for single hepatocellular carcinoma. Hepatology 2001; 33:1124–1129.

93. Napier D, Dodd G, Hubbard L, Chintapalli K, Chopra S, Medina D. Postablation syndrome following thermal ablation of liver lesions. Presented at the 29th annual meeting of the Society of Gastrointestinal Radiology, Kauai, Hawaii, March 12, 2000.

94. Zagoria RJ. Imaging of small renal masses: a medical success story. AJR 2000; 175: 945–955.

95. Macari M, Bosniak MA. Delayed CT to evaluate renal masses incidentally discovered at contrast enhanced CT: demonstration of vascularity with de-enhancement. Radiology 1999; 213:674–680.

Index